*Todarānanda–Āyurveda Saukhyam Series No. 8*

# FIVE SPECIALISED THERAPIES OF AYURVEDA (PANCA-KARMA)

BASED ON

AYURVEDA SAUKHYAM OF TODARANANDA

VAIDYA BHAGWAN DASH
D.A.M.S., H.P.A., M.A., Ph.D.
former Deputy Adviser (Āyurveda)
Ministry of Health and Family Welfare
Govt. of India
and
Consultant in Traditional Medicine
World Health Organisation (1979)

VAIDYA LALITESH KASHYAP
B.I.M.S., Ph.D.
Medical Superintendent
Ayurvedic Hospital
Central Govt. Health Scheme
Directorate General of Health Ser
New Delhi



CONCEPT PUBLISHING COMPANY, NEW DELHI-110059

ISBN 81-7022-024-6 (Set)
ISBN 81-7022-397-0 (No. 8)

First Published 1992
Reprinted 2003



*Published and Printed by*
Ashok Kumar Mittal
**Concept Publishing Company**
A/15-16. Commercial Block. Mohan Garden
NEW DELHI-110059 (India)

*Phones* : 25351460, 25351794
*Fax* : 091-11-25357103
*Email* : publishing@conceptpub.com

*Dedicated*

*to*

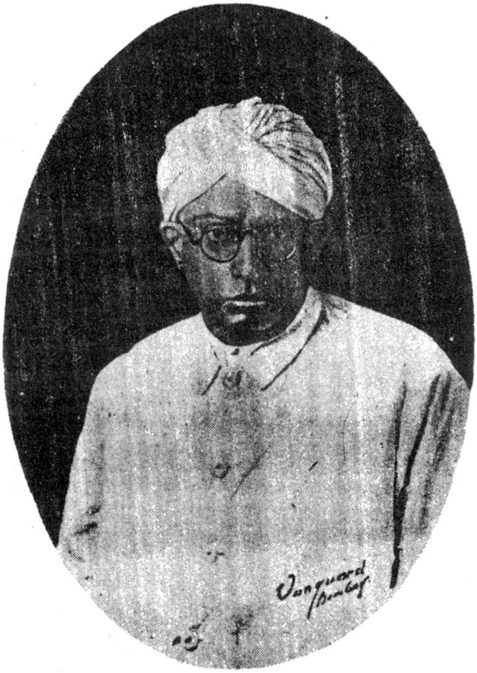

*Late Vaidya Yadavji Trikamji Acharya*

whose profound scholarship and devotion to salvage and publish Ayurvedic literature provided us inspiration to undertake this work.

# PREFACE

Āyurveda has eight specialised branches (Skt. *Aṣṭāṅga*) as follows:

(1) *Kāyacikitsā* or Internal medicine;
(2) *Śalyatantra* or Surgery;
(3) *Śālākyatantra* or Treatment of diseases of Eye, Ear, Nose and Throat;
(4) *Bhūtavidyā* or Psychiatry;
(5) *Kaumārabhṛtya* or Paediatrics including Gynaecology and Maternity;
(6) *Agadatantra* or Treatment of different types of Poisoning;
(7) *Rasāyana* or Rejuvenation therapy; and
(8) *Vājikaraṇatantra* or Aphrodisiac therapy including Geriatrics.

In the earlier volumes of this Series (nos. 1 to 7), the former four specialised branches have already been described. The present volume deals with the remaining four specialised branches. In addition, a group of five specialised and classical therapies called *Pañca-karma* are also described in detail in this volume.

Procreation is a normal physiological process in all living beings including humanbeings, animals and plants. But animals and plants, because of their sublatent and latent mental faculty are incapable of exercising their power of discrimination and indulge in sexual union as a matter of natural instinct. As a result, they procreate offsprings which may be useful or harmful and healthy or diseased. On the other hand, humanbeings are endowed with the power of discrimination, fully developed mental faculty and wisdom. Being a social animal, they instinctively do not desire to have a child who will be a liability to themselves and harmful to the society. To procreate a healthy child who will be an asset to their family, society, country and humanity as a whole is in their own hands. It is left to them if they want to use this naturally gifted power or not. The present day disorder in the social fabric of Man which has culminated in crime, violence, terrorism, abuse of drugs and AIDS is the result of his misuse of his power of discrimination. Āyurveda stands for a healthy and peaceful society, and therefore, has prescribed several dos and don'ts for procreating a healthy and socially useful offsprings. While taking care of the child, it is necessary to take care of the mother and her ailments. These measures are described in the Chapters I to VII of this volume.

In nature, some plants, animals and metals including minerals are provided with such properties which when used indiscriminately produce harmful effects on the human body. These substances are poisons. Some other substances, though non-poisonous in nature, produce adverse effects on the human beings because of some physico-changes, they undergo as a result of exposure to rain, sun, etc. At times, human beings misuse their power of discrimination and indulge in rivalry. They want to inflict injury upon their enemies and artificially prepare poisonous stuff. Therefore, a person, specially a Ruler should be careful about it. If such poisoning effects are inflicted in spite of all precautions, then the ailments are to be treated by the Physician. These are described in the Chapter-VIII of this volume.

Diseases, when already manifested, are no doubt to be treated. But what is important from Ayurvedic point of view is to prevent occurrence of such diseases. According to Ayurveda, simple freedom from disease is not Health. For a person to be called healthy, he should be mentally and spiritually happy. Death can not be prevented. But what can be prevented is the invalidating old age which impairs the sensasory and motor functions of the individual and which leads to several diseases like Heart disease, High Blood pressure, Cancer, Asthma and Arthritis. A person should not be a liability to the family and society during his old age but should be an asset with his accumulated experience. To prevent the aging process and to preserve as well as promote his positive health certain measures are prescribed in Āyurveda. These *Rasāyana* or Rejuvenation therapies are detailed in the Chapter-IX of this volume.

To take food for enabling the body to function, to sleep for giving rest to the body and the mind, to defend himself from injuries and evil designs of others and to have sexual union for procreation and satisfaction of the carnal desires are the natural instincts of all living beings. If a person fails to satisfy the sexual desire, he leads a miserable life and ultimately loses interest in his life. This gives rise to several family and social problems. Timely use of Aphrodisiacs and proper management of the geriatric problems are the *sine qua non* for a healthy and happy society. The specialised branch of Ayurveda dealing with such problems and their remedies is called *Vājikaraṇa-tantra*. It is elaborated in the Chapter-X of this volume.

Six Specialised Therapies, called in Ayurvedic parlance *Pañca-karma*, play an important role in Ayurvedic therapeutics inasmuch as even one of these, viz., *Basti* or Medicated enema therapy is described in *Caraka saṃhitā* as half of all the therapeutic measures described in this system. Apart from curing several obstinate and otherwise incurable diseases, these specialised therapies are capable of rejuvenating the body for preservation and promotion of Positive health and prevention of diseases. These are as follows:

(1) *Vamana* (Emetic therapy);
(2) *Virecana* (Purgation therapy);
(3) *Nirūha basti* (A type of Medicated Enema therapy);
(4) *Anuvāsana basti* (Another type of Medicated Enema therapy); and
(5) *Nasya* (Inhalation therapy).

Suśruta of the School of Surgeons, has replaced the fifth one by *Rakta-mokṣaṇa* or Blood-letting therapy. Before administering these therapies, the body of a person has to be specially processed to accept these therapies for obtaining excellent results. These are called *Pūrva-karma* or Preparatory measures. These include *snehana* or Oleation therapy and *svedana* or Fomentation therapy. In addition, several minor but important therapies like *gaṇḍūṣa* or gargling therapy are also included in this category. All these are described in the Chapters XI to XVI of this volume.

Because of the importance of these "Five Specialised Therapies of Ayurveda" in practice, the title of the present volume is designed accordingly not withstanding other topics included in it.

The Chapter numbers of this volume, like the previous ones, are given by us. Different manuscripts of this work, we have consulted, have different chapter numbers and these are furnished in the foot-notes and colophons of each chapter. As we are coming to the end of this Series, gradually, we are facing more and more of grammatical and syntactical errors in these manuscripts. Within limits, we have made efforts to correct some of these, and some others are intentionally left out untouched for fear of unauthorised interpolations. This is not a literature but a scientific work with practical implications. With all humility at our command, we therefore, seek the indulgence of our esteemed readers.

Ṭoḍaramalla, the author of this work was a versatile genius and had the unique privilege to collect the most authentic and time tested recipes and therapeutic measures. He had at his disposal the services of reputed scholars and libraries to compile and interpret textual material. Because of the wealth of material contained in it, this volume will be equally useful for Ayurvedic physicians, doctors of Modern medicine of this country as well as abroad and for the research workers in the fields of health and humanities.

A-71, Swasthya Vihar
New Delhi-110092
8th October 1991

BHAGWAN DASH
LALITESH KASHYAP

## ACKNOWLEDGEMENTS

We are extremely thankful to Ku. Kanchan Gupta, M.A. M.Ed. for her valuable assistance in the preparation and publication of this work . We wish her happy, healthy and long life.

BHAGWAN DASH
LALITESH KASHYAP

## INDO-ROMANIC EQUIVALENTS OF DEVANĀGARĪ

| | | | | | | | |
|---|---|---|---|---|---|---|---|
| अ | a | क | ka | ढ | ḍha | र | ra |
| आ | ā | ख | kha | ण | ṇa | ल | la |
| इ | i | ग | ga | त | ta | व | va |
| ई | ī | घ | gha | थ | tha | श | śa |
| उ | u | ङ | ṅa | द | da | ष | ṣa |
| ऊ | ū | च | ca | ध | dha | स | sa |
| ऋ | ṛ | छ | cha | न | na | ह | ha |
| ए | e | ज | ja | प | pa | | |
| ऐ | ai | झ | jha | फ | pha | | |
| ओ | o | ञ | ña | ब | ba | | |
| औ | au | ट | ṭa | भ | bha | | |
| अं | ṁ/ṃ | ठ | ṭha | म | ma | | |
| अः | ḥ | ड | ḍa | य | ya | | |

# CONTENTS



---

1. * Numbers given in the square brackets of Contents indicate the verse/paragraph number of the concerned chapter.

**Chapter VIII**

## Chapter XI



## Chapter XII

## Chapter XIV



## Chapter XV

## Chapter XVI

# CHAPTER I

## ॥ अथ असृग्दरनिदानं चिकित्सा च ॥

*(Diagnosis and Treatment of Menorrhagia)*

"विरुद्धमद्याध्यशनादजीर्णाद् गर्भप्रपातादतिमैथुनाच्च ।
यानाध्वशोकादतिकर्षणाच्च भाराभिघाताच्छयनाद् दिवा च ॥१॥

***Etiology***

[All the varieties of menorrhagia] are caused by the following factors:

(1) intake of mutually contradictory food & drinks;
(2) intake of alcoholic drinks;
(3) intake of food before the previous meal is digested;
(4) indigestion;
(5) abortion and miscarriage;
(6) sexual intercourse in excess;
(7) excessive emaciation because of riding over animals and vehicles or walking a long distance or grief;
(8) injury because of carrying excessive weight; and
(9) sleep during the day time.

असृग्दरं भवेत्सर्वं साङ्गमर्दं सवेदनम् ।
तस्यातिवृत्तौ[2] दौर्बल्यं भ्रमो[3] मूर्च्छामदस्तृषः ॥
दाहः प्रलापः पाण्डुत्वं तन्द्रा रोगाश्च वातजाः ॥२॥

***Signs and Symptoms in General***

All the varieties of menorrhagia are associated with malaise and pain. If there is excessive bleeding, then the patient suffers from weakness, giddiness, fainting, feeling as if intoxicated, morbid thirst, burning sensation, delirium, anemia, drowsiness and diseases caused by *vāyu.*

तं श्लेष्मपित्तानिलसन्निपातैश्चतुःप्रकारं[4] प्रदरं वदन्ति ॥३॥

***Varieties***

*Asṛgdara* (menorrhagia) is of four types, viz., *kaphaja, paittika, vātika* and *sānnipātika.*

आमं सपिच्छाप्रतिमं[5] सपाण्डु पुलाकतोयप्रतिमं कफाच्च ।
सपीतनीलासितरक्तमुष्णं पित्तार्तियुक्तं भृशवेगि पित्तात् ॥
रूक्षारुणं फेनिलमल्पमल्पं वातार्तियुक्तं पिशितोदकाभम् ॥४॥

***Signs and Symptoms of Kaphaja, Paittika and Vātika Asṛgdara***

In *kaphaja* type of *asṛgdara,* the secretion is mucoid, slimy, pale-yellow and like rice-water (wash).

In *paittika* type of *asṛgdara,* the secretion is yellow, blue, black or red in colour and hot. It is associated with *paittika* symptoms like burning sensation and the secretion takes place with great force.

In *vātika* type of *asṛgdara,* the secretion is ununctuous, reddish and frothy, the secretion takes place frequently in small quantities and it is associated with *vātika* symptoms like pain. The secretion looks like water in which flesh is washed.

सक्षौद्रसर्पिर्हरितालवर्णं मज्जप्रकाशं कुणपं त्रिदोषात् ।
तच्चाप्यसाध्यं[6] प्रवदन्ति तज्ज्ञाः न तत्र कुर्वीत भिषक् चिकित्साम् ॥५॥

### *Signs and Symptoms of Sānnipātika Asṛgdara*

In *sānnipātika* type of *asṛgdara*, the secretion is of the colour of honey, ghee, *haritāla* (yellow orpiment) or bone-marrow. It has a smell of dead body. This type of *asṛgdara* is incurable and the physician should not treat such cases.

मासान्निष्पिच्छदाहार्त्ति- पञ्चरात्रानुबन्धि च ।
नैवातिबहुलात्यल्पमार्त्तवं शुद्धमादिशेत् ॥६॥
शशासृक्प्रतिमं यच्च यद्वा लाक्षारसोपमम् ।
तदार्त्तवं प्रशंसन्ति यद्वासो[७] न विरंजयेत् ॥७॥

### *Normal Menstruation*

The menstrual bleeding which takes place after a month, which continues for five nights, which is free from sliminess, burning sensation and pain and which is neither excessively more not excessively less in quantity is to be considered as pure (normal).

The menstrual fluid which is like rabbit's blood or like the lac-water and which does not leave any stain on the cloth (after washing) is to be treated as normal.

शश्वत् स्रवन्तीमास्रावं तृष्णादाहज्वरान्विताम् ।
क्षीणरक्तां दुर्बलां च तामसाध्यां विवर्जयेत्[८] ॥८॥
॥ असृग्दरनिदानं[९] ॥

(माधवनिदान : प्रदररोगनिदान : १-७)

### *Prognosis*

If the menstrual bleeding continues constantly (without interruption), if it is associated with morbid thirst, burning sensation and fever, if the patient is anemic and weak, then she is incurable. Such a patient should not be treated.

Thus, ends the diagnosis of menorrhagia.

### *Soma Roga (Polyuria)*

"स्त्रीणामतिप्रसङ्गाद्वा[१०] शोकाच्चापि श्रमादपि ।
अभिचारिकयोगाद्वा[११] गरदोषात्तथैव च ॥९॥

आपः सर्वशरीरस्थाः क्षुभ्यन्ति प्रस्रवन्ति च ।
तस्यास्ताः प्रच्युताः स्थानान्मूत्रमार्गं प्रविश्य[१२] हि ॥१०॥
प्रसन्ना विमलाः शीता निर्गन्धा नीरुजः सिताः ।
स्रवन्ति चातिमात्रं तु[१३] न शक्नोति सुदुर्बला ॥
'वेगं[१४] धारयितुं तासां न विंदति सुखं क्वचित्' ॥११॥

### *Etiology and Pathogenesis*

Because of excessive sexual intercourse, grief, exhaustion, *abhicāra* (infliction of spell) or *garadoṣa* (administration of artificially prepared poisons), the watery element in the entire body of the lady gets excited and exudes. Being displaced, this watery element enters into the urinary channel and comes out. The urine, thus voided, is transparent, clear, cool, free from any foul smell or pain and white in colour. There is excessive discharge of this urine and the patient who is weak becomes incapable of retaining such urine flow. As a result of this she always feels uncomfortable.

शिरसः शिथिलत्वं च मुखतालुविशोषणम्[१५] ।
मूर्च्छा जृम्भा प्रलापश्च त्वग्रूक्षा चातिमात्रतः[१६] ॥१२॥
भक्ष्यैर्भोज्यैश्च पेयैश्च तुष्टिं न लभते सदा।
(योगरत्नाकर : सोमरोगनिदान : पृष्ठ ४०२)
सोमरोग इति ख्यातो देहक्षयकरः परः ॥१३॥

### *Signs and Symptoms*

The patient suffering from *soma roga* (polyuria) exhibits the following signs and symptoms :

(1) Unstability (lit. looseness) of the head, dryness of mouth and palate, fainting, yawning, delirium and excessive dryness of the skin; and

(2) she does not feel satisfied in spite of taking food (chewables and eatables) and drinks in adequate quantity.

This is called *soma roga* which causes extreme emaciation of the body.

शरीरधारणाच्चापि सोम इत्यभिधीयते ।
तस्मात्सोमक्षयाद्देहो निश्चेष्टश्च भवेत्सदा ॥१४॥
॥ इति सोमनिदानम्[१७] ॥

### *Soma*

It is called *soma* because of its attributes to sustain the body. Excretion of this *soma* makes the body incapable of performing its activities.

Thus, ends the diagnosis of *soma roga*.

"दध्ना[१८] सौर्वचलाजाजीमधुकं नीलमुत्पलम्' ।
पिबेत्क्षौद्रयुतं नारी वातासृग्दरपीडिता ॥१५॥
(योगरत्नाकर : प्रदरचिकित्सा : पृष्ठ ३९७)

### *Treatment of Menorrhagia*

*Sauvarcala, ajājī, madhuka* and *nīla utpala* should be added to curd. Intake of this potion along with honey makes the woman free from *vātika* type of menorrhagia.

पिबेदैणेयकं[२०] रक्तं शर्करामधुसंयुतम्" ॥१६॥
(भैषज्यरत्नावली : स्त्रीरोगाधिकार : १-२)
"वासकस्य[२१] रसं पित्ते गुडूच्या रसमेव वा" ॥१७॥
(भैषज्यरत्नावली : स्त्रीरोगाधिकार : १४)

### *Recipes*

Intake of deer-blood along with sugar and honey cures menorrhagia.

Intake of the juice of *vāsaka* or *guḍūcī* (along with sugar and honey) cures *paittika* type of menorrhagia.

"रोहीतकान्मूलकल्कं पाण्डुरेऽसृग्दरे पिबेत् ।
जलेनामलकीबीजकल्कं वा ससितामधु ॥१८॥
धातक्याश्चाक्षमात्रं[२२] वा आमलक्या मधुद्रवम् ।
काकजानुकमूलं वा मूलं कार्पासमेव वा ।
पाण्डुप्रदरशान्त्यर्थं पिबेत्तण्डुलवारिणा" ॥१९॥
(भैषज्यरत्नावली : स्त्रीरोगाधिकार : ११-१२)

In *kaphaja* type of menorrhagia, the patient should take the paste of the root of *rohītaka* in the form of a drink along with sugar and honey.

Seed-pulp of *āmalakī* should be made to a paste by triturating with water. Intake of this potion by adding sugar and honey cures *kaphaja* type of menorrhagia.

Intake of the paste of *dhātakī* (one *akṣa*) or *āmalakī* along with honey cures *pāṇḍura* (*kaphaja*) type of menorrhagia. *Kākajaṅghā* or *kārpāsa* should be made to a paste. Intake of this paste along with rice-water (wash) cures *kaphaja* type of *pradara*.

"अशोकवल्कलक्वाथशृतं दुग्धं सुशीतलम् ।
यथाबलं पिबेत्प्रातस्तीव्रासृग्दरनाशनम्" ॥२०॥

(भैषज्यरत्नावली : स्त्रीरोगाधिकार : ५)

*Use of Aśoka*

A decoction should be prepared out of the bark of *aśoka*. Milk should be boiled by adding this decoction. This medicated milk should be cooled and taken early in the morning in appropriate quantity depending upon the strength of the patient which cures *vātika* type of menorrhagia.

दार्वीरसाञ्जनकिरातवृषाब्दबिल्व-
भल्लातकैरवकृतो मधुना[२३] कषायः ।
पीतो जयत्यतिबलं प्रदरं सशूलं[२४]
पीतासितारुणविलोहितनीलशुक्लम् ॥२१॥

(भैषज्यरत्नावली : स्त्रीरोगाधिकार : ४)

***Recipe***

The decoction of *dārvī rasāñjana* (solid extract of *dāru haridrā*), *kirāta tikta, vāsaka, mustā, bilva* and *bhallātaka* should be mixed with honey. Intake of this potion cures acute form of menorrhagia associated with colic-pain and discharge of yellow, black, reddish, red, blue or white colour.

"रसाञ्जनं तण्डुलकस्य मूलं
क्षौद्रान्वितं तण्डुलतोयपीतम् ।
असृग्दरं सर्वभवं निहन्ति
श्वासं च भार्गी सहनागरेण" ॥२२॥

(योगरत्नाकर : प्रदरचिकित्सा : पृष्ठ ३९८)

*Rasāñjana* (solid extract of *dāru haridrā*) and root of *taṇḍulīyaka* should be made to a paste by adding honey. Intake of this potion along with rice-wash cures *sānnipātika* type of menorrhagia. If the above mentioned potion is added with *bhārgi* and *nāgara*, then it cures dyspnoea associated with this condition.

"कुशमूलं समुद्धृत्य पेषयेत्तण्डुलाम्बुना ।
एतत्पीत्वा त्र्यहान्नारी प्रदरात्परिमुच्यते" ॥२३॥

(भैषज्यरत्नावली : स्त्रीरोगाधिकार : २)

The root of *kuśa* should be made to a paste by triturating with rice-water (wash). Intake of this potion for three days makes the woman free from menorrhagia.

"भूम्यामलकमूलं तु पीतं तण्डुलवारिणा ।
द्वित्रिरेव[२५] दिनैर्नार्याः प्रदरं दुस्तरं जयेत्"[२६] ॥२४॥

(भैषज्यरत्नावली : स्त्रीरोगाधिकार : १६)

The root of *bhūmyāmalakī* should be made to a paste by triturating with rice-wash. Intake of this potion for two or three days cures serious type of menorrhagia in a woman.

"क्षौद्रयुक्तं फलरसं काष्ठदुम्बरजं पिबेत् ।
असृग्दरविनाशाय सशर्करपयोन्नभुक्[२७]" ॥२५॥

(योगरत्नाकर : प्रदरचिकित्सा : पृष्ठ ३९८)

The juice of the fruit of *kāṣṭhodumbara* should be mixed with honey. Intake of this potion cures menorrhagia. During the period of treatment, the patient should take rice along with sugar and milk.

"प्रदरं हन्ति बलाया मूलं दुग्धेन मधुयुतं[२८] पीतम् ।
कुशवाट्यालकमूलं तण्डुलतोयेन[२९] रक्ताख्यम्" ॥२६॥

(भैषज्यरत्नावली : स्त्रीरोगाधिकार : ६७)
(योगरत्नाकर : प्रदरचिकित्सा : पृष्ठ ३९८)

Root of *balā* should be boiled with milk. Intake of this medicated milk along with honey cures menorrhagia. Similarly, intake of the paste of *kuśa* and *vāṭyālaka* along with rice-wash cures menorrhagia.

वंशपत्रकपित्थस्य क्वाथं पीत्वा सशर्करम् ।
सप्ताहान्नात्र संदेहो रक्तासृग्दरनाशनम् ॥२७॥

Decoction of bamboo-leaf and *kapittha* should be added with sugar. Intake of this potion with sugar for one week undoubtedly cures menorrhagia.

"पाठाजम्ब्वाम्रयोर्मध्यं शिलोद्भेद[३०]रसाञ्जनम् ।
अम्बष्ठकी[३१] मोचरसः समङ्गा पद्मकेशरम् ॥२८॥
वाह्लीकातिविषे[३२] मुस्तं बिल्वं लोध्रं सगैरिकम् ।
कट्फलं मरिच[३३] शुण्ठीमृद्वीका रक्तचन्दनम् ॥२९॥
कट्वङ्गवत्सकानन्ता धातकी मधुकार्जुनम् ।
पुष्येणोद्धृत्य तुल्यानि श्लक्ष्णचूर्णानि कारयेत् ॥३०॥
तानि क्षौद्रेण संयोज्य पाययेत्तण्डुलाम्बुना ।
अर्शःसु[३४] चातिसारेषु रक्तं यच्चोपविश्यते ॥३१॥
दोषागन्तुकृता ये च बालानां तांश्च नाशयेत् ।
योनिदोषं रजोदोषं श्वेतं नीलं सपीतकम् ॥३२॥
स्त्रीणां श्यावारुणं यच्च तत्प्रसह्य निवर्त्तयेत् ।
चूर्णं पुष्यानुगं नाम हितमात्रेयपूजितम्[३५] ॥३३॥

॥ पुष्यानुगचूर्णम् ॥

(भैषज्यरत्नावली : स्त्रीरोगाधिकार : ४६-५१)

***Puṣyānuga Cūrṇa***

During *puṣya* constellation, the physician should collect *pāṭhā*, seed pulp of *jambū* and *āmra*, *śilodbheda*, *rasāñjana*, *ambaṣṭhakī*, *mocarasa*, *samaṅgā*, *padma keśara*, *vāhlīka*, *ativiṣā*, *mustā*, *bilva*, *lodhra*, *gairika*, *kaṭphala*, *marica*, *śuṇṭhī*, *mṛdvīkā*, *rakta candana*, *kaṭvaṅga*, *vatsaka*, *anantā*, *dhātakī*, *madhuka* and *arjuna*. All these drugs, taken in equal quantities should be made to fine power. Administration of this potion along with rice-wash and honey effectively cures piles, diarrhoea, passage of blood in the stool, diseases of children caused by vitiated *doṣas* and extraneous factors, diseases of the female genital tract and menstrual disorders having white, blue, yellow, brown and reddish discharge. This is called *Puṣyānuga cūrṇa* and it is propounded by Lord Ātreya.

"शतावरीरसप्रस्थं क्षोदयित्वा[३६] च पीडितम् ।
घृतप्रस्थसमायुक्तं क्षीरद्विगुणितं भिषक् ॥३४॥
अतः कल्कानिमान्दद्यात्स्थूलोदुम्बरसम्मितान्[३७] ।
'जीवनीयानि तान्यष्टौ[३८] यष्टीचन्दनपद्मकैः ॥३५॥
श्वदंष्ट्रा चात्मगुप्ता च बला नागबला तथा'[३९] ।
शालिपर्णी[४०] पृश्निपर्णी विदारी सारिवाद्वयम् ॥३६॥
शर्करा च समा देया काश्मर्याश्च फलानि[४१] च ।
सम्यक् सिद्धं तु विज्ञाय तद्घृतं चावतारयेत्[४२] ॥३७॥
रक्तपित्तविकारेषु वातपित्तकृतेषु च ।
वातरक्तं क्षयं श्वासं हिक्कां कासं च दुस्तरम्[४३] ॥३८॥
अङ्गदाहं शिरोदाहं रक्तपित्तसमुद्भवम् ।
असृग्दरं सर्वभवं मूत्रकृच्छ्रं च दारुणम् ।
एतान्रोगान् शमयति भास्करस्तिमिरं यथा" ॥३९॥

॥ शतावरीघृतम् ॥

(भारतभैषज्यरत्नाकर : पञ्चमभाग : पृष्ठ ४३-४४)

***Śatāvarī Ghṛta***

Roots of *śatāvarī* should be crushed by pounding and squeezed to take out the juice. One *prastha* of this juice should be added with one *prastha* of ghee and two *prasthas* of milk. To this, the pastes of eight drugs belonging to *Jīvanīya* group, *yaṣṭi madhu, candana, padmaka, śvadaṃṣṭrā, ātmaguptā, balā, nāga balā, śāliparṇī, pṛśniparṇī, vidārī, sārivā, ananta mūla*, sugar and fruits of *kāśmarī*, each taken in quantities equal to a big fruit of *udumbara*, should be added and cooked. After it is properly cooked, the medicated ghee should be taken out of the oven and strained through a cloth. As the sun dispels darkness, so also the administration of this medicated ghee cures *rakta pitta* (a disease characterised by bleeding from different parts of the body), diseases caused by *vāyu* and *pitta, vāta rakta* (gout), consumption, asthma, hiccup, bronchitis of serious nature, burning sensation in the limbs and head caused by the vitiation of *rakta* as well as *pitta*, all varieties of menorrhagia and serious type of dysuria.

"मुद्गमाषस्य निर्यूहे[४४] रास्नाचित्रकनागरैः[४५] ।
सिद्धं सपिप्पलीबिल्वैः सर्पिः श्रेष्ठमसृग्दरे ॥४० ॥
॥ मुद्गादिघृतम्[४६] ॥
(भारतभैषज्यरत्नाकर : चतुर्थभाग : पृष्ठ ८९)

*Mudgādi Ghṛta*

Ghee cooked with the decoctions of *mudga* and *māṣa* added with the pastes of *rāsnā, citraka, nāgara, pippalī* and *bilva* is excellent in curing menorrhagia.

तण्डुलोदकसंपीतं बालं वा कदलीफलम् ।
रुणद्धि योषितां योनेः रक्तस्रावमतिद्रुतम् ॥४१ ॥

*Use of Kadalī*

Tender fruits of *kadalī* should be made to a paste by triturating with rice-wash. Intake of this potion stops excessive bleeding from the genital tract of the woman.

"कुमुदं पद्मकोशीरं[४७] गोधूमो[४८] रक्तशालयः ।
मुद्गपर्णी पयस्या च काश्मरी मधुयष्टिका ॥४२ ॥
'बलातिबलयोर्मूलमुत्पलं[४९] तालमस्तकम् ।
विदारी शतपुष्पा च शालपर्णी सजीरका[५०] ॥४३ ॥

'फल'[11] त्रपुषबीजानि प्रत्यग्रं कदलीफलम् ।
एषामर्द्धपलान् भागान् गव्यक्षीरं चतुर्गुणम् ॥४४॥
पानीयं द्विगुणं दत्त्वा घृतप्रस्थं विपाचयेत् ।
प्रदरे रक्तगुल्मे च रक्तपित्ते हलीमके ॥४५॥
बहुरूपञ्च'[12] यत्पित्तं कामलायां सशोणितम्'[13] ।
अरोचके ज्वरे जीर्णे पाण्डुरोगे मदे[14] भ्रमे ॥४६॥
तरुणी चाल्पपुष्पा च या च गर्भं न विन्दति ।
अहन्यहनि च स्त्रीणां भवति प्रीतिवर्द्धनम्'[15] ।
शीतकल्याणकं नाम परमुक्तं रसायनम् ॥४७॥
॥ शीतकल्याणकं घृतम् ॥
(भैषज्यरत्नावली : स्त्रीरोगाधिकार : ३०-३५)
(भारतभैषज्यरत्नाकर : पंचमभाग : पृष्ठ ४९)

### *Śīta Kalyāṇaka Ghṛta*

One *prastha* of ghee should be cooked by adding two *prasthas* of water, four *prasthas* of cow's milk and the paste of half *pala* of each of *kumuda, padmaka, uśīra, godhūma,* red variety of *śāli, mudga parṇī, payasyā, kāśmarī, madhuyaṣṭi,* roots of *balā* and *atibalā, utpala, tāla mastaka* (top of *tāla* tree), *vidārī, śatapuṣpā, śāla parṇī, jīraka, phala* (*mṛdvīkā*), seeds of *trapuṣa,* and upper portion of the fruits of *kadalī.* This medicated ghee is useful in menorragia, *rakta gulma* (tumour in the uterus), *rakta pitta* (a disease characterised by bleeding from different parts of the body), *halīmaka* (a serious type of jaundice), different morbid conditions of *rakta* and *pitta,* jaundice, anorexia, chronic fever, anemia, giddiness, less of menstrual flow in young girls and female sterility. Intake of this potion makes ladies lovable. This is called *Śīta kalyāṇaka* and it is an excellent rejuvenating recipe.

"चन्द्रप्रभाख्या'[16] गुटिका शिवासंज्ञा च शस्यते' ।
हितश्चात्र विशेषेण लेहो यः कुटजाष्टकः ॥४८॥

### *Use of Candraprabhā*

In the treatment of menorrhagia, *Candraprabhā guṭikā, Śivā* (*guṭikā*) and *Kuṭajāṣṭaka leha* are specially useful.

"कदलीनां"[५७] फलं पक्वं धात्रीफलरसं मधु ।
शर्करासहितं पेयं[५८] सोमधारणमुत्तमम् ॥४९॥

*Treatment of Soma Roga*
*Use of Kadalı*

Ripe banana fruit and *āmalakı* juice mixed with honey and sugar are useful for curing *soma roga.*

माषचूर्णं च मधुकं[५९] विदारीमधुशर्कराम् ।
पयसा पाययेत्प्रातस्त्वपां[६०] धारणमुत्तमम् ॥५०॥

*Recipe*

Powder of *māṣa, madhukā* and *vidārī* should be added with honey and sugar. Intake of this potion in the morning with milk is excellent for stopping excessive urination.

जलेनाऽऽमलकीबीजकर्कंधुमधुशर्करम्[६१] ।
पिबेद्दिनत्रयेणैव श्वेतप्रदरनाशनम् ॥५१॥

*Recipes for Treatment of Leucorrhoea*

Intake of the seed pulp of *āmalakı, karkandhu,* honey and sugar with water for three days cures leucorrhoea.

तक्रौदनाहाररता सन्पिबेन्नागकेशरम् ।
त्र्यहं तक्रेण संपिष्टं श्वेतप्रदरनाशनम् ॥५२॥
(योगरत्नाकर : सोमरोगचिकित्सा : पृष्ठ ४०२)

*Nāga kešara* should be made to a paste by triturating with butter-milk. Intake of this potion for three days cures leucorrhoea. The patient should take rice with butter-milk as food during the period of treatment.

॥ तत्रैव मूत्रातिसारचिकित्सा ॥

सोमरोगे चिरं जाते यदा मूत्रमतिस्रवेत् ।
मूत्रातिसारं तं प्राहुर्बलविध्वंसनं परम् ॥५३॥

### *Mūtrātisāra (Serious type of Polyuria)*

When *soma roga* becomes chronic and the patient voids urine in excessively large quantity, then the condition is called *mūtrātisāra.*

"तालकन्दश्च खर्जूरं मधुकं च विदारिकाम् ।
शर्करामधुसंयुक्तं[६७] मूत्रातीसारनाशनम् ॥५४॥

### *Treatment*

*Tāla kanda* (soft pith at the top of *tāla* tree), *kharjūra, madhuka* and *vidārikanda* should be added with sugar and honey. Intake of this potion cures *mūtrātisāra.*

चक्रमर्दकमूलं तु संपष्टिं तण्डुलाम्बुना ।
प्रभातसमये पीतं जलप्रदरनाशनम्" ॥५५॥
(योगरत्नाकर : सोमरोगचिकित्सा : पृष्ठ ४०३)

Root of *cakra marda* should be made to a paste by triturating with rice-wash. Intake of this potion early in the morning cures *jala pradara* (*mutratisara*).

'सगुडः[६३] श्यामतिलानां क्वाथः पीतः सुशीतलो नार्य्याः ।
जनयति कुसुमं सहसा गतमपि सुचिरं निरातङ्कम् ॥५६॥

### *Emmenagogue Recipes*

Decoction of black sessame should be cooled and added with jaggery. Intake of this instantaneously induces menstruation, even if it had ceased since long. This is safe for use.

तिलशेलुकारवीणां क्वाथं पीत्वापि[६४] नष्टरजाः ।
सगुडं शिशिरं वनिता[६५] जनयति कुसुमं न सन्देहः ॥५७॥

Ladies who are not having menstruation should take the decoction of *tila, śelu* and *kāravī* after cooling it and after adding jaggery. This undoubtedly causes menstruation.

"इक्ष्वाकुबीजदन्तीचपलागुडमदनफलकिण्वयावशूकैः[६६] ।
सस्नुक्क्षीरैर्वर्त्तिर्योनिगता कुसुमसञ्जननी" ॥५८॥

(भैषज्यरत्नावली : स्त्रीरोगाधिकार : १५०)
(योगरत्नाकार : योनिव्यापचिकित्सा : पृष्ठ ४०६)

A *varti* (suppository) prepared of the seeds of *ikṣvāku, dantī, capalā, guḍa, madanaphala, kiṇva, yava kṣāra* and milky-latex of *snuhī* should be inserted into the genital tract which induces menstrual bleeding.

क्वाथस्तिलानां विनिधाय पीतं कटुत्रिकब्राह्मणयष्टिचूर्णम् ।
निहन्ति सद्यः कुसुमावरोधं स्त्रीणामसंजातमतिप्रवृद्धम् ॥५९॥

Intake of the decoction of *tila* by adding the powders of *śuṇṭhī, pippalī, marica* and *brahmaṇa yaṣṭi* instantaneously cures amenorrhoea in women of long standing nature.

निम्बपत्रभुजंगत्वक् श्लेष्मान्तकदलान्वितम् ।
वराङ्गं धूपयेन्नारी रजःपतनाकांक्षिणी ॥६०॥

A woman desirous of getting menstruation should fumigate her vagina with the smoke of neem leaves, scales of snake and leaves of *śleṣmāntaka.*

"भूम्यामलकमूलं[६७] तु पीतं तण्डुलवारिणा ।
तद्दिनाद्द्वितयेनैव[६८] प्रदरं दुस्तरं जयेत्" ॥६१॥

(योगरत्नाकर : प्रदरचिकित्सा : पृष्ठ ३९८)

Root of *bhūmyāmalakī* should be made to a paste by triturating with the rice-wash (*taṇḍula-vāri*). Intake of this potion cures even serious type of menorrhagia in two days.

रक्तोत्पलशिफाखण्डशालूकं मधुनान्वितम् ।
गर्भिणीरक्तविस्रावे देयमेतन्महौषधम् ।
रक्तं च स्तंभ्यते तेन गर्भो नैव विनश्यति ॥६२॥

If a pregnant woman gets bleeding, then she should take the [powder of the] root of *raktotpala*, sugar and *śālūka* along with honey. This is an effective recipe. By its administration, bleeding will stop and there will be no harm to the foetus.

"जीरकं[६९] हपुषा धान्यं शताह्वा बदराणि च ।
यवानी[७०] अक्षका[७१] हिङ्गुपत्रिका कासमर्दकम् ।
पिप्पली पिप्पलीमूलमजमोदाऽथ वार्षिका[७२] ॥६३॥
चित्रकं च पलांशानि तथान्यच्च[७३] चतुःपलम् ।
कशेरुकं नागरं च कुष्ठं दीप्यकमेव च ॥६४॥
गुडस्य च शतं दद्यात् घृतप्रस्थं तथैव च ।
क्षीरद्विप्रस्थसंयुक्तं शनैर्मृद्वग्निना पचेत् ॥६५॥
पञ्चजीरक इत्येव सूतिकानां प्रशस्यते ।
गर्भार्थिनीनां नारीणां बृंहणीये समारुते ॥६६॥
विंशतिव्यापदो योनेः कासं श्वासं स्वरक्षयम्[७४] ।
हलीमकं पाण्डुरोगं दौर्गन्ध्यं कृच्छ्रमूत्रताम्[७५] ॥६७॥
हन्ति[७६] पीनोन्नतकुचाः पद्मपत्रायतेक्षणाः ।
उपयोगात् स्त्रियो नित्यमलक्ष्मीमलवर्जिताः" ॥६८॥

॥ इति पञ्चजीरकगुडावलेहः[७७] ॥

(भैषज्यरत्नावली : स्त्रीरोगाधिकार : ४००-४०६)

**Pañca-jīraka-guḍāvaleha**

One *pala* of each of *jīraka, hapuṣā, dhānya, śatāhvā, badara, yamānī, akṣakā, hiṅgupatrikā, kāsamarda, pippalī, pippalī mūla, ajamodā, vārṣikā* and *citraka*, four *palas* of each of *kaseruka, nāgara, kuṣṭha* and *dīpyaka*, one hundred *palas* of jaggery, one *prastha* of ghee and two *prasthas* of milk should be slowly cooked together over mild fire. This recipe is called *Pañcajīraka* and it is useful for ladies after delivery. In ladies desirous of conception, it provides nourishment and alleviates *vāyu*. It cures twenty diseases of *yoni* (genital tract including uterus), cough, asthma, suppression of voice, *halīmaka* (a type of jaundice), anemia, foul smell coming out of the body and dysuria. By the use of this recipe, the breasts of ladies become plumpy and elevated, the eyes become wide like the leaf of lotus and ladies become free from inauspiciousness and dirt.

Note : The purpose for which the prefix '*pañca*' meaning 'five' used in the name of this recipe is not clear.

"जीरकं प्रस्थमेकं तु क्षीरं द्व्याढकमेव[७८] च।
घृतप्रस्थार्द्धसंयुक्तं[७९] शनैर्मन्दाग्निना[८०] पचेत् ॥६९॥
सुशीते[८१] शर्करा प्रस्थद्वयं वापि विनिक्षिपेत् ।
चातुर्जातं कृष्णाविश्वमजाजीं[८२] च घनं जलम् ॥७०॥
दाडिमं रसजं धान्यं रजनी कंटवासकम् ।
वंशजातं[८३] तवक्षीरं प्रत्येक तु पलार्द्धकम् ॥७१॥
जीरकस्यावलेहोऽयं[८४] प्रदरापहरः[८५] परम् ।
ज्वरप्रमेहतृड्दाहकृच्छ्रक्षवथुनाशनः"[८६] ॥७२॥

॥ जीरकावलेहः ॥

इति श्रीमहाराजाधिराजटोडरमल्लविरचिते टोडरानन्दे आयुर्वेदसौख्ये असृग्दरनिदानचिकित्सा[८७]कथनं नाम एकसप्ततितमो हर्षः ।

***Jīrakāvaleha***

One *prastha* of *jīraka*, two *āḍhakas* of milk and half *prastha* of ghee should be slowly cooked over mild fire. After it cools down, two *prasthas* of sugar should be added to it. To this, half *pala* of each of *tvak, elā, patra, nāgakesara, pippalī, śuṇṭhī, ajājī, ghana, jala, dāḍima, rasaja, dhānya, rajanī, kaṇṭa-vāsaka* and *vaṃśalocana* should be added. This recipe is called '*Jīrakāvaleha*'. It is an excellent recipe for the cure of menorrhagia. It also cures fever, *prameha* (obstinate urinary disorders), morbid thirst, burning sensation, dysuria and sneezing.

Thus, ends the 71st chapter dealing with the diagnosis and treatment of menorrhagia in *Āyurveda saukhya* of *Ṭoḍarānanda* composed by the great king Ṭoḍaramalla.

## NOTES AND REFERENCES

१. (क) This is the beginning of seventy fifth chapter of *Āyurveda saukhya* in *Todarānanda* and invocation reads as follows :

मल्लोत्सवं द्रष्टुं समुत्सुको यः सुरंगरागेण पुरं प्रयातः ।
पुनर्दिवा पातु सुपुत्रमित्रं श्रीटोडरं विप्रदरिद्रतारिम् ॥
मदाघूर्णितनेत्राय रेवती कण्ठलंबिने ।
स्खलते पादविन्यासे कस्मैश्चिन्महसे नमः ॥

(ख) 'मल्लोत्सवं ..... नमः' पाठोऽयं चतुर्थषष्ठपुस्तकयोः नोपलभ्यते ।

२. तस्याभिवृद्धौ इति प्रथमपुस्तके पाठः ।

३. श्रमो इत प्रथमपुस्तके पाठः ।

४. (क) प्रकारं प्रवदन्ति तज्ज्ञाः इति प्रथमपुस्तके पाठः ।
(ख) प्रकारं प्रवदन्ति मालमतज्ञाः इति पंचमपुस्तके पाठः ।

५. सपिच्छप्रथमं इति प्रथमपुस्तके पाठः ।

६. तं चाप्यसाध्यं इति आकरे पाठः ।

७. यच्चासु न विरंजयेत् इति षष्ठपुस्तके पाठः ।

८. तामसाध्यां विनिर्दिशेत् इति षष्ठपुस्तके पाठः ।

९. इति प्रदराधिकारः अथ सोमरोगनिदानं इति षष्ठपुस्तके पाठः ।

१०. "स्त्रीणाम् ..... भवेत्सदा" पाठोऽयं प्रथमपुस्तके नोपलभ्यते ।

११. अतिसारिक. इति चतुर्थपुस्तके पाठः ।

१२. व्रजन्ति हि इति आकरे पाठः ।

१३. ताः सा न शक्नोति दुर्बला इति आकरे पाठः ।

१४. 'वेगं ..... क्वचित्' पाठोऽयं पंचमपुस्तके नोपलभ्यते ।

१५. च शुष्यति इति आकरे पाठः ।

१६. अतिमात्रकः पंचमपुस्तके पाठः ।

१७. असृग्दरसोमरोगनिदानम् इति चतुर्थषष्ठपुस्तकयोः पाठः ।

१८. 'दध्ना ..... नीलमुत्पलम्' पाठोऽयं षष्ठपुस्तके नोपलभ्यते ।

१९. वातासृग्दरनाशीनी इति षष्ठपुस्तके पाठः ।

२०. पिबेदैणयकरक्तं इति षष्ठपुस्तके पाठः ।

२१. वासकस्वरसै पैत्ते इति आकरे पाठः ।

२२. धातक्याः कोलमात्रं इति आकरे पाठः ।

२३. मधु सकषायः इति षष्ठपुस्तके पाठः ।

२४. सुशीतलं इति प्रथमपुस्तके पाठः ।

२५. दिनत्रयान्तरेणैव स्त्रीरोगं नाशयेद्ध्रुवम् इति आदर्शपुस्तकेषु पाठः ।

२६. 'भूम्यामलकमूलं ..... जयेत्' पाठोऽयं प्रथमपुस्तके नोपलभ्यते ।

२७. 'दध्ना च औषधीपिष्टां लोहितप्रदरी पिबेत्' पाठोऽयं चतुर्थषष्ठपुस्तकयोः अधिकमुपलभ्यते ।

२८. (क) मधुना युतम् इति षष्ठपुस्तके पाठः ।
(ख) मधुना संयुतं पीतम् इति आकरे पाठः ।

२९. तण्डुलसलिलेन इति आकरे पाठः ।

३०. शिलाभेदं इति आकरे पाठः ।

३१. अवष्टिकी इति प्रथमपुस्तके पाठः ।

३२. .विषा इति आकरे पाठः ।

३३. मधुकं इति षष्ठपुस्तके पाठः ।

३४. असृग्दरातिसारेषु इति आकरे पाठः ।

३५. अम्बष्ठा दक्षिणे ख्याता गृह्णन्त्यन्ये तु लक्ष्मणाम् पाठोऽयं आकरे अधिकमुपलभ्यते ।

३६. क्षोदयित्वाऽवपीडयेत् इति आकरे पाठः ।

३७. सन्निभान् इति प्रथमपुस्तके पाठः ।

३८. यान्यष्टौ इति आकरे पाठः ।

३९. 'जीवनीयानि ..... तथा' पाठोऽयं षष्टपुस्तके नोपलभ्यते ।

४०. शालपर्णी पृष्ठिपर्णी इति आदर्शपुस्तकेषु पाठः ।

४१. समानि च इति षष्ठपुस्तके पाठः ।

४२. चावचारयेत् इति आकरे पाठः ।

४३. क्षयं तथा इति षष्ठपुस्तके पाठः ।

४४. निर्यूहै इति प्रथमपुस्तके पाठः ।

४५. .मुस्तकैः इति आकरे पाठः ।

४६. मुद्गाद्यं घृतम् इति प्रथमचतुर्थषष्ठपुस्तकेषु पाठः ।

४७. यमकोशीरं इति चतुर्थपुस्तके पाठः ।

४८. गोधूमं इति आकरे पाठः ।

४९. 'बलाति ..... सजीरका' पाठोऽयं प्रथमपुस्तके नोपलभ्यते ।

५०. संजीवकम् इति आदर्शपुस्तकेषु पाठः ।

५१. 'फलं ..... द्विगुणं' पाठोऽयं चतुर्थपुस्तके नोपलभ्यते ।

५२. बहुरूपे च यत्पित्ते इति चतुर्थषष्ठपुस्तकयोः पाठः ।

५३. सशोणिते इति चतुर्थषष्ठपुस्तकयोः पाठः ।

५४. मदात्यये इति चतुर्थषष्ठपुस्तकयोः पाठः ।

५५. प्रीतिदर्शनम् इति षष्ठपुस्तके पाठः ।

५६. 'चन्द्रप्रभाख्या ..... शस्यते' पाठोऽयं प्रथमपुस्तके नोपलभ्यते ।

५७. "कदलीनां ..... श्वेतप्रदरनाशनम्" पाठोऽयं प्रथमपुस्तके नोपलभ्यते ।

५८. खादेत्सोमधारणमुत्तमम् इति आकरे पाठः ।

५९. समधुकं इति आकरे पाठः ।

६०. पाययेत्प्रातः सोमधारणमुत्ततम् इति आकरे पाठः ।

६१. बीजकल्कं समधुशर्करम् इति आकरे पाठः ।

६२. सितामधुयुतां खादेन्मूत्रातिसारनाशनम् इति आकरे पाठः ।

६३. 'सगुडः ..... पतनकांक्षिणी' पाठोऽयं प्रथमषष्ठपुस्तकयोः नोपलभ्यते ।

६४. गतरजा महिला इति आकरे पाठः ।

६५. त्रिदिनाज्जनयति इति आकरे पाठः ।

६६. किण्वयष्ट्याह्वैः इति आकरे पाठः ।

६७. "भूम्यामलकमूलं ..... विनश्यति" पाठोऽयं पंचमपुस्तके अधिकमुपलभ्यते ।

६८. (क) द्वित्रैरेव दिनैर्नार्याः प्रदरं दुस्तरं जयेत् इति आकरे पाठः ।

(ख) तद्दिनद्वितयेनैव स्त्री वरांगं वासयेद् ध्रुवम् इति पंचमपुस्तके पाठः ।

६९. "जीरकं ..... जीरकगुडावलेहः" पाठोऽयं प्रथमपंचमपुस्तकयोः नोपलभ्यते ।

७०. यमानी इति आकरे पाठः ।

७१. (क) पक्षका इति षष्ठपुस्तके पाठः ।

(ख) क्रुष्टिको इति आकरे पाठः ।

७२. (क) वाष्पिका इति आकरे पाठः ।

(ख) वात्थिका इति षष्ठपुस्तके पाठः ।

७३. तथा धान्यं इति षष्ठपुस्तके पाठः ।

७४. ज्वरं क्षयम् इति आकरे पाठः ।

७५. (क) मूत्रकृच्छ्रताम् इति आकरे पाठः ।

(ख) कृच्छ्रमूत्रणम् इति आकरे पाठः ।

७६. घ्नन्ति इति आकरे पाठः ।

७७. पंचजीरकगुडः इति आकरे पाठः ।

७८. तु क्षीरराष्णाढकमेव च इति प्रथमपुस्तके पाठः ।

७९. प्रस्थार्धं लोध्रघृत्योः पचेन्मन्देन वह्निना इति आकरे पाठः ।

८०. शनैर्मृद्वग्निना इति षष्ठपुस्तके पाठः ।

८१. (क) सशीते इति षष्ठपुस्तके पाठः ।

(ख) लेहीभूतेथ शीतेऽत्र सितप्रस्थं विनिक्षिपेत् इति आकरे पाठः ।

८२. जाजीमुस्तबालकम् इति आकरे पाठः ।

८३. वंशजं च तवक्षीरी प्रत्येकं शुक्तिसम्मितम् इति आकरे पाठः ।

८४. जीरकस्यावलेहः तु इति षष्ठपुस्तके पाठः ।

८५. प्रमेहप्रदरापहः इति आकरे पाठः ।

८६. ज्वरवल्यरुचिश्वासतृष्णादाहक्षयापहः इति आकरे पाठः ।

८७. (क) प्रदरनिदानचिकित्सा इति चतुर्थपुस्तके पाठः ।

(ख) सोमरोगनिदानचिकित्सा इति षष्ठपुस्तके पाठः ।

# CHAPTER II

## ।। अथ योनिव्यापद्योनिकन्दनिदानं चिकित्सा च ।।

*(Diagnosis and Treatment of Diseases of Female Genital Tract and Prolapse Uterus)*

"विंशतिर्व्यापदो[१] योनेनिर्दिष्टा रोगसंग्रहे ।
मिथ्याचारेण[२] ता स्त्रीणां प्रदुष्टेनाऽऽर्त्तवेन च ।।
जायन्ते बीजदोषाच्च दैवाद्वा शृणु ताः पृथक् ।।१।।

(योगरत्नाकर : योनिरोगधिकार : पृष्ठ ४०४)

*Varieties and Etiology*

Diseases of the female genital tract are described to be of twenty varieties. These diseases are caused by the following factors :

(1) Wrong regimens;
(2) vitiation of menstrual flow including ovum;
(3) defects in genes; or
(4) providential causes.

Different types of these diseases are described here under.

सा फेनिलमुदावर्त्ता रजः कृच्छ्रेण मुञ्चति ।

*Udāvartā Yoni*

In *udāvartā*, the woman voids frothy menstrual blood and the menstruation is associated with pain.

वन्ध्यां नष्टार्त्तवां विद्यात् विप्लुतां नित्यवेदनाम् ॥२॥

***Vandhyā & Viplutā***

Cessation of menstruation in a woman is called *vandhyā*.

Constant pain [in the pelvic region] in a woman is called *viplutā*.

परिप्लुतायां भवति ग्राम्यधर्मेण रुग् भृशम् ।
वातला कर्कशा स्तब्धा शूलनिस्तोदपीडिता ॥
चतसृष्वपि चाद्यासु भवन्त्यनिलवेदनाः ॥३॥

***Paripluta & Vātalā***

In *pariplutā*, the woman gets excruciating pain during sexual intercourse.

Roughness, stiffness and colic pain in the genital tract are the characteristic features of *vātala*.

The first four varieties, viz., *udāvartā, vandhya, viplutā*, and *paripluta* of *yoni roga*, are also associated with different types of pain caused by aggravated *vāyu*.

सदाहं क्षीयते रक्तं यस्या सा लोहितक्षया ।

***Lohitakṣayā***

If there is excessive bleeding during menstruation and if it is associated with burning sensation in the genital tract, then the ailment is called *lohitakṣayā*.

सवातमुद्गिरेत् बीजं वामिनी रजसा युतम् ॥४॥

***Vāminī***

If the woman expels the *bīja* (sperm and ovum) along with menstrual blood and flatus, then the condition is called *vāminī*.

प्रस्रंसिनी स्रंसते च क्षोभिता दुष्प्रजायिनी ।

*Prasraṃsinī*

If there is excruciating pain during menstruation and delivery, then the condition is called *prasraṃsinī.*

स्थितं स्थितं हन्ति गर्भं पुत्रघ्नी रक्तसंक्षयात् ॥५॥

*Putraghnī*

Repeated conceptions followed by repeated abortions accompanied by loss of blood is called *putraghnī.*

अत्यर्थं पित्तला योनिर्दाहपाकज्वरान्विता ।
चतसृष्वपि चाद्यासु[४] पित्तलिङ्गोच्छ्रयो[५] भवेत् ॥६॥

*Pittalā*

Excessive burning sensation and suppuration in the genital tract and association of high fever are the characteristic features of *pittala* type of *yoniroga.*

The earlier four varieties, viz., *lohitakṣayā, vāminī, prasraṃsinī* and *putraghnī* are also associated with the signs and symptoms of aggravated *pitta.*

अत्यानन्दा न सन्तोषं ग्राम्यधर्मेण गच्छति ।

*Atyānandā*

In *atyānandā* variety of *yoniroga,* the woman does not draw satisfaction even after (appropriate) sexual intercourse.

कर्णिभ्यां कर्णिका योनौ श्लेष्मासृग्भ्यां[६] च जायते ॥७॥

*Karṇinī*

In *karṇinī*, a *karṇikā* (ring like mass) appears in the genital tract because of the vitiation of *kapha* and *rakta* (blood).

मैथुनाचरणात्पूर्वं[७] पुरुषादतिरिच्यते[८] ।
बहुशश्चातिचरणा तयोर्बीजं न विन्दति ॥८॥

*Acaraṇā and Aticaraṇā*

If the woman gets orgasm before the man during sexual intercourse then she is called *acarṇā.*

If the woman gets orgasm only after excessive (repeated) sexual intercourse, then she is called *aticaraṇā.*

Both these types of women do not conceive as a result of sexual intercourse.

श्लेष्मला पिच्छिला योनिः कण्डूग्रस्ताऽतिशीतला[९] ।
'चतसृष्वपि[१०] चाद्यासु श्लेष्मलिङ्गोच्छ्रयो भवेत् ॥९॥

*Śleṣmalā*

If the genital tract is slimy, itchy and excessively cold, then the condition is called *ślcṣmala.*

The earlier mentioned four varieties, viz., *atyānanda, karṇinī, acaraṇā* and *aticaraṇa* are associated with the signs and symptoms of excessively aggravated *kapha.*

अनार्त्तवाऽस्तनी षण्डी खरस्पर्शा च मैथुने ।

*Ṣaṇḍī*

The woman who does not get menstruation, whose breasts are not developed and whose genital tract remains rough during the act of coitus is called *ṣaṇḍī.*

अतिकायगृहीतायास्तरुण्यास्त्वण्डिनी भवेत् ॥१०॥

*Aṇḍinī*

If a young woman enters into sexual intercourse with a person having robust body, the resultant change in her genital tract is called *aṇḍinī.*

विवृतातिमहायोनिः[११] सूचीवक्त्राऽतिसंवृता ।
सर्वलिङ्गसमुत्थाना सर्वदोषप्रकोपजाः ॥
चतसृष्वपि चाद्यासु सर्वलिङ्गस्य[१२] दर्शनम् ॥११॥

*Vivṛtā and Sūcīvaktrā*

The woman whose vaginal tract is very wide is called *vivṛtā*.

The woman whose vaginal tract is very narrow is called *sūcīvaktrā*.

*Sānnipātika Yoniroga*

In *sānnipātika* type of *yoniroga*, signs and symptoms of all the three *doṣas*, viz., *vāyu*, *pitta* and *kapha* are manifested.

The earlier mentioned four varieites, viz., *ṣaṇḍī*, *aṇḍinī*, *vivṛtā* and *sūcīvaktrā* are also associated with the signs and symptoms of excessively aggravated *vāyu*, *pitta* and *kapha*.

पञ्चासाध्या भवन्ति हि योनयः सर्वदोषजाः ॥१२॥
(माधवनिदान : योनिरोगनिदान : ६२:१-१३)

*Prognosis*

The five varieties of *yoniroga*, viz., *ṣaṇḍī*, *aṇḍinī*, *vivṛtā*, *sūcīvaktrā* and *sānnipātika* which are caused by the simultaneous aggravation of all the three *doṣas*, are incurable.

"दिवास्वप्नादतिक्रोधाद् व्यायामादतिमैथुनात् ।
क्षताच्च नखदन्ताद्यैर्वाताद्याः कुपिता यदा ॥१३॥
पूयशोणितसंयुतं[१३] निकुचाकृतिसन्निभम्[१४] ।
उत्पद्यते[१५] तदा योनौ नाम्ना कन्दस्तु[१६] योनिजः ॥१४॥

*Yonikanda (Prolapse Uterus)*

*Etiology and Pathogenesis*

Prolapse of uterus takes place because of the following factors :

(1) Sleep during the day time;

(2) excessive anger and exercise;

(3) excessive sexual intercourse; and
(4) injury by nails and teeth.

Because of the above mentioned factors, *vāyu*, etc., get aggravated, and in the vaginal tract, a growth like the fruit of *nikuca*, smeared with pus and blood, appears which is called *yonikanda*.

Note : Although, *yonikanda* generally refers to prolapse of uterus, some physicians interprete this term as a vaginal tumour or polyp.

रूक्षं विवर्णं स्फुटितं वातिकं तं विनिर्दिशेत्।
दाहरागज्वरयुतं विद्यात् पित्तात्मकं च तम् ॥१५॥
नीलपुष्पप्रतिकाशं कण्डूमन्तं कफात्मकम् ।
सर्वलिङ्गसमायुक्तं सन्निपातात्मकं वदेत्[१७] ॥१६॥
॥ योनिव्यापद्योनिकन्दनिदानम् ॥

(माधवनिदान : योनिकन्दनिदान : ६३ : १-४)

*Varieties and Their Signs and Symptoms*

In *vātika* type of *yonikanda*, the growth is ununctuous, discoloured, and cracked.

If the growth is associated with burning sensation, redness and fever, then it is to be determined as *paittika yonikanda*.

If the growth appears like a blue flower and itchy, then it is *kaphaja* type of *yonikanda*.

If the signs and symptoms of all the three *doṣas*, viz., *vāyu*, *pitta* and *kapha* are manifested in the growth, then it is of *sannipātika* type.

Thus, ends the diagnosis of *yonivyapat* and *yonikanda*.

योनिव्यापत्सु भूयिष्ठं[१८] शस्यते कर्म वातजित् ।
बस्त्यभ्यङ्गपरीषेकप्रलेपाः पिचुधारणम् ॥१७॥

*Line of Treatment*

In *yoniroga*, therapies, which predominantly alleviate *vāyu*, like *basti* (medicated enema), *abhyaṅga* (massage), *pariṣeka* (sprinkling of medicated water), *pralepa* (external application of drugs in the form of paste) and *picudhāraṇa* (keeping medicine-smeared cotton pads in the vagina) are useful.

वचोपकुञ्चिकाजाजी-कृष्णा-वृषकसैन्धवम्[१९] ।
अजमोदायवक्षारचित्रकं शर्करान्वितम् ॥१८॥
पिष्ट्वा प्रसन्नयालोड्य खादेत्तु[२०] घृतभर्जितम् ।
योनिपाश्वर्ार्त्तिहृद्रोगगुल्माशोर्ं[१] विनिवृत्तये ॥१९॥
(भैषज्यरत्नावली : स्त्रीरोगाधिकार : १२३-१२५)

*Recipes*

*Vacā, upakuñcikā, ajāji, kṛṣṇā, vṛṣaka*, rock-salt, *ajamodā, yavakṣāra* and *citraka* mixed with sugar should be made to a paste by triturating. This paste should be mixed with *prasannā* type of wine and taken after sizzling with ghee. This cures pain in the female genital tract and sides of the chest, heart diseases, *gulma* (phantom tumour) and piles.

कर्पासबीजसाधितं घृतमुंदुरुमांसतैलं वा ।
भगभरणेन तदीयं सूतायाः शूलमपनयति ॥
"रास्नास्वदंष्ट्रावृषकैशृंतं[२२] शूलहरं पयः ॥२०॥
(योगरत्नाकर : योनिव्यापच्चिकित्सा : पृष्ठ ४१०)

The genital tract of the woman should be filled with the following recipes :

(1) medicated ghee prepared by boiling with cotton-seed; or
(2) medicated oil prepared by boiling with the flesh of *unduru* (mouse).

These recipes cure colic pain in the vaginal canal of a woman after delivery.

Intake of the milk boiled with *rāsnā, svadaṃṣṭrā* and *vṛṣaka* cures colic pain in the vaginal canal of a woman.

अपामार्गस्य कल्कं तु योनिमध्ये विधारयेत् ।
योनिपीडा शमं यान्ति गर्भिन्यां न च कारयेत् ॥२१॥

Keeping the paste of *apāmārga* in the vaginal canal cures pain (of the vaginal canal). This recipe should not, however, be administered if the lady is pregnant.

पिष्ट्वा लिप्ते योनौ मूलेन खरमञ्जरीपुनर्नवयोः ।
नवसूतायाः सकलं योनिगतं शूलमपनयति ॥२२॥

The vaginal canal of a freshly delivered woman should be smeared with the paste of the root of *kharamañjarī* and *punarnavā* which cures her pain in the genital tract.

"गुडूचीत्रिफलादन्तीक्वाथैश्च परिषेचनम् ॥२३॥

Sprinkling of the vaginal canal with the decoction of *guḍūcī, harītakī, bibhītaka, āmalakī* and *dantī* cures pain of the female genital tract.

नतवार्त्ताकिनीकुष्ठसैन्धवामरदारुभिः[२३] ।
तैलात् प्रसाधिताद्धार्यः पिचुर्योनौ रुजापहः[२४] ॥२४॥

*Treatment of Vātika Yoniroga*

Oil should be cooked with *nata, vārtākinī, kuṣṭha, saindhava* and *devadāru*. Keeping a cotton pad smeared with this medicated oil in the vaginal canal cures pain.

पित्तलानान्तु योनिनां सेकाभ्यङ्गपिचुक्रियाः ।
कार्याः सर्वाः प्रयत्नेन स्नेहनार्थं घृतानि च ॥२५॥

*Treatment of Paittika Yoniroga*

For the cure of *pittala* types of *yoniroga* one should carefully use ghee for oleation in the form of *seka* (sprinkling), *abhyaṅga* (massage) and *picukriyā* (application of medicated cotton pad in the genital tract).

योन्यां बलासदुष्टायां सर्वरूक्षोष्णमौषधम् ॥२६॥
पिप्पलीमरिचैर्माषैः शताह्वाकुष्ठसैन्धवैः ।
वर्त्तिस्तुल्या प्रदेशिन्या धार्या योनिविशोधिनी ॥२७॥

(भैषज्यरत्नावली : स्त्रीरोगाधिकार : १२६-१३०)

***Treatment of Kaphaja Yoniroga***

In *kaphaja* tyes of *yoniroga*, medicines which are ununctuous and hot should be used.

A *varti* (suppository) of the size and shape of index finger should be prepared of *pippalı, marica, māṣa, śatāhvā, kuṣṭha* and *saindhava*. Keeping this *varti* in the vaginal canal helps in the cleansing of the tract.

'मूषकं क्वाथकल्काभ्यां मांसं तैले विपाचयेत् ।
योनिकन्दहरस्त्रीणां सर्वशूलविनाशनम् ॥२८॥

***Use of Mouse-flesh***

The flesh of mouse, in the form of decoction and paste should be cooked in oil. Application of this medicated oil cures *yonikanda* and all types of pain in the vaginal canal.

पुष्योद्धृतं लक्ष्मणाया मूलं पिष्टं च कन्यया ।
ऋत्वन्ते घृतदुग्धाभ्यां पीत्वाप्नोति बला सुतम् ॥२९॥

***Use of Lakṣmaṇā***

Root of *lakṣmaṇā* should be collected during *puṣya* constellation and made to a paste by triturating with the juice of *kumarı*. Intake of this potion along with ghee and milk after the cessation of menstrual flow helps in the procreation of a male offspring.

रोहितपित्तकणाघृतविमलाञ्जनसैन्धवैरथवा ।
भगलेपः सौभाग्यं जनयति न संदेहः ॥३०॥

The paste of the bile of *rohita, pippalı*, ghee, *vimala, añjana* and *saindhava* should be applied over the vagina. This undoubtedly endows auspiciousness.

दाडिमपंचागैर्वा सिद्धं सिद्धार्थकतैलम् ।
मालतीकाकुसुमैर्वा गुह्याभ्यङ्गेन सौभाग्यम् ॥३१॥

Mustard oil cooked with either the five parts (flower, fruit, leaf, stem and root) of pomegranate (*dāḍima*) or the flower of *mālatı* should be applied over the vagina which endows auspiciousness.

"पत्रमेकं[२५] पलाशस्य गर्भिणी पयसान्वितम् ।
पीत्वा च लभते पुत्रं वीर्यवन्तं न संशयः ॥३२॥

*Use of Palāśa*

If a pregnant woman takes one leaf of *palāśa* triturated with milk she undoubtedly gets son endowed with strength.

बस्तमूत्रं च सघृतं नवनीतं तु माहिषम् ।
रात्रत्रयं पिबेन्नारी अपि वन्ध्या प्रसूयते ॥३३॥

Intake of goat's urine along with the ghee or butter collected from buffalo-milk for three nights helps in the conception of even a sterile woman.

आखोर्मांसं दृषदि बहुधा सूक्ष्मखण्डीकृतं तत् ।
तैले पाच्यं चलति नियतं यावदेतन्न सम्यक्।
तत्तैलाक्तं वसनमनिशं योनिदेशे दधाना ।
सत्यं व्रीडाजनकमबलायोनिकन्दं निहन्ति ॥३४॥

Flesh of mouse should be finely minced and properly cooked in oil. A piece of cloth should be smeared with the oil and kept in the vaginal canal. This cures the humiliating *yonikanda* of women.

इति श्रीमहाराजाधिराजश्रीटोडरमल्लविरचिते टोडरानन्दे
आयुर्वेदसौख्ये योनिव्यापद्योनिकन्दनिदान-चिकित्साकथनं
नाम द्विसप्ततितमो हर्षः ।

Thus ends the 72nd chapter dealing with the diagnosis and treatment of *yoniroga* and *yonikanda* in *Āyurveda saukhya* of *Ṭodarānanda* composed by the great king Ṭodaramalla

## NOTES AND REFERENCES

१. (क) This is the beginning of seventy sixth chapter of *Āyurveda saukhya* in *Ṭoḍarānanda* and the invocation reads as follows :
'मदोत्कटद्वारिससादिकुञ्जरं निहत्य रङ्गस्य रणोत्सुकं स्थितम् ।
तद्दन्तरक्तोद्भवविंदुभिर्यो रेजे सदीप्तिं विदधातु भूपे' ॥

(ख) 'मदो. ...........भूपे' पाठोऽयं चतुर्थपंचमपुस्तकयोः नोपलभ्यते ।

२. (क) मिथ्यापचारैस्ता इति प्रथमपुस्तके पाठः ।
(ख) मिथ्योपचारिस्ता इति षष्ठपुस्तके पाठः ।

३. (क) वेदनम् इति प्रथमपुस्तके पाठः ।
(ख) वेदना इति चतुर्थपुस्तके पाठः ।

४. चैतासु इति आदर्शपुस्तकेषु पाठः ।

५. पित्तलिङ्गोच्छ्रितो इति षष्ठपुस्तके पाठः ।

६. प्रजायते इति आकरे पाठः ।

७. मैथुनेऽचरणा पूर्वं इति आकरे पाठः ।

८. .तिरित्यति इति चतुर्थपुस्तके पाठः ।

९. सूचिव्रक्राति संवृता इति प्रथमपुस्तके पाठः ।

१०. 'चतसृष्वपि....मैथुने' पाठोऽयं प्रथमपुस्तके नोपलभ्यते ।

११. विवृता च इति आकरे पाठः ।

१२. सर्वलिङ्गोच्छ्रयो भवेत् इति आकरे पाठः ।

१३. संकाश इति आकरे पाठः ।

१४. लकुचाकृति. इति प्रथमपुस्तके पाठः ।

१५. जनयन्ति यदा योनौ इति आकरे पाठः ।

१६. कन्दः स इति आकरे पाठः ।

१७. (क) विदुः इति आकरे पाठः ।
(ख) भवेत् इति षष्ठपुस्तके पाठः ।

१८. निर्दिष्टं इति षष्ठपुस्तके पाठः ।

१९. धवोपकुञ्जिकाजाजीगौंडीवासकसैन्धवम् इति चतुर्थपुस्तके पाठः ।

२०. (क) खादेत्तद् इति आकरे पाठः ।
(ख) प्रसन्नया लोध्रं खादेत्तु इति षष्ठपुस्तके पाठः ।

२१. योनिव्यापत्ति हृद्रोग. इति आकरे पाठः ।

२२. रास्नाश्वगन्धावृषकैर्योनि. इति आकरे पाठः ।

२३. नववार्त्तकिनोकुष्ठं इति चतुर्थपुस्तके पाठः ।

२४. 'क्वाथस्तिलानां विनिधाय पीतं कटुत्रिकं ब्राह्मणयष्टिचूर्णम् ।
निहन्ति सद्यः कुसुमावरोधं स्त्रीणामसंजातमपि प्रवृद्धम् ॥
निम्बपत्रभुजंगत्वक् श्लेष्मातकदलान्वितम् ।
वरांगं धूपयेत् नारी रजः पतनकांक्षिणी ॥
नासयास्येन वा पीतं वटशृंगाष्टकं नवम् ।
वारिणा शुक्लपक्षे हि पुष्पितं तु समाहृतम् ॥
एरण्डस्य तु बीजानि मातुलुङ्गस्य चैव हि ।
सर्पिषा परिपिष्टानि पिबेद् गर्भप्रदानि तु ॥
गोघृतेन सह नागकेशरं श्लक्ष्णचूर्णकमृतौ ।
नितम्बिनी गव्यदुग्धनिरता प्रपिवेद्यदि ॥
सातटानियतमेव वीरसूः ।
पत्रमेकं पलाशस्य गर्भिणी पयसाचितम् ।
पीत्वा च लभते पुत्रं वीर्यवन्तं न संशयः ॥
पुष्ये पुत्तलकं कृत्वा हैमं वह्निप्रतापितम् ।
नी (क्षी) रे निर्वापयेत्तपृं पिबेत्तत्पलकाष्टकम् ॥
पुत्रं जनयते नारि महाबलपराक्रमः ।
वस्तमूत्रं च संवृत्तम् नवनीतं तु माहिषम् ॥
पलत्रयं पिवेन्नारी अपि वन्ध्या प्रसूयते ।
क्षौद्रं वृषं चन्दनसिंधुजातं महैन्द्रमाता पयसा निपिष्टम् ॥
गर्भं च रक्तं प्रतिहन्ति सर्वं योगोयमुक्तो हरमेखलायाम् ।
क्वाथेन हयगंधाया साधितं या पयोघृतम् ॥
ऋतुस्नाता पिबेन्नारी गर्भं धते न संशयः ।
माधवात् लक्ष्मणा लक्षणम् -
गोक्षीरसदृशैः पुष्पैवन्र्ष्णीरोमसमन्विता ।
रक्तविन्दुस्तु तल्यन्ते लक्ष्मणाकन्द उच्यते ॥
लिंगकारं लक्ष्मणायास्तन्मूलम् ।
यागे लब्धं सर्पिषा नस्ययोगात् ॥
पीत्वा सूते पुत्रमत्यन्तवीर्यम् ।
पश्चादन्यान (म)प्यमन्दांगयष्टि ॥
आखोर्मांसं दृषदि बहुधा सूक्ष्मखण्डीकृतं तत् ।
तैले पाच्यं चलति नियतं यावदेतन्न सम्यक् ॥

तत्तैलाक्तं वसनमनिशं योनिभागे दधाना ।
हन्ति ब्रीडाकरभगफलं नात्र संदेहबुद्धिः ॥
योषितः सततं यस्या गर्भवत्याः स्रवेदसृक् ।
पारावतपुरीषं च पाययेत्तंदुलांबुना ॥
॥ राजमार्त्तण्डात्' ॥
पाठोऽयं चतुर्थषष्ठपुस्तकयोः अधिकमुपलभ्यते ।

२५. "पुत्रमेकं .... निहन्ति" पाठोऽयं पंचमपुस्तके अधिकमुपलभ्यते ।

# CHAPTER III

## ॥ अथ मूढगर्भनिदानं चिकित्सा च ॥

*(Diagnosis and Management of Abnormal Pregnancy)*

"भयाभिघातात्[१] तीक्ष्णोष्णपानाशननिषेवणात् ।
गर्भे पतति रक्तस्य सशूलं दर्शनं भवेत् ॥१॥

***Etiology***

Abortion accompanied by bleeding from the genital tract and colic pain, is caused by the following factors :

(1) Fear;

(2) injury (assult);

(3) intake of food and drinks which are *tīkṣṇa* (having sharp attribute) and hot.

आचतुर्थात्ततो मासात् प्रस्रवेद्गर्भविद्रवः[२] ।
ततः स्थिरशरीरस्य[३] पातः पञ्चमषष्ठयोः[४] ॥२॥

*Abortion and Miscarriage*

If it takes place during the first four months of pregnancy when the foetus is a fluid-state, then it is called *garbhasrāva* (abortion). If it occurs during the fifth and sixth months of pregnancy when the foetus has acquired a stable physique, then it is called *garbhapāta* (miscarriage).

गर्भोऽभिघातविषमाशनपीडनाद्यैः
पक्वद्रुमादिव फलं पतति क्षणेन ।
मूढः करोति पवनः खलु मूढगर्भं
शूलं च योनिजठरादिषु मूत्रसङ्गम् ॥३॥

*Pathogenesis*

Because of injury, irregular and inappropriate food and pressure on the abdomen, the foetus comes out of the genital tract instantaneously as a ripe fruit falls down from the tree. Alternatively, the aggravated *vāyu* causes immobility of the foetus in the uterus giving rise to colic pain in the genital tract, pelvis (abdomen), etc., resulting in the urinary obstruction.

भुग्नोऽनिलेन विगुणेन ततः स गर्भः
संख्यामतीत्य बहुधा समुपैति योनिम् ।
द्वारं निरुध्य शिरसा जठरेण कश्चित्
कश्चिच्छरीरपरिवर्तितकुब्जदेहः ॥४॥
एकेन कश्चिदपरस्तु भुजद्वयेन
तिर्यगतो भवति कश्चिदवाङ्मुखोऽन्यः ।
पार्श्वापवृत्तगतिरेति तथैव कश्चि-
दित्यष्टधा गतिरियं ह्यपरा चतुर्धा ॥५॥
संकीलकः प्रतिखुरः परिघोऽथ बीज-
स्ते पृष्ठबाहुचरणैः शिरसा च योनिम् ।
संकीलको भवति कीलकवत् स कीलः
दृश्यैः खुरैः प्रतिखुरं स हि कायसङ्गी ॥६॥

गच्छेद्भुजद्वयशिरः स च बीजकाख्यो
योनौ स्थितः स परिघः परिघेण तुल्यः ॥७॥

### *Different Abnormal Presentations*

The aggravated *vāyu* causes impairment in the foetus as a result of which innumerable types of abonormal foetal presentations are caused in the genital tract.

By these abnormal presentations, the cervical opening of the uterus gets obstructed by different parts of the foetus which are as follows :

(1) Head;
(2) abdomen;
(3) retroverted and squeezed body;
(4) one hand;
(5) both the hands;
(6) body in an oblique position;
(7) face in an extended position; and
(8) twisted chest.

In addition to the above mentioned eight, four more abnormal presentations also occur commonly which are as follows :

(1) *Sankīlaka* : In this, the cervical opening of the uterus gets obstructed by the back, hands, legs and head like a peg;

(2) *Pratikhura* : In this, the cervical opening of the uterus gets obstructed by the body of the foetus with its limbs projecting out through the vaginal canal (like the hoof of horse);

(3) *Bījaka* : In this, the cervical opening of the uterus gets obstructed by the projecting head and two hands of the foetus; and

(4) *Parigha* : In this, the cervical opening of the uterus gets obstructed by the body of the foetus (in transverse position) like a bolt in the door.

अपविद्धशिरा[१] या तु शीताङ्गी निरपत्रपा ।
नीलोद्धतसिरा हन्ति सा गर्भं[०] स च तां तथा ॥८॥

### *Prognosis*

If the enceinte is unable to hold her head straight, if her body is cold, if she loses her natural bashfulness and if blue veins appear prominently in her body, then both the mother and the child succumb to death.

गर्भास्पन्दनमावीनां प्रणाशः श्यावपाण्डुता ।
भवेदुच्छ्वासपूतित्वं[११] शूनताऽन्तर्मृते[१२] शिशौ ॥९॥

***Signs & Symptoms of Foetal Death***

Following are the signs and symptoms of foetal death inside the womb of the mother :

(1) Absence of foetal movement;
(2) cessation of labour pain;
(3) gray or pale yellow coloration of the skin;
(4) emission of foul smell from the body and the mouth of the enceinte; and
(5) oedema in the body, specially in the abdomen.

मानसागन्तुभिर्मातुरुपतापैः प्रपीडितः ।
गर्भो व्यापद्यते कुक्षौ व्याधिभिश्च निपीडितः ॥१०॥

***Causes of Foetal Death***

Foetal death in the womb of the mother takes place because of the following factors :

(1) Mental tension;
(2) extraneous injury; and
(3) occurence of diseases.

योनिसंवरणं[१३] सङ्गः कुक्षौ मक्कल्ल एव च ।
हन्युः स्त्रियं मूढगर्भा[१४] यथोक्ताश्चाप्युपद्रवाः ॥११॥
॥ इति मूढगर्भनिदानम् ॥

(माधवनिदान : मूढगर्भ : ६४ : १-१०)

***Causes of Maternal Death***

The enceinte having abnormal presentation of foetus succumbs to death because of the following factors :

(1) Stuffing of the vaginal tract by the foetus;
(2) retention of the (dead foetus) in the womb (pelvic region);
(3) appearance of *makalla* (a type of colic pain which occurs after delivery); and

(4) manifestation of other complications.

Thus, ends the diagnosis of abnormal presentation of foetus.

परूषकशिफालेपः स्थिरामूलकृतोऽथवा ।
नाभिबस्तिभगाद्येषु[१५] मूढगर्भोपकर्षणम् ॥१२॥

*Recipe for Mūḍhagarbha*

The root of *parūṣaka* or *sthirā* should be made to a paste by triturating with water. Application of this paste in the umbilical region, region of urinary bladder and over vagina facilitates delivery of the abnormally presented foetus.

(मासानुमासिकाः योगाः)
"मधुकशाकबीजश्च पयस्या सुरदारु च ।
अश्मन्तकं[१६] कृष्णतिलास्ताम्रवल्ली[१७] शतावरी ॥१३॥
वृक्षादनी[१८] पयस्या च तथैवोत्पलशारिवा ।
अनन्ता शारिवा रास्ना पद्मा मधुकमेव च ॥१४॥
बृहतीद्वयकाश्मर्यक्षीरीशुङ्गस्त्वचा[१९] घृतम् ।
पृथक्पर्णी-बला-शिग्रु श्वदंष्ट्रा मधुयष्टिका ॥१५॥
शृङ्गाटकं बिसं[२०] द्राक्षा कसेरु मधुकं सिता[२१] ।
इत्येते[२२] सप्तयोगाः स्युरर्द्धश्लोकसमापनाः ।
यथाक्रमं प्रयोक्तव्या गर्भस्रावे[२३] तु योषिताम् ॥१६॥
कपित्थबिल्वबृहतीपटोलेक्षुनिदिग्धिका-
मूलानि क्षीरसिद्धानि[२४] दापयेद् भिषगष्टमे ॥१७॥
नवमे मधुकानन्तापयस्याशारिवाः[२५] पिबेत् ।
पयस्तु दशमे शुण्ठ्याः शृतशीतं प्रशस्यते ॥१८॥
सक्षीरा वा हिता शुण्ठी मधुकं देवदारु च ।
एवमापूर्यते[२६] गर्भस्तीव्रा रुक् चोपशाम्यति[२७]" ॥१९॥

(भैषज्यरत्नावली : स्त्रीरोगाधिकार : २८७-२९४)

***Treatment of Abortion During Different Months of Pregnancy***

In threatened abortion during different months of pregnancy, the enceinte should be given recipes containing the following drugs :

First month :

*Madhuka, śākabīja, payasyā* and *devadāru*;

Second month :

*Aśmantaka, kṛṣṇatila, tāmravallī* and *śatāvarī*;

Third month :

*Vṛkṣādanī, payasyā* and *utpalasārivā*;

Fourth Month :

*Anantā, śārivā, rāsnā, padmā* and *madhuka*;

Fifth month :

*Bṛhatī, kaṇṭakārī, kāśmarya, śṛṅga*, bark of *kṣīrī vṛkṣas* and ghee;

Sixth month :

*Pṛthakparṇī, balā, śigru, śvadaṃṣṭrā* and *yaṣṭimadhu*;

Seventh month :

*Śṛṅgāṭaka, bisa, drākṣā, kaseru, madhuka* and sugar.

Eighth month :

Milk boiled with the roots of *kapittha, bilva, bṛhatī, paṭola, ikṣu* and *nidigdhikā*;

Ninth month :

[Milk boiled with] *madhuka, anantā, payasyā* and *śārivā*;

Tenth month :

Milk boiled with ginger and cooled. Alternatively, milk boiled with *śuṇṭhī, madhuka* and *devadāru*.

With the above mentioned receipe, the foetus gets fully matured and excruciating pain gets subsided.

'क्षीरिकामुत्पल[२८] दुग्धं समंगामूलकं शिवम् ।
पिबेदेकादशे मासे गर्भिणी शूलशान्तये ॥२०॥

***Recipe for Eleventh month***

During the eleventh month, the enceinte should be given milk boiled with *kṣīrikā, utpala*, root of *samaṅgā* and *harītakī* for relief of pain.

सिता विदारी काकोलीक्षीरं चैव मृणालकम् ।
गर्भिणी द्वादशे मासि पिबेत् शूलघ्नमौषधम् ॥
एवमाप्यायते गर्भस्तीव्रा रुक् चोपशम्यति ॥२१॥

*Recipe for Twelfth Month*

During the twelfth month, the enceinte should be given milk boiled with *vidārī, kākolī* and *mṛṇāla* and added with sugar. It relieves pain.

Thus, the foetus gets nourished and excruciating pain of the enceinte gets subsided.

मतान्तरेण सप्तमासचिकित्सा लिख्यते—
मासि प्रथमे गर्भे मधूकसुरदारुपद्मकं बिसम् ।
पयसि क्वथितं देयं सशर्करं वेदनाहरणम् ॥२२॥
लोध्रः कार्पासकुसुमं गुडूची तिलमल्लिका ।
द्वितीये मासे दुग्धेन देयः क्वाथं सुशर्करः ॥२३॥
लोध्रं रसालबलितं क्षीरिका शर्करा बला ।
तृतीये सरुजे गर्भे देयं पिष्ट्वा सशर्करम् ॥२४॥
रास्ना ससारिवानन्ता मधूकं पद्मकं मधु ।
संक्वाथ्य पानं पातव्यं चतुर्थे मासि वेदने ॥२५॥
वैणवं बृहतीयष्टीकाश्मर्यतृटिसंयुतम् ।
पंचमे पयसा पिष्ट्वा देयं क्षौद्रघृतान्वितम् ॥२६॥
शालिपर्णी बलाशिग्रुयष्टीगोक्षुरगोस्तनीः ।
षष्ठे मासि प्रदातव्यः क्वाथः शूलनिवारणः ॥२७॥
कसेरुकं गोक्षुरगोस्तनीकं सजीरकं यष्टिघृतप्लुतं च ।
क्षीरेण पिष्ट्वातिशयं निहन्ति शूलं च गर्भेषु च सप्तमेषु ॥२८॥

॥ इति सप्तमासचिकित्सा ॥

अष्टममासेन सह सम्बन्धम्' ॥२९॥

***Treatment During Seven Months of Pregnancy—An Alternative View***

According to some physicians the following receipes should be used during the first seven months of pregnancy:

First month :

Milk boiled with *madhuka, devadāru, padmaka* and bisa, and added with sugar should be given for the relief of pain.

Second month :

The decoction of *lodhra*, flower of *kārpāsa, guḍūcī, tila* and *mallikā*, and milk added with adequate quantity of sugar should be given.

Third month :

The paste of *lodhra, rasālabalita, kṣīrikā*, sugar and *balā* mixed with (more of) sugar should be given to relieve pain.

Fourth month :

If there is pain during this month, then the enceinte should be given the decoction of *rāsnā, sārivā, anantā, madhūka* and *padmaka* along with honey to drink.

Fifth month :

The enceinte should be given the paste of *vaṃśalocana, bṛhatī, yaṣṭimadhu, kāśmarya* and *tṛti* prepared by triturating with milk, along with honey and ghee.

Sixth month :

The decoction of *śāliparṇī, balā, śigru, yaṣṭimadhu, gokṣura* and *gostanī* should be given for the relief from pain.

Seventh month :

Excruciating pain in the seventh month of pregnancy is cured by the intake of the paste of *kaseruka, gokṣura, gostanī, jīraka* and *yaṣṭimadhu* prepared by triturating with milk and added with ghee.

Thus, ends the treatment of ailments during the first seven months of pregnancy.

During eight month onwards, receipes described in verse nos. 17-21 should be used.

"समधुच्छागदुग्धेन[२९] कुलालकरमृत्तिका[३०] ।
अवश्यं स्थापयेद् गर्भं चलितं पानयोगतः" ॥३०॥

(भैषज्यरत्नावली : स्त्रीरोगाधिकार : २९७)

***Recipes***

Intake of the mud used by a blacksmith along with honey and goat's milk certainly corrects threatened abortion.

"कुशकाशोरुबूकाणां मूलैर्गोक्षुरकस्य च ।
शृतं दुग्धं सितायुक्तं गर्भिण्याः शूलनुत्परम् ॥३१॥

Milk boiled with the roots of ***kuśa, kāśa,*** *urubūka* and *gokṣura* and added with sugar corrects colic pain in a pregnant woman.

कशेरुशृंगाटकजीवनीयपद्मोत्पलैरण्डशतावरीभिः ।
सिद्धं पयः शर्करया विमिश्रं संस्थापयेद् गर्भमुदीर्णवेगम्[३१] ॥३२॥
(भैषज्यरत्नावली : स्त्रीरोगाधिकार : २९५-२९६)

Milk boiled with *kaśeru, śṛṅgāṭaka, jīvanīya, padma, utpala, eraṇḍa* and *śatāvarī,* and mixed with sugar cures even serious type of threatening abortion.

"कशेरुशृंगाटकपद्मकोत्पलं समुद्गपर्णी मधुकं सशर्करम् ।
सशूलगर्भस्रुतिपीडिताङ्गना पयोविमिश्रं[३२] पयसान्तभुक् पिबेत्" ॥३३॥
(भैषज्यरत्नावली : स्त्रीरोगाधिकार : २९८)

Paste of *kaśeru, śṛṅgāṭaka, padmaka, utpala, mudgaparṇī, yaṣṭimadhu* and sugar should be taken added with milk if the woman is suffering from threatening abortion associated with colic pain. While taking this recipe she should use milk and rice as food.

"आम्रजम्बूत्वचः[३३] क्वाथं लेहयेल्लाजशक्तुभिः ।
अनेन लीढमात्रेण गर्भिणी ग्रहणीं जयेत् ॥३४॥

Flour prepared of fried rice should be made to a paste by mixing with the decoction of the barks of *āmra* and *jambū.* Use of this linctus instantaneously cures *grahaṇī* (sprue syndrome) in a pregnant woman.

(ह्रीबेरादिक्वाथः)

"ह्रीबेररलुरक्तचन्दनबलाधान्याकवत्सादनी-
मुस्तोशीरयवासपर्पटविषाक्वाथं पिबेद् गर्भिणी ॥३५॥

नानावर्णरुजातिसारकगदे रक्तस्रुतौ वा ज्वरे
योगोऽयं मुनिभिः पुरा निगदितः सूत्यामयेषूत्तमः" ॥३६॥

(भैषज्यरत्नावली : स्त्रीरोगाधिकार : ३०४-३०५)

*Hrīberādi Kvātha*

Decoction of *hrībera, aralu, rakta candana, balā, dhānyaka, vatsādanī, mustā, uśīra, yavāsā, parpaṭa* and *ativiṣā* should be taken by a pregnant woman if she is suffering from diarrhoea associated with different colours of the stool and different types of pain. This receipe is also useful curing bleeding and fever of the pregnant woman. This is an excellent receipe described by the sage of the yore for the treatment of ailments in a pregnant woman.

ॐ नमः शान्तिदेवत्यै गर्भरलस्यै (गर्भपातालस्यै)
गर्भस्रावं रक्ष रक्ष स्वाहा ॥
अनेन मन्त्रेणाभिमन्त्रितं पयः पाययेत् ॥३७॥

Water should be consecrated by reciting the incantation "*Oṃ namaḥ śāntidaivatyai garbharalasyai garbhasravaṃ rakṣa rakṣa svāhā.* This consecrated water should be given to the pregnant woman to drink to prevent abortion.

"पाठासुरससिंहास्यमयूरकजटाः पृथक् ।
नाभिबस्तिभगलेपात् सुखं नारी प्रसूयते" ॥३८॥

(भैषज्यरत्नावली : स्त्रीरोगाधिकार : ३५०)

The paste of the root of either *pāṭhā, surasā, siṃhāsya* or *mayūraka* should be applied over the umbilical region, region of urinary bladder and vagina which helps in easy delivery.

पिष्ट्वा दंष्ट्रां वराहस्य जलेनैवांजयेत् दृशौ ।
सद्यः प्रसूयते[34] नारी सर्ज्जत्वग्धूपनादपि[35] ॥३९॥

The tooth of wild boar should be rubbed over a stone by adding water.

This paste should be applied in the eyes as collyrium which causes instant delivery. Fumigation of the vaginal tract with the smoke of *sarjarasa* also helps in instant delivery.

"मातुलुङ्गस्य मूलानि मधुकं मधुसंयुतम् ।
घृतेन सह पातव्यं सुखं नारी प्रसूयते"[३६] ॥४०॥

(भैषज्यरत्नावली : स्त्रीरोगाधिकार : ३५२)
(योगरत्नाकर : स्त्रीगर्भचिकित्सा : पृष्ठ ४२३)

Root of *mātuluṅga* and *yaṣṭimadhu* should be added with honey and ghee. Intake of this potion helps in easy delivery.

'तुषांबुपरिपिष्टेन[३७] मूलेन परिलेपयेत्' ॥४१॥

(This line appears to be incomplete; hence left untranslated).

"एरण्डमूलममृता[३८] मंजिष्ठा रक्तचन्दनम् ।
दारुपद्मसमः क्वाथो गर्भिण्या ज्वरशान्तये"[३९] ॥४२॥

(भैषज्यरत्नावली : स्त्रीरोगाधिकार : ३०२)

Decoction of the root of *eraṇḍa, amṛtā, mañjiṣṭhā, raktacandana, devadāru* and *padma* cures fever in a pregnant woman.

"चन्दनं शारिवा लोध्रं मृद्वीकाशर्करान्वितम् ।
क्वाथं कृत्वा प्रदातव्यं गर्भिण्या ज्वरशान्तये"[४०] ॥४३॥

॥ चन्दनादि क्वाथः ॥

(भैषज्यरत्नावली : स्त्रीरोगाधिकार : ३००)

***Candanādi Kvātha***

Intake of the decoction of *candana, sārivā, lodhra* and *mṛdvīkā* mixed with sugar cures fever in a pregnant woman.

"इहामृतश्च सोमश्च चित्रभानुश्च भामिनी ।
उच्चैःश्रवाश्च तुरगो मन्दिरे निवसन्तु ते ॥४४॥
इदममृतमपां समुद्धृतं वै भव लघु गर्भमिमं विमञ्चतु स्त्री ।
तदनलपवनार्कवासवास्ते सह लवणाम्बुधरैर्दिशन्तु शान्तिम् ॥४५॥
मुक्ताः पाशा विपाशाश्च मुक्ताः सूर्येण रश्मयः[४१] ।
मुक्तः सर्वभयाद् गर्भ एह्येहि मा चिरं स्वाहा ॥४६॥
जलं च्यवनमन्त्रेण सप्तवाराभिमन्त्रितम् ।
पीत्वा प्रसूयते नारी दृष्ट्वा चोभयत्रिंशकम् ॥४७॥

(भैषज्यरत्नावली : स्त्रीरोगाधिकार : ३५३-३५६)

नाडी[४२] १६ ऋतु ६ बसवः ८ पक्ष २ दिक् १० अष्टादश
१८ अर्क १२ भुवन १८ अब्धिसहितैरुभयत्रिंशकेनाश्चर्यम् ॥४८॥

[उभयत्रिंशक यन्त्र]

| | | |
|---|---|---|
| १६ | ६ | ८ |
| २ | १० | १८ |
| १२ | १४ | ४ |

(भैषज्यरत्नावली : स्त्रीरोगाधिकार : ३५८)

### *Tantra & Yantra*

Water should be consecrated with the above incantation (*Cyavana mantra*) for seven times and given to the enceinte for drinking. Simultaneously, she should see the above described *yantra* called *Ubhayatriṃśaka* which helps in easy delivery.

कटुतुम्ब्यहिनिर्मोककृतवेधनसर्षपैः[४३] ।
कटुतैलान्वितैर्योनिधूपः[४४] पातयतेऽ[४५]ऽपराम् ॥४९॥

### *Recipe For Placenta*

Fumigation with the smoke of *kaṭu tumbī*, slough of snake, *kṛta vedhana* and *sarṣapa* added with mustard oil helps in the fall of placenta.

कचवेष्टितयाङ्गुल्या घृष्टे कण्ठे सुखं पतत्यपराम्[४६]।
मूलेन लाङ्गलिक्याः संलिप्ते पाणिपादे[४७] वा ॥५०॥
(भैषज्यरत्नावली : स्त्रीरोगाधिकार : ३६३-३६५)

Tinglining of the throat with the finger surrounded with hair helps in easy removal of placenta.

Similarly, application of the paste of *lāngalī*-root in the palms and soles of feet helps in easy removal of placenta.

"उपकुञ्चिकां पिप्पलीञ्च मदिरां लाभतः पिबेत् ।
सौवर्चलेन संयुक्तां योनिशूलनिवारणीम्"[४८] ॥५१॥
(भैषज्यरत्नावली : स्त्रीरोगाधिकार : ३६७)

*Upakuñcikā* and *pippalī* mixed with adequate quantity of alcohol and sonchal-salt cures colic pain in the genital tract.

इति श्रीमहाराजाधिराजश्रीटोडरमलल्लविरचिते टोडरानन्दे आयुर्वेदसौख्ये मूढगर्भनिदानचिकित्साकथनं नाम त्रिसप्ततितमो हर्षः ॥

Thus, ends the 73rd chapter dealing with the diagnosis and management of *mūḍhagarbha* (abnormal presentation of foetus) in the *Āyurveda saukhya* of *Ṭoḍarānanda* composed by the great king Ṭoḍaramalla.

## NOTES AND REFERENCES

१. (क) This is the beginning of seventy seventh chapter of *Āyurveda saukhya* in *Ṭoḍarānanda* and the invocation reads as follows :
'रौद्रादिप्रेमान्तरसीजनानां रंगेस्थितानां च तथाविधानाम् ।
तथा तथा यो विवभौ तादानीं कुर्यान्नृपे भावररंगयातः' ॥
(ख) 'रौद्रादि. ....... भावररंगयातः' पाठोऽयं चतुर्थषष्ठपुस्तकयोः नोपलभ्यते ।

(ग) भाराभिघातात् इति चतुर्थपुस्तके पाठः ।

२. स्रवेयुर्गर्भविदंवः इति षष्ठपुस्तके पाठः ।

३. स्थितः इति षष्ठपुस्तके पाठः ।

४. तत् उद्धर्वं प्रसूतिः स्यादिति प्रोक्तं महर्षिभिः पाठोऽयं चतुर्थषष्ठपुस्तकयोः अधिकमुपलभ्यते ।

५. सहसा इति षष्ठपुस्तके पाठः ।

६. तिर्यग्मुखो इति चतुर्थपुस्तके पाठः ।

७. बीजस्तेषूर्ध्वबाहुचरणैः इति आकरे पाठः ।

८. सङ्गी च यो भवति कीलकवत् सकीलो इति आकरे पाठः ।

९. प्रविध्यति शिराया तु इति पंचमपुस्तके पाठः ।

१०. स्रवतां तथा इति प्रथमपुस्तके पाठः ।

११. भवन्त्युच्छ्वास इति पंचमपुस्तके पाठः ।

१२. शूलांतर्मृते इति प्रथमपुस्तके पाठः ।

१३. योनिसंचरणं इति प्रथमपुस्तके पाठः ।

१४. (क) मूढगर्भाः इति प्रथमपुस्तके पाठः ।

(ख) मूढगर्भो इति षष्ठपुस्तके पाठः ।

१५. .भगलेपा इति षष्ठपुस्तके पाठः ।

१६. अस्मंतकः इति प्रथमपुस्तके पाठः ।

१७. .ताम्रपर्णो इति चतुर्थपुस्तके पाठः ।

१८. वृक्षादनं इति षष्ठपुस्तके पाठः ।

१९. (क) कास्मर्यक्षीरिसुंगात्त्वचो इति प्रथमपुस्तके पाठः ।

(ख) क्षीरासुंगात्त्वचो इति पंचमपुस्तके पाठः ।

(ग) क्षीरिशृङ्गीत्वचो इति चतुर्थषष्ठपुस्तकयोः पाठः ।

२०. विषं इति पंचमपुस्तके पाठः ।

२१. (क) मासेषु इति आकरे पाठः ।

(ख) सप्तैते इति षष्ठपुस्तके पाठः ।

२२. रक्तस्रावे पयोयुताः इति आकरे पाठः ।

२३. रक्तस्रावे पयोयुताः इति आकरे पाठः ।

२४. क्षीरपिष्टानि इति आकरे पाठः ।

२५. .पयस्यामाद्रिचाः पिबेत् इति प्रथमपुस्तके पाठः ।

२६. 'एवमापूर्यते ..... चोपशाम्यति' पाठोऽयं चतुर्थषष्ठपुस्तकयोः नोपलभ्यते ।

२७. रुक् च प्रशाम्यतिं इति आकरे पाठः ।

२८. 'क्षीरिकामुत्पल ..... सम्बन्धम्' पाठोऽयं चतुर्थषष्ठपुस्तकयोः अधिकमुपलभ्यते ।

२९. मधुना इति आकरे पाठः ।

३०. (क) कुलालकरकर्दमः इति आकरे पाठः ।
(ख) कुलालकरमृत्तिका इति चतुर्थषष्ठपुस्तकयोः पाठः ।

३१. गर्भमुदीर्णशूलम् इति प्रथमपुस्तके पाठः ।

३२. पयोन्नमिश्रं इति षष्ठपुस्तके पाठः ।

३३. "आम्रजम्बूत्वचः ..... पाययेत्" पाठोऽयं प्रथमपुस्तके नोपलभ्यते ।

३४. प्रसूतये इति चतुर्थपुस्तके पाठः ।

३५. (क) सर्पत्वग्धूपनादपि इति पंचमपुस्तके पाठः ।
(ख) सर्जस्तत् धूपनादपि इति चतुर्थषष्ठपुस्तकयोः पाठः ।

३६. प्रसूतयेत इति पंचमपुस्तके पाठः ।

३७. 'तुषांबु. ........परिलेपयेत्' पाठोऽयं चतुर्थषष्ठपुस्तकयोः नोपलभ्यते ।

३८. "एरण्डमूलम. ........ज्वरशान्तये" पाठोऽयं प्रथमपुस्तके नोपलभ्यते ।

३९. ज्वरनाशनः इति आकरे पाठः ।

४०. ज्वरनाशनम् इति आकरे पाठः ।

४१. सुर्येन्दुरश्मयः इति आकरे पाठः ।

४२. 'नाड्यर्तुवसुभिः सह पक्षदिगष्टांशभिरेव च ।
अर्कभुवनाब्धिसहितैरुभयत्रिंशकमाश्चर्यम् ॥'
इति आकरे पाठः ।

४३. 'हिमवान् दक्षिणे पार्श्वे सरसा नाम यक्षिणी ।
तस्या नूपुरशब्देन विशल्या भव गर्भिणी ।'
पाठोऽयं षष्ठपुस्तके अधिकमुपलभ्यते ।

४४. कटुतैलान्वितैर्धूपो योनेः इति आकरे पाठः ।

४५. पातयतेऽमराम् इति आकरे पाठः ।

४६. कण्ठे पतत्यमरा इति आकरे पाठः ।

४७. हस्तपादे च इति आकरे पाठः ।

४८. 'लाङ्गल्या वापामार्गस्येन्द्रवारुणकस्य च ।
मूलं योनिगतं स्त्रीणां पुष्परोधहरं भवेत् ।
सकांजिकं जयापुष्पं भृष्टं ज्योतिष्मतीदलम् ।
दूर्वापिष्टं दश प्राश्य वनितार्त्तुमती भवेत् ।
ॐ नमः शान्त्रि दैवत्यै गर्भस्रावं रक्ष रक्ष स्वाहा

अनेन मन्त्रेणाभिमंत्रितं पयः पाययेत् ।
इक्ष्वाकुबीजदन्तीएरण्ड-गजामदनयष्टयकैः ।
सस्नुक्क्षीरैः वर्तिः योनिगता कुसुमसंजननी ।
पिबति प्रसूनसमये जया प्रसूनं विमर्द्य कांजिकायाम् ।
न विभर्ति सा प्रसूनं धृतेऽपि तस्या न गर्भः स्यात् ।
धूपितेन योनिरंध्रं निम्बकाष्ठेन युक्तितः ।
ऋत्वंते तेन सा स्त्री स्याद्गर्भदुःखेन वर्ज्जिता ।
धत्तूरमूलिका पुष्पे गृहीत्वा कीटसंस्थिता ।
गर्भं निवारयत्येव रण्डावेश्यादियोषिताम् ।
तन्दुलियकमूलं तु पिष्ट्वा तन्दुलवारिणा ।
ऋत्वंते तु त्र्यहं पीतं वन्ध्या च कुरुते स्त्रियम् ।
कृत्वा च सप्तखण्डं गुञ्जामूलं निबन्ध्य कटिदेशेषु ।
सूत्रैः सप्तभिरचिरात्सुखसूतिं भामिनी लभते ।
पिष्ट्वा पाठापत्रं नारीक्षीरेण या पिबेदबला ।
सामूढगर्भजनिते व्यथया प्रतिमुच्यते झटति ।
तुम्बीपत्रं सलोध्रं च समभागं च कारयेत् ।
दध्ना लेपं भगस्येदं प्रसूता अक्षता भवेत् ।
पलाशोन्दुम्बरफलं तिलतैलसमन्वितम् ।
मधुना योनिमालिप्य गाढीकरणमुत्तमम् ।
तुषाम्बुपरिपिष्टेन मूलेन परिलेपयेत् ।
लाङ्गल्याश्चरणौ सूते क्षिप्रमापन्नगर्भिणी ।
आरण्ये वसते काको गंगातीरमुपस्थितः ।
दूतः पिबति पानीयं विशल्या भव गर्भिणी ।'
पाठोऽयं चतुर्थपंचमपुस्तकयोः अधिकमुपलभ्यते ।

# CHAPTER IV

## ॥ अथ सूतिकारोगनिदानं चिकित्सा च ॥

*(Diagnosis and Treatment of Puerperal Diseases)*

"वायुः[१] प्रकुपितः कुर्यात् संरुध्य रुधिरं च्युतम्।
सूताया हृच्छिरोबस्तिशूलं मक्कल्लसंज्ञितम्" ॥१॥
(योगरत्नाकर : स्त्रीरोगचिकित्सा : पृष्ठ ४२६)

***Makalla***

The aggravated *vāyu* obstructs the flowing blood (in the genital tract) of the woman after delivery to cause colic pain in the regions of heart, head and urinary bladder. This is called *Makkalla.*

"अङ्गमर्दो ज्वरः कम्पः पिपासा गुरुगात्रता ।
शोथः शूलातिसारौ च सूतिकारोगलक्षणम् ॥२॥

***Signs & Symptoms of Puerperal Diseases***

Malaise, fever, tremors, morbid thirst, heaviness of the body, oedema, colic pain and diarrhoea—these are the signs and symptoms of puerperal diseases.

मिथ्योपचारात् संक्लेशाद्विषमाजीर्णभोजनात् ।
सूतिकायाश्च ये रोगा जायन्ते दारुणा[2] स्मृताः ॥३॥

*Etiology*

Puerperal diseases occur in a woman after delivery as a result of the following factors :

(1) Adoption of wrong regimens;
(2) physical strain; and
(3) intake of irregular meals and intake of meals before the previous food is undigested;

The ailments which appear in a woman after delivery because of the above mentioned factors are of serious nature.

ज्वरातिसारं शोथश्च शूलानाहबलक्षयाः ।
तन्द्रारुचिप्रलापाद्याः[3] कफवातामयोद्भवाः ॥४॥
कृच्छ्रसाध्या हि ते रोगाः क्षीणमांसबलान्विताः ।
ते सर्वे सूतिकानाम्ना रोगास्ते चाप्युपद्रवाः ॥५॥
॥ इति सूतिकारोगनिदानम् ॥

(माधवनिदान : सूतिकारोग : ६५ : १-४)

*Enumeration of Puerperal Diseases*

Fever, diarrhoea, oedema, colic pain, *ānāha* (abdominal distension), loss of strength, drowsiness, anorexia, delirium and other diseases caused by the vitiation of *kapha* as well as *vāyu* appear during puerperium. These are difficult of cure because of the diminution of muscle tissue and strength in the woman during puerperal period. All these are called *Sūtikā roga*. These are the disease-entities and they might also appear as complications of other ailments.

Thus, ends the section on the diagnosis of *sūtikā* (puerperal) diseases.

क्षुद्रैरण्डजटाशुण्ठीकणामुण्डीसुखास्पृशा[4] ।
सूतिकारोगशान्त्यर्थं निःक्वाथ्य मधुना पिबेत् ॥६॥

*Recipe*

For the alleviation of *sūtikā* (puerperal) diseases the woman should take the decoction of *kaṇṭakārī*, root of *eraṇḍa, śuṇṭhī, pippalī, muṇḍī* and *sukhāspṛśā* along with honey.

"पृथिव्यां पतिते गर्भे योनौ[५] पिडनमिष्यते ।
अप्रवेशो यथा वायोस्तथा संरक्षणक्रिया"[६] ॥७॥
(योगरत्नाकर : सूतिकारोगाधिकार : पृष्ठ ४२६)

*Post-partum Management*

After the delivery of the foetus, pressure should be applied over the uterine region so as to prevent the access of *vāyu* into the genital tract.

"यवक्षारं पिबेत्तत्र सर्पिषोष्णोदकेन वा ।
पिप्पल्यादिगणक्वाथं पिबेद्वा लवणान्वितम्" ॥८॥
(भैषज्यरत्नावली : स्त्रीरोगाधिकार : ३६९-३७०)

*Recipes*

After delivery, the enceinte should take *yavakṣāra*, along with ghee or warm water. She should also take the decoction of drugs belonging to *Pippalyādi* group along with salt.

"अमृतानागरसहचरभद्रोत्कटपञ्चमूलजलदजलम् ।
शृतशीत[७] मधुसहितं निवारयति[८] सूतिकातङ्कम्" ॥९॥
(भैषज्यरत्नावली : स्त्रीरोगाधिकार : ३७३)
(योगरत्नाकर : स्त्रीरोगचिकित्सा : पृष्ठ ४२८)

Decoction should be prepared of *amṛtā, nāgara, sahacara, bhadra mustā, utkaṭa (itkaṭa), kaṇṭaka pañca mūla, mustā* and *hrībera*. This decoction should be cooled and added with honey. Intake of this potion prevents *sūtikā* diseases.

'हिंस्राभीरुस्वदंष्ट्रा[९] च सैरेयं करमर्दकम् ।
एभिरेकत्र संयुक्तमुत्कटं मूलपञ्चकम्' ॥१०॥

**Kaṇṭaka Pañcamūla**

*Hiṃsrā, abhīru* (*śatāvarī*), *śvadaṃṣṭrā, saireya, karamardaka*—roots of all these five drugs, taken together, constitute *kaṇṭaka pañcamūla.*

देवदारुवचामुस्तधान्यपर्पटकं[10] शिवा ।
नागरातिविषे चैव क्वाथं वै सूतिकाहितम् ।
गर्भशूलप्रशमनं वेदनायाश्च निग्रहम् ॥११॥

**Recipe**

Decoction of *devadāru, vacā, musta, dhānya, parpaṭaka, śivā, nāgara* and *ativiṣā* is useful in curing puerperal diseases. Intake of this potion cures pain in the uterine region and prevents occurence of such pain.

"देवदारु वचा कुष्ठं पिप्पली विश्वभेषजम् ।
कट्फलं मुस्तं भूनिम्बतिक्ताधान्यहरीतकी ॥१२॥
गजकणा[11] च दुःस्पर्शा गोक्षुरो[12] धन्वयासकम् ।
बृहत्यतिविषा छिन्ना कर्कटं कृष्णजीरकम् ॥१३॥
समभागान्वितैरेतैः सिन्धुरामठसंयुतम् ।
क्वाथमष्टावशेषं तु प्रसूतां पाययेत्स्त्रियम् ॥१४॥
शूलकासज्वरश्वासमूर्च्छाकम्पशिरोऽर्त्तिभिः ।
युक्तं प्रलापतृड्दाहतन्द्रातीसारिणे[13] तथा ।
निहन्ति सूतिकारोगं वातपित्तकफान्वितम्[14] ॥१५॥
॥ देवदार्वादिः क्वाथः" ॥

(भैषज्यरत्नावली : स्त्रीरोगाधिकार : ३८०-३८४)

**Devadārvādi Kvātha**

Decoction should be prepared of *devadāru, vacā, kuṣṭha, pippalī, viśvabheṣaja, kaṭphala, mustā, bhūnimba, tiktā, dhānya, harītakī, gaja pippalī, duḥsparśā, gokṣura, dhanvayāsaka, bṛhatī, ativiṣā, guḍūcī, karkaṭa* and *kṛṣṇa jīraka*, all taken in equal quantities, boiled by adding water and reduced to one eighth. Intake of this decoction by adding rock-salt and *hiṅgu* by the woman, after delivery, cures colic pain, cough, fever, asthma, fainting, tremor, headache, delirium, morbid thirst, burning sensation, drwosiness, diarrhoea and other puerperal diseases associated with *vāyu*, *pitta* and *kapha*.

"सहचरपुष्करवेतसमूल[१५] वैकंकतदारुकुलत्थसमम्[१६] ।
जलमधुसैंधवहिंगुयुतं[१७] सद्योज्वरसूतिकाशूलहरम्" ॥१६॥
(भैषज्यरत्नावली : स्त्रीरोगाधिकार : ३७४)

Decoction should be prepared of *sahacara, puṣkara*, root of *vetasa, vaikaṅkata, devadāru* and *kulattha*, all taken in equal quantities. Intake of this decoction along with the powder of *hrībera*, honey, rock-salt and *hiṅgu* cures freshly occuring fever and colic pain during puerperium.

"पञ्चमूलस्य वा क्वाथं तप्तलोहेन संगतम् ।
सूतिकारोगनाशाय पिबेद्वा तद्युतां सुराम्" ॥१७॥
(योगरत्नाकर : स्त्रीरोगचिकित्सा : पृष्ठ ४२८)

A hot iron rod should be immersed into the decoction of *pañcamūla*. Intake of this decoction cures puerperal diseases. Similarly, intake of the alcohol into which a hot iron rod is immersed is useful in curing puerperal diseases.

"पिप्पली पिप्पलीमूलं चव्यं शुण्ठी यमानिका ।
जीरके द्वे हरिद्रे द्वे विडं सौवर्चलं तथा ॥१८॥
एतैरवौषधैः पिष्टैरारनालं विपाचयेत् ।
आमवातहरं[१८] वृष्यं कफघ्नं वह्निदीपनम् ॥१९॥
काञ्जिकं[१९] वज्रकं नाम स्त्रीणां बलविवर्द्धनम्[२०] ।
मक्कल्लशूलशमनं परं क्षीराभिवर्द्धनम्[२१] ॥२०॥
॥ वज्रकाञ्जिकम्" ॥
(भैषज्यरत्नावली : स्त्रीरोगाधिकार : ३८५-३८७)

*Vajra Kāñjika*

*Pippalī, pippalī mūla, cavya, śuṇṭhī, yamānī, śveta jīraka, kṛṣṇa jīraka, haridrā, dāru haridrā, viḍa* and *sauvarcala* should be made to a paste. *Āranāla* (a type of vinegar) should be cooked by adding this paste. Intake of this potion cures *āmavāta* (rheumatism), it is aphrodisiac, it alleviates *kapha* and it stimulates the power of digestion. It is called *Vajra kāñjika.* It promotes strength of ladies and cures *makalla* type of colic pain. It also promotes lactation.

"नागरस्य[२२] पलान्यष्टौ घृतस्य पलविंशतिः ।
क्षीरद्विप्रस्थसंयुक्तं खण्डस्यार्धशतं[२३] तथा ॥२१॥
व्योषं त्रिजातकं चैव[२४] पलांशमुपकल्पयेत् ।
निदध्याच्चूर्णितं तत्र खादेदग्निबलं प्रति ॥२२॥
कासश्वासारुचिहरं बलपुष्टिविवर्द्धनम् ।
वृष्यमायुष्यमोजस्यं वलीपलितनाशनम्" ॥२३॥
॥ सौभाग्यशुण्ठी[२५] ॥

*Saubhāgya Śuṇṭhī*

Eight *palas* of the powder of *śuṇṭhī*, twenty *palas* of ghee, two *prasthas* of milk and fifty *palas* of sugar should be cooked together. To this, one *pala* of each of *śuṇṭhī, pippalī, marica, tvak, elā* and *patra* should be added in powder form. Depending upon the power of digestion, this should be taken in appropriate dose. It cures cough, asthma and anorexia. It promotes strength and plumpness of the body. It promotes virility, longevity and *ojas* (essence of all the tissue elements). It cures wrinkling of the skin and graying of hair.

'वचा[२६] चातिबला चैव बृहती कण्टकारिकाम् ।
कटुरोहिणीका चैव तैलमेभिर्विपाचयेत् ॥२४॥
सर्वव्याधिहरं चैव गर्भिण्याः नात्र संशयः ।
अष्टौ दोषास्तु नारीणां नवमं पुरुषस्य च ॥२५॥
रक्तं पित्तं तथा वातं कफं चैव त्रिदोषजम् ।
ग्रहदोषविकारे च देवतानां प्रकोपनम् ॥२६॥

अभिचारकृते चैव रेतोहीनपुंसां तथा ।
मृतवत्साकाकबन्ध्या च गर्भस्रावी तु या स्त्रीयः ॥
आदि वन्ध्या च क्षीयन्ते योगैरेभिर्न चान्यथा ॥२७॥

*Recipe of Medicated Oil*

Oil should be cooked by adding *vacā, atibalā, bṛhati, kaṇṭakāri* and *kaṭurohiṇī*. This medicated oil cures eight female diseases and one of the male diseases (impotency). It cures *raktapitta* (a disease characterised by bleeding from different parts of the body), diseases caused by vitiated *vāyu, pitta* and *tridoṣa* (simultaneous vitiation of all the three *doṣas*), diseases caused by the seizure of evil spirits and ill-disposed gods (super natural bodies), diseases caused by *abhicāra* (employment of spells for a malevolent purpose), impotency in males, *mṛtavatsā* (giving birth to dead foetus), *kāka-vandhyā* (those who become sterile after the first conception), *garbhasrāva* (abortion) and *ādivandhyā* (those who are sterile right from the beginning). One should not doubt about the therapeutic efficacy of this recipe.

पुष्पं च जायते तस्याः फलं तस्या न विद्यते ।
तस्माद्दोषविकारांश्च ज्ञात्वा कर्म समाचरेत् ॥२८॥

*Need For Proper Examination*

At times, inspite of proper menstruation (*puṣpa*), a woman is incapable of conception because of the absence of ovum (*phala*). Therefore, the physician should initiate treatment of such cases after careful examination with special reference to the vitiated *doṣas* and the nature of the disease.

शिफाकुकुरमर्दस्य दन्तपुन्ना धृता मुखे ।
स्तन्यवृद्धिकरा स्त्रीणां स्तनकीलकनाशनी ॥२९॥

*Recipe for Lactation*

Keeping the root of *kukuramarda* or *dantapunnā* in the mouth helps the lady in lactation and in curing of *stanakīla* (polyp like growth in the breasts).

धात्रीकुमारश्च पिबेत्क्वाथयित्वा सशर्करम् ।
त्रिफला मुस्तकं निम्बं पटोलं कटुरोहिणी ॥३०॥

Decoction of *harītakī, bibhītaka, āmalakī, mustā, nimba, paṭola* and *kaṭurohiṇī* should be added with sugar and given to the wet-nurse and the child [for curing diseases caused by the intake of vitiated milk].

कफदुष्टे घृतं पीत्वा यष्टीसैन्धवसंयुतम् ।
राठपुष्पो स्तनौ लिप्ते शिशोश्च दशनच्छदौ ।
सुखमेव वमेद्बालस्तीक्ष्णैर्धात्रीं च वामयेत् ॥३१॥

*Recipe for Child's Disease*

If the child is suffering from diseases caused by vitiated *kapha*, then he should be given ghee mixed with the powder of *yaṣṭimadhu* and rock-salt. In addition, the nipples of the mother's breast and the gums of the child should be smeared with the paste of the flower of *rāṭha*. This causes emesis of the child [and cures his diseases]. The wet-nurse should be given strong emetic drugs [to cleanse her breast-milk].

स्तन्यं त्रिदोषदुष्टे च शकृदामं जलोपमम् ।
नानावर्णरुजा चाक्षं विट्बद्धमुपवेश्यते ।
धात्री क्षीरविशुद्ध्यर्थं मुद्गयूषरसाशिनी ॥३२॥

*Diagnosis and Correction of Defective Lactation*

If the breast-milk is afflicted by the simultaneous vitiation of all the three *doṣas*, then the child voids stool mixed with mucus, the stool becomes watery, different types of colour and pain appears in the eyes and at times he passes hard stool. In such event the mother or wet-nurse should be given appropriate therapies and soup of mung dal to drink for the cleansing of the breast-milk.

'नागरं[१७] खंडशः कृत्वा प्रस्थमात्रं[१८] भिषग्वरः ।
अजादुग्धाढकद्वंद्वे विपचेन्मंदवह्निना ॥३३॥

घनीभूते तु पयसि शुण्ठी[29] तस्मात्समुद्धरेत् ।
अतिसूक्ष्मं पेषितव्यं शोषयेदातपे दिनम् ॥३४॥
घृतमाणीं समावाप्य तद्‌दुग्धं तु पुनः पचेत् ।
यावत्स्थिरत्वमायाति[30] ततस्तच्च विमिश्रयेत् ॥३५॥
चातुर्ज्जातं तुगां वेल्लं धान्यकं जीरकद्वयम् ।
मिसि कुस्तुंबुरुं कुष्ठं लवंगं च शतावरी ॥३६॥
तालमूलीं त्रिकटुकं कपिकच्छूं च षड्दः[31] ।
जातिफलं जातिकोषं शृंगाटं वृद्धदारकम् ॥३७॥
त्रिवृतं पद्मबीजं च त्रिफलां च बलात्रयम् ।
जलं सेव्यं वाजिगन्धां चन्दनागरुकारवी ॥३८॥
कंकोलमजगंधा च द्राक्षामक्षोडचारं तम् ।
अजमोदां च बादामं नारिकेलगरं तथा ॥३९॥
कर्पूरमभ्रकं लोहं वंगं ताम्रं शिलाजतु ।
स्वर्णमाक्षिका पच्येत् प्रत्येकं कर्षसंमितम् ॥४०॥
चूर्णीकृत्य क्षिपेत्तत्र पाणिभ्यां मर्दयेद् दृढम् ।
ततः खण्डतुलां पक्त्वा व्यातं च चक्रिकां चरेत् ॥४१॥
खंडनागरकं नाम्ना भैषज्यमिदमुत्तमम् ।
यथाबलमिदं खादेत्प्रातर्नक्तं च भेषजम् ॥४२॥
स्त्रीणामतिहितं नात्र पथ्यापथ्यविचारणा ।
क्षये पाण्डौ ज्वरे कासे श्वासे मंदानले तथा ॥४३॥
संग्रहण्यां रक्तगुल्मे प्रदरे सोमरोगके ।
रक्तपित्ते चाम्लपित्ते सर्ववातामयेषु च ॥४४॥
पित्तरोगेषु सर्वेषु वातपित्तगदेषु च ।
धातुशोषे प्रमेहे च रजोदोषे स्वरक्षये ॥४५॥
दुग्धक्षये मूत्ररोगे कामलायां मलग्रहे ।

सूतिकापवनव्याधौ शस्तमेतन्न संशयः ॥४६॥
अश्विभ्यां पूर्वमुदितं शच्यै योगमनुत्तमम् ।
एषा सौभाग्यदा शुण्ठी स्त्रिणां पुत्रप्रदा शुभा ॥४७॥
॥ इति बृहत् सौभाग्यशुण्ठी ॥

(भारतभैषजरत्नाकर : पञ्चम भाग : पृष्ठ ३९५)

***Bṛhat Saubhāgya Śuṇṭhī (Nāgara Khaṇḍa)***

One *prastha* of *śuṇṭhī* should be cut into small pieces and boiled with two *āḍhakas* of goat's milk over mild fire till the milk becomes thick. The pieces of *śuṇṭhī* should be filtered out, made to a fine paste by grinding and dried by exposing to the sun for one day. This paste should again be added to the earlier milk. To this, one *māṇi(kā)* of ghee should be added and boiled till the whole thing becomes semi-solid. To this, one *karṣa* of the powders of each of *tvak, elā, patra, nāgakesara, tugā, vella, dhanyaka, śveta jīraka, kṛṣṇa jīraka, misi, kustumburu, kuṣṭha, lavaṅga, śatavarī, tālamūlī, śuṇṭhī, pippalī, marica, kapikacchū, ṣahṛda (?), jātiphala, jātikoṣa, śṛṅgāṭa, vṛddhadāru, trivṛt,* seeds of *padma, harītakī, bibhītaka, āmalakī, balā, mahābalā, nāgabalā, hrībera, uśīra, vājigandhā, candana, aguru, kāravī, kaṅkola, ajagandhā, drākṣā, akṣoḍa, cāra, ajamodā, bādāma,* pulp of *nārikela, karpūra, abhraka bhasma, lauha bhasma, vaṅga bhasma, tāmra bhasma, śilājatu and svarṇa mākṣika* should be added and kneaded by the hands for one day. This should then be cooked in the syrup of one *tulā* of sugar. From out of this, small cakes should be prepared. This is called *Khaṇḍa nāgaraka*. Depending upon the strength, the patient should take this potion in appropriate dose, both during the day and the night. It is exceedingly useful for ladies and its administration does not involve any diet restriction. It undoubtedly cures *kṣaya* (consumption), anemia, fever, cough, asthma, suppression of the power of digestion, *saṅgrahaṇī* (sprue syndrome), *rakta gulma* (tumour caused by the vitiation of blood), menorrhagia, *soma roga* (diabetes insipidus), *rakta pitta* (a disease characterised by bleeding from different parts of the body), *amla pitta* (hyper acidity), all types of *vāta rogas*, all types of *pitta rogas*, all types of diseases caused by the simultaneous vitiation of *vāyu* and *pitta*, emaciation of tissue elements, *prameha* (obstinate urinary disorders), menstrual disorders, *svara kṣaya* (diminution of voice), lack of lactation, urinary disorders, jaundice, *galagraha* (obstruction in the throat) and puerperal diseases caused by the vitiated *vāyu*. This excellent recipe was disclosed in the days of yore to Śacī (wife of Lord Indra) by the Aśvins. This preparation of *śuṇṭhī* (called *Saubhāgya śuṇṭhī*) endows women with male progeny and auspiciousness.

"जीरकस्य पलान्यष्टौ धान्यकस्य पलत्रयम् ।
शतपुष्पा यमानीं च कृष्णजीरं पलं[32] तथा ॥४८॥
क्षीरं द्विप्रस्थसंयुक्तं खण्डस्यार्द्धतुलां तथा ।
घृतस्य च पलान्यष्टौ शनैर्मृद्वग्निना[33] पचेत् ॥४९॥
व्योषं त्रिजातकञ्चैव विडङ्गं चव्यचित्रकम् ।
मुस्तकञ्च लवङ्गञ्च पलांशं तु प्रकल्पयेत् ॥५०॥
सर्वयोषिद्विकारणां[34] नाशनं वह्निकारकम्[35] ।
गर्भार्थिनी[36] च या नारी या च गर्भं न विंदति ॥५१॥
अल्पायुषं या जनयेत् या वा जनयते मृतम्।
या च कन्या प्रसूयेत वयःस्थापनमेव च ॥५२॥
॥ बृहज्जीरकावलेहः[37] ॥
(भैषज्यरत्नावली : स्त्रीरोगाधिकार : ४३०-४३३)

***Bṛhat Jīrakāvaleha***

Eight *palas* of *jīraka*, three *palas* of *dhānyaka*, one *pala* of each of *śatapuṣpā*, *yamānī* and *kṛṣṇa jīraka*, two *prasthas* of milk, half *tulā* of sugar and eight *palas* of ghee should be gradually cooked together over mild fire. To this, one *pala* of each of *śuṇṭhī*, *pippalī*, *marica*, *tvak*, *elā*, *patra*, *viḍaṅga*, *cavya*, *citraka*, *mustā* and *lavaṅga* should be added. It cures all the diseases of ladies. It promotes digestion. The woman who desires to have a progeny, who, after conception, does not retain the foetus till maturity, who gives birth to offsprings having small life span, who gives birth to dead foetus and who gives birth to female offsprings only are all benefitted by this recipe. In addition, it promotes longevity of the woman.

"पिप्पली पिप्पलीमूलं चित्रको हस्तिपिप्पली ।
चव्यं सरजनी[38] रास्नाभद्रमुस्तावचाभयाः ॥५३॥
धान्यकमजमोदा च सपञ्चलवणानि च ।

भद्रदारुयवानी च भार्ङ्गीकुटजतण्डुला ॥५४॥
कण्टकार्यास्तथा मूलं बृहती बिल्वपेशिका ।
विडङ्गमरिचयासकल्कैरेतैश्च पाटकैः ॥५५॥
यवकोलकुलित्थानां तथा क्वाथैश्चतुर्गुणे ।
साधयेत्तत्[39] घृतं प्रस्थं प्रस्थं प्रस्थं पयो दधि ॥५६॥
क्षिप्त्वानलेन[40] मृदुना सिद्धमेतत्समाचरेत् ।
एतस्याभ्यङ्गपानाभ्यां कर्णपूरणतस्तथा ॥५७॥
विंशतिर्योनिजा रोगा वातिकाः सान्निपातिकाः ।
पैत्तिकाः श्लैष्मिकाः सद्यसूतिकोपद्रवास्तथा ॥५८॥
लभन्ते सहसा नाशं निधयो नात्र संशयः ।
पिप्पल्याद्यघृतं ख्यातमिदमुक्तं रसायनम् ॥५९॥
॥ पिप्पल्याद्यं घृतम्' ॥

(भारतभैषज्यरत्नाकर : तृतीयभाग : पृष्ठ ३५७)

***Pippalyādya Ghṛta***

One *prastha* of ghee should be cooked by adding one *prastha* of each of milk and curd, four *prasthas* of the decoctions of *yava, kola* and *kulattha* and the paste (1/4th *prastha* in total) of *pippalī, pippalī mūla, citraka, gaja pippalī, cavya, haridrā, rāsnā, bhadra mustā, vacā, abhayā, dhānyaka, ajamodā, viḍa, sāmudra lavaṇa, saindhava lavaṇa, sauvarcala lavaṇa, audbhida lavaṇa, bhadra dāru, yamānī, bhārgī*, seeds of *kuṭaja*, root of *kaṇṭakārī, bṛhatī*, pulp of *bilva, viḍaṅga, marica* and *yavāsaka*. Cooking should be performed over mild fire. This medicated ghee should be used for massage, *pāna* (internal use), *karṇa pūraṇa* (pouring into the ears) by which twenty varieties of *yoniroga* (diseases of the female genital tract) caused by vitiated *vāyu, sannipāta* (simultaneous vitiation of all the three *doṣas*), *pitta and kapha*, and freshly occuring puerperal complications get instantaneously cured and there is no doubt about the therapeutic efficacy of this recipe. This rejuvenating recipe is called *Pippalyādya ghṛta*.

शतपुष्पाणि शिवा वा हपुषा कृमिहा तथा ।
सवत्सकश्चेंद्रयवक्षारपंचकमेव च ॥६०॥

षट्निंब-हिंगु-शिवाटि-तुम्बरु-त्वक्-फलानि च ।
एभिः संसाधितं सर्पिः पयसा योनिदोषजित् ॥६१॥
मूत्रकृच्छ्रार्त्तिशूलघ्नं वन्ध्यानामापि पुत्रदम् ।
ग्रहण्यर्शः - पाण्डुरोगप्लीहागुल्मोदरापहम् ॥६२॥
॥ शतपुष्पाद्यघृतम्' ॥

***Śatapuṣpādya Ghṛta***

Ghee cooked with milk by adding *śatapuṣpā, śivā, hapuṣā, kṛmihā, vatsaka, indrayava,* five varieties of alkalies, six parts of *nimba, hiṅgu, śivāṭi* and bark as well as fruits of *tumburu*, cures dysuria. It gives male progeny even to a sterile woman. It also cures *grahaṇī* (sprue syndrome), piles, anemia, splenic disorders, *gulma* (phantom tumour) and *udara* (obstinate abdominal disorders including ascites).

इति श्रीमहाराजाधिराजश्रीटोडरमल्लविरचिते टोडरानन्दे
आयुर्वेदसौख्ये सूतिकारोगनिदानचिकित्साकथनं नाम
चतुःसप्ततितमो हर्षः ॥

Thus, ends the 74th chapter dealing with the diagnosis and treatment of puerperal diseases in the *Āyurveda saukhya* of *Ṭodarānanda* composed by the great king Ṭodaramalla.

## NOTES AND REFERENCES

१. (क) This is the beginning of seventy eighth chapter of *Āyurveda saukhya* in *Ṭodarānanda* and the invocation reads as follows :
'नेत्रैः स्वरूपं पिबतो विलोक्य लोकान् कथां संवदतः स्वलग्नैः ।
चित्रां च चाणरमुखान् निहन्यान्नृपानरीन् च दयया मुरारिः ॥'
(ख) 'नेत्रैः ..... मुरारिः' पाठोऽयं चतुर्थषष्ठपुस्तकयोः नोपलभ्यते ।

२. दारुणास्तु ते इति आकरे पाठः ।

३. तन्द्रारुचिप्रसेकाद्याः इति आकरे पाठः ।

४. (क) स्पर्श इति पंचमपुस्तके पाठः ।
(ख) स्युणा इति षष्ठपुस्तके पाठः ।

५. योनि इति प्रथमपुस्तके पाठः ।
६. (क) संरक्षणी क्रिया इति पंचमपुस्तके पाठः ।
(ख) संरक्षणा क्रिया इति षष्ठपुस्तके पाठः ।
७. पीतं मधुसंयुक्तं इत आकरे पाठः ।
८. शमयत्यचिरेण इति योगरत्नाकरे पाठः ।
९. 'हिंस्रा ...... मूलपञ्चकम्' पाठोऽयं पंचमपुस्तके अधिकमुपलभ्यते ।
१०. 'धान्य' पाठोऽयं प्रथमपुस्तके नोपलभ्यते ।
११. गजकृष्णा सदुःस्पर्शा इति आकरे पाठः ।
१२. गोक्षुरैर्धन्वयासकम् इति आदर्शपुस्तकेषु पाठः ।
१३. (क) तन्द्रातीसारवान्तिभिः इति आकरे पाठः ।
(ख) तन्द्रातीसारसंयुतम् इति चतुर्थषष्ठपुस्तकयोः पाठः ।
१४. कफोद्भवम् इति आकरे पाठः ।
१५. दारुशृङ्गघनयासतिक्तकंकुष्ठनागरसकट्फलं विषाम् ।
कृष्णजीरककणाहरीतकीचव्यहिंगुसकिरातधान्यकम् ॥
सैन्धवेन च पिवन्ति युवत्यः सूतिकागदनिषूदनं भवेत् ।
पाठोऽयं चतुर्थषष्ठपुस्तकयोः अधिकमुपलभ्यते ।
१६. विकङ्कतदारु. इति आकरे पाठः ।
१७. जलमत्र ससैन्धवहिंगुयुतं इति आकरे पाठः ।
१८. एतदामहरं इति आकरे पाठः ।
१९. कांजिकां कांजिकं तङ्चलोहनिवापितां वज्र कांजिक इति चतुर्थपुस्तके पाठः ।
२०. स्त्रीणामग्निविवर्द्धनम् इति आकरे पाठः ।
२१. क्षीरपाकविधानेन काञ्जिकस्यापि साधनम् इति आकरे पाठः ।
२२. द्रष्टव्यम्—भारतभैषज्यरत्नाकर : पंचमभाग : पृष्ठ १८० ।
२३. खण्डं सार्द्धशतं न्यसेत् इति प्रथमपुस्तके पाठः ।
२४. द्रव्यं प्रत्येकं च पलं पलम् इति प्रथमपुस्तके पाठः ।
२५. (क) नागराद्योऽवलेहः इति आकरे पाठः ।
(ख) लघुसौभाग्यशुण्ठी इति षष्ठपुस्तके पाठः ।
२६. 'वचाचातिबला....रसाशिनी' पाठोऽयं पंचमपुस्तके अधिकमुपलभ्यते ।
२७. (क) 'नागरं ..... शतपुष्पाद्यघृतम्' पाठोऽयं चतुर्थषष्ठपुस्तकयोः अधिकमुपलभ्यते ।
(ख) नागचं इति षष्ठपुस्तके पाठः ।

२८. मानं मिठाग्दरः इति षष्ठपुस्तके पाठः ।

२९. शुद्धी इति चतुर्थपुस्तके पाठः ।

३०. यावत्पिण्डत्वमायाति इति षष्ठपुस्तके पाठः ।

३१. षट्क इति षष्ठपुस्तके आकरे च पाठः ।

३२. पलं पलम् इति आकरे पाठः ।

३३. धान्यकस्य च पलत्रये । सर्वस्थितान्यौषधानिं शनैर्मृद्वग्निना पचेत् इति षष्ठपुस्तके पाठः ।

३४. 'मन्देन वह्निना पक्त्वा मोदकं कारयेत् भिषक्' पाठोऽयं आदर्शपुस्तकेषु नोपलभ्यते ।

३५. वह्निदीपनम् इति आकरे पाठः ।

३६. 'गर्भार्थिनी ...... च' पाठोऽयं आकरे नोपलभ्यते ।

३७. जीरकादि मोदकम् इति आकरे पाठः ।

३८. चव्यञ्च रजनी देया भद्रमुस्तकवचाभयाः इति आकरे पाठः ।

३९. दधिप्रस्थं पयः प्रस्थं दत्त्वा प्रस्थं घृतं पचेत् इति आकरे पाठः ।

४०. 'वातिकान्पैत्तिकांश्चैव श्लैष्मिकान्सन्निपातिकान् ।
सूतिकोपद्रवान्सर्वानभ्यङ्गादेव नाशयेत् ।' इति आकरे पाठः ।

# CHAPTER V

## ॥ अथ स्तनरोगनिदानं चिकित्सा च ॥

*(Diagnosis and Treatment of Breast-Diseases)*

"सक्षीरौ चाप्यदुग्धौ वा दोषाः प्राप्य स्तनौ स्त्रियाः ।
प्रदूष्य मांसरुधिरे स्तनरोगाय कल्पते ॥१॥

***Pathogenesis***

Aggravated *doṣas* having entered into the breasts during the period of lactation or otherwise (when there is no lactation) afflict the *māṃsa* (muscle tissue) and *rakta* (blood) of the locality and give rise to diseases of the breasts.

पञ्चानामपि तेषां हि रक्तजं विद्रधिं विना ।
लक्ष्णानि समानानि बाह्यविद्रधिलक्षणैः" ॥२॥

॥ स्तनरोगनिदानम् ॥

(योगरत्नाकर : स्त्रीरोगचिकित्सा : पृष्ठ ४३१)

***Varieties, Signs and Symptoms***

Breast-diseases are of five varieties, viz., *vātaja, pittaja, kaphaja, sānnipātika* and *kṣataja* (caused by external injury). Their signs and symptoms are similar to the respective varieties of *bāhya* (external) *vidradhis* (abscesses or swollen growths). There is a sixth variety of *bāhya vidradhi*, viz., *raktaja vidradhi* (abscess caused by the primary vitiation of blood; in the breast-diseases blood gets secondarily vitiated) which does not occur in the breasts.

"शोथं स्तनोत्थिमवेक्ष्य[१] भिषग्विदध्याद्
यद्विद्रधावभिहितं बहुधा विधानम् ।
आमे विदह्यति तथैव गते च पाकं
तस्याः[२] स्तनौ सततमेव च निर्गृहीतम्"[३] ॥३॥

(योगरत्नाकर : स्त्रीरोगचिकित्सा : पृष्ठ ४३२)
(भैषज्यरत्नावली : स्त्रीरोगाधिकार : ५०८)

### Line of Treatment

If there is swelling in the breasts, the physician should administer various therapies prescribed for the treatment of *vidradhis* (abscesses) in their different stages, viz., *āma* (immature stage when there is the beginning of the swelling), *vidagdha* (when there is inflammation but no suppuration) and *pakva* (when there is suppuration). The breasts should always be squeezed to remove the accumulated milk.

"विशालामूललेपस्तु हन्ति पीडां स्तनोत्थिताम्" ॥४॥

(भैषज्यरत्नावली : स्त्रीरोगाधिकार : ५०९)

### External Application

Application of the paste of *viśālā*-root cures pain in the breasts.

'जलौकाभिर्हरेद्रक्तं[४] विम्लानमुपनाहनम् ।
पित्तघ्नानि तु शीतानि द्रव्याणि च सुभोजयेत्' ॥५॥

### Blood-letting, Etc.

The patient having breast-diseases should be given blood-letting therapy with the help of leeches. Ointments (warm) should be applied for dissolving the inflammed mass. She should be administered cooling drugs for the alleviation of *pitta* and appropriate cooling food should be given to her.

कारयेद् व्रणवत्सर्वगतिं संरक्ष्य पाचयेत् ॥६॥

The physician should treat breast-diseases on the lines suggested for the treatment of ulcer. Therapies should be administered for the suppuration of inflammed mass. Care should, however, be taken to see that there is no sinus formation in the breasts.

पिप्पल्यास्तप्तलोहेन निर्वाप्य सलिलं पिबेत् ॥७॥

The patient should take water added with the powder of *pippalı* and immersed with a hot piece of iron.

तृणकाष्ठो भवति व नेमकुष्ठदलसंनिभः ।
लेपाद्यैः कुचशोथेषु विधेयः सहसैन्धवः ॥८॥

[The meaning of this verse is not clear; hence left untranslated.]

वनकर्पासकेक्षूणां मूलं सौवीरकेन वा ।
विदारीकन्दं सुरसां पिबेद्वा स्तन्यवर्द्धनम् ॥९॥

***Recipe for Promoting Lactation***

Intake of the root of *vanyakārpāsa* and *ikṣu* along with *sauvīra* (a type of vinegar) promotes lactation. Similarly, intake of *vidārīkanda* and *surasā* helps in the promotion of lactation.

इति टोडरानन्दे स्तनरोगनिदानचिकित्साकथनं
नाम पंचसप्ततितमो हर्षः ॥

Thus, ends the 75th chapter dealing with the diagnosis and treatment of breast-diseases in the *Āyurveda saukhya* of *Ṭoḍarānanda* composed by the great king Ṭoḍaramalla.

## NOTES AND REFERENCES

१. रक्तमांसं च संदूष्य इति आकरे पाठः ।

२. यस्या इति आकरे पाठः ।

३. (क) निर्गृहीतौ इति योगरत्नाकरे पाठः ।
   (ख) निदुर्हीत इति भैषज्यरत्नावलीपाठः ।

४. द्रष्टव्यम्—योगरत्नाकर : स्त्रीरोगाधिकार : पृष्ठ ४३२ ।

५. संरक्ष कारयेत् इति पंचमपुस्तके पाठः ।

६. तृणकष्णो भवनेन कुष्ठदलसंनिभः इति षष्ठपुस्तके पाठः ।

७. पाठोऽयं षष्ठपुस्तके उपलभ्यते । इतरेषु "स्तनरोगनिदानचिकित्साधिकारः" इति पाठः ।

# CHAPTER VI

## ॥ अथ स्तन्यदुष्टिनिदानं चिकित्सा च ॥

*(Diagnosis and Treatment of Polluted Breast-Milk)*

"गुरुभिर्विविधैरन्नैर्दुष्टैर्दोषैः प्रदूषितम् ।
क्षीरं धात्र्याः कुमारस्य नानारोगाय कल्पते ॥१॥

### *Etiology*

The breast-milk of the *dhātrī* (wet-nurse) gets polluted because of the affliction by aggravated *doṣas* as a result of the intake of various types of heavy food-articles. Intake of this polluted milk produces several types of ailments in the child.

कषायं सलिलप्लावि स्तन्यं मारुतदूषितम् ।
कट्वम्ललवणं पीतराजिमत् पित्तसंज्ञितम् ॥२॥
कफदुष्टं घनं तोये निमज्जति सुपिच्छिलम् ।
द्विलिङ्गं द्वन्द्वजं विद्यात् सर्वलिङ्गं त्रिदोषजम् ॥३॥
अदुष्टं चाम्बुनि क्षिप्तमेकीभवति पाण्डुरम् ॥४॥
(योगरत्नाकर : स्त्रीरोगचिकित्सा : क्षीरदोषचिकित्साः पृष्ठ ४३३)

### *Signs of Pollution*

If the breast-milk is polluted by the aggravated *vāyu*, then the taste of the milk becomes astringent and the milk floats on water when added to it.

If the breast-milk is polluted by aggravated *pitta*, then taste of the milk becomes pungent, sour or saline and milk looks surrounded by yellow-lines.

If the breast-milk is polluted by aggravated *kapha*, then it becomes thick and slimy; when poured into the water the milk does not get mixed up but settles down at the bottom of the vessel.

If the breast-milk is afflicted by the simultaneous vitiation of two *doṣas* (viz., *vāyu-pitta*, *vāyu-kapha* and *kapha-pitta*) and of all the three *doṣas*, then the respective signs of the vitiated *doṣas* are manifested in the milk.

The unpolluted breast-milk is *pāṇḍura* (yellowish white) and when added to water, it gets mixed up quickly.

रसः प्रसादो मधुरः पक्वाहारनिमित्तजः ।
कृत्स्नदेहमनुप्राप्तः स्तन्यमित्यभिधीयते[२,३] ॥५॥

### *Process of Milk Formation*

After the digestion of food, *rasa* (nutrient fraction of food) is formed. A part of it, which is sweet in taste, circulates in the whole body [and gets accumulated in the breasts] which is called *stanya* (breast-milk).

"हरिद्रादिं[४] वचादि वा पिबेत् स्तन्यविशुद्धये" ॥६॥

### *Line of Treatment*

For the purification of the polluted breast-milk, the wet-nurse or mother should be given the decoction of drugs belonging to *Haridrādi* or *Vacādi* group.

"तत्र वातात्मिके स्तन्ये दशमूलीजलं[५] पिबेत् ॥७॥

### *Recipe for Pollution by Vāyu*

If the breast-milk is polluted by aggravated *vāyu*, then the wet-nurse should be given the decoction of *daśamūla*.

पित्तदुष्टेऽमृताभीरुपटोलं निम्बचन्दनम् ।
धात्री कुमारश्च पिबेत्क्वाथयित्वा सशर्करम् ॥८॥

*Recipe for Pollution by Pitta*

If the breast-milk is polluted by aggravated *pitta*, then both the wet-nurse and the child should be given the decoction of *amṛtā, abhīru, paṭola, nimba* and *candana* mixed with sugar.

कफदुष्टे घृतं पीत्वा यष्टीसैन्धवसंयुतम् ।
राठपुष्पैः स्तनौ लिम्पेच्छिशोश्च दशनच्छदौ ।
सुखमेवं वमेद्बालः कफकोपश्च शाम्यति ॥९॥

*Recipe for Pollution by Kapha*

If the breast-milk is polluted by *kapha*, then the wet-nurse should take ghee mixed with *yaṣṭimadhu* and *saindhava*. Her nipples and the gums of the child should be smeared with the paste of the flowers of *madana*. This causes easy emesis as a result of which the aggravated *kapha* in the child gets alleviated.

स्तन्ये त्रिदोषसंदुष्टे शकृदामं जलोपमम् ।
नानावर्णरुजं चार्धविबद्धमुपवेश्यते ॥१०॥

(योगरत्नाकर : स्त्रीरोगचिकित्सा : क्षीरदोषचिकित्सा : पृष्ठ ४३३)

*Pollution by All Three Doṣas*

If the breast-milk is polluted by all the three *doṣas*, then the stool of the child contains mucus, and he voids watery stool with variegated colours and associated with different types of pain. Sometimes he voids semisolid stool also.

धात्रीक्षीरविशुद्ध्यर्थं मुद्गयूषरसाशिनी ।
भार्ङ्गीदारुवचापाठाः पिबेत्सातिविषाः शृताः ॥११॥

(भैषज्यरत्नावली : स्त्रीरोगाधिकार : ५०६)

*Recipe for Purification of Breast-Milk*

Intake of the decoction of *bhārṅgī, devadāru, vacā, pāṭhā* and *ativiṣā* corrects faults in the breast-milk. While taking this recipe, the wet-nurse (or mother) should use the soup of *mudga* and meat soup as diet.

मागधिकायाः कर्षं सप्ताहं वापि परिपिष्टम् ।
श्रावणपयोधराभौ तस्याः सुपयोधरौ भवतः ॥१२॥

*Recipes for Increasing Lactation*

Intake of the paste of *pippalī* (one *karṣa* each dose) for one week promotes lactation in the wet-nurse (or mother) and makes the breasts plumpy like the rain (cloud) in the month of *śrāvaṇa*.

या जीरकं द्विशाणं पिष्टं दुग्धेन पिबति गतदुग्धा ।
सप्ताहादपि तस्याः स्यातां घटदुग्धदौ सुकुचौ ॥१३॥

If there is no lactation, then the mother should take the paste of *jīraka* (two *śāṇas* each dose) along with milk for one week. This promotes lactation inasmuch as jarful of milk comes out of her breasts and her breasts become beautiful.

शतावरीरसं पीतं सघृतं स्तन्यवर्द्धनम् ।
पिप्पली सघृतां पीत्वा नारीदुग्धं स्रवेदिति ॥१४॥

Intake of the juice of *śatāvarī* along with ghee promotes lactation. Similarly, intake of the decoction of *pippalī* along with ghee promotes lactation.

"जीरकं हपुषा धान्यं शताह्वा बदराणि च ।
यवानी मेथिका[९] हिंगुपत्रिकामम्लवृक्षकम्[१०] ॥१५॥
पिप्पलीपिप्पलीमूलमजमोदाऽथ वाष्पिका ।
चित्रकं च पलांशानि तथैव[११] च चतुष्पलम् ॥१६॥
कसेरुकं[१२] नागरं च कृष्णजीरकमेव[१३] च ।
गुडस्यार्द्धशतं[१४] दद्याद् घृतप्रस्थं तथैव च ॥१७॥

क्षीरद्विप्रस्थसंयुक्तं शनैर्मृद्वग्निना पचेत् ।
'शीतीभूते[१५] च तस्मिंस्तु चातुर्जातपलं क्षिपेत् ॥
पंचजीरक इत्येष सूतिकानां प्रशस्यते ।
गर्भार्थिनीनां नारीणां बृंहणीये समारुते ॥१८॥
विंशतिर्व्यापदो योनेः कासं श्वासं क्षतक्षयम्[१६] ।
हलीमकं पाण्डुरोगं दौर्गन्ध्यं मूत्रकृच्छ्रताम् ॥१९॥
हंति[१७] पीनोन्नतिं कुर्यात् पद्मपत्रायतेक्षणाः ।
उपयोगात् स्त्रियो भांति शरच्चंद्रनिभाननाः"[१८] ॥२०॥
॥ पञ्चजीरकावलेहः[१९] ॥
(भैषज्यरत्नावली : स्त्रीरोगाधिकार : ४००-४०६)

*Pañcajīrakāvaleha*

One *prastha* of ghee, fifty *palas* of jaggery and two *prasthas* of milk should be cooked by adding the powders of one *pala* of each of *jīraka, hapuṣā, dhānyaka, śatāhva, badara, yavānī, methikā, hiṅgupatrikā, amlavṛkṣa, pippalī, pippalīmūla, ajamoda, vāṣpikā* and *citraka*, and four *palas* of each of *kaseruka, nāgara* and *kṛṣṇajīraka*. Cooking should be performed gradually over mild fire. After the preparation cools down, the powders of four *palas* of each of *tvak, ela, patra* and *nāgakesara* should be added and mixed well. This preparation is called "*Pañcajīraka*" and it is useful in puerperal diseases. It is nourishing and it alleviates *vāyu* of ladies desirous of conception. It cures twenty varieties of diseases of the female genital tract, cough, asthma, phthisis, consumption, *halīmaka* (a type of jaundice), anemia, foul smell emitting from the body and dysuria. It promotes the plumpness and hardness of the breasts and makes the eyes wide like a lotus petal. It promotes the complexion of ladies and they appear beautiful like the full-moon of the autumn.

"मंजिष्ठा[२०] मधुकं कुष्ठं त्रिफला शर्करा बला ।
मेदा पयस्या काकोली मूलञ्चैवाश्वगन्धजम् ॥२१॥
अजमोदा हरिद्रे द्वे हिंगु कटुकरोहिणी ।
उत्पलं कुमुदं द्राक्षाकाकोल्यौ चन्दनद्वयम् ॥२२॥

एतेषां कार्षिकैर्भागैर्घृतप्रस्थं विपाचयेत् ।
शतावरीरसक्षीरं घृताद्देयं चतुर्गुणम् ॥२३॥
सर्पिरेतन्नरः पीत्वा नित्यं स्त्रीषु वृषायते ।
पुत्रान् सञ्जनयेन्नारी मेधाढ्यान् प्रियदर्शनान् ॥२४॥
या चैवास्थिरगर्भां स्याद्या च वा जनयेन्मृतम् ।
अल्पायुषं वा जनयेद् या च कन्यां प्रसूयते ॥२५॥
योनिदोषे रजोदोषे परिस्रावे च शस्यते ।
प्रजावर्द्धनमायुष्यं सर्वग्रहनिवारणम् ॥२६॥
नाम्ना फलघृतं ह्येतदश्विभ्यां परिकीर्त्तितम् ।
अनुक्तं लक्ष्मणामूलं क्षिपन्त्यत्र चिकित्सकाः ॥२७॥
जीवद्वत्सैकवर्णाया घृतमत्र तु गृह्यते ।
आरण्यगोमयेनापि वह्निज्वाला तु दीयते" ॥२८॥

॥ फलघृतम्[21] ॥

(भैषज्यरत्नावली : स्त्रीरोगाधिकार : १६४-१७९)

***Phala Ghṛta***

One *prastha* of ghee, four *prasthas* of the juice of *śatāvarī* and four *prasthas* of milk should be cooked by adding the pastes of one *karṣa* of each of *mañjiṣṭhā, madhuka, kuṣṭha, harītakī, bibhītaka, āmalakī*, sugar, *balā, medā, payasyā, kākolī*, root of *aśvagandhā, ajamodā, haridrā, dāruharidrā, hiṅgu, kaṭukī, utpala, kumuda, drākṣā, kākolī, kṣīrakākolī, candana* and *rakta candana*. Intake of this medicated ghee promotes the virility in men inasmuch as they successfully indulge in sex with ladies every day. This recipe helps a lady to give birth to the male progeny endowed with intellect and good complexion. It is useful for ladies who suffer from habitual abortion, who habitually give birth to dead foetus, who give birth to short-lived children and who habitually give birth to female progeny. It is useful in the diseases of the female genital tract, in menstrual disorders and in polyuria. It promotes progeny and longevity and cures afflictions by all evil spirits. It is called "*Phala ghṛta*" and it is propounded by the Aśvins.

Some physicians add the root of *lakṣmaṇā* into this recipe though it is not mentioned here. The ghee to be used in this recipe is to be collected from the milk of the cow who is uniformly of one colour and who has live-calves. For cooking this recipe, the fire of the cowdung cake collected from the forest should be used.

"शतं पक्त्वाश्वगन्धायाः जलद्रोणेंऽशशेषिते ।
विस्राव्य विपचेत्तैलं क्षीरं दत्त्वा चतुर्गुणम् ॥२९॥
कल्कैर्मृणालपद्मकैर्बिसकिञ्जल्कमालती[२२]-
पुष्पैर्ह्रीबेरमधुकैः शारिवापद्मकेशरैः ॥३०॥
मेदापुनर्नवाद्राक्षामञ्जिष्ठाबृहतीद्वयैः ।
त्वगेलात्रिफला-पत्रमुस्तचन्दनपद्मकैः[२३] ॥३१॥
पक्वं रक्ताशयं वातं रक्तपित्तमसृग्दरम् ।
हन्यात्पुष्टिबलं कुर्यात् कृशानां मांसवर्द्धनम् ॥३२॥
वातयोनिविकारघ्नं[२४] व्रणदोषापकर्षणम् ।
षण्ढानपि वृषान् कुर्यात् पानाभ्यङ्गावगाहनैः'[२५] ॥३३॥
॥ अश्वगन्धाद्यं[२६] तैलम् ॥
(भारतभैषज्यरत्नाकर : प्रथमभाग : पृष्ठ ६८)

***Aśvagandhādya Taila***

One hundred *palas* of *aśvagandhā* should be boiled by adding one *droṇa* of water and reduced to one fourth. This should then be filtered, and to this decoction, oil and four times of milk should be added. This should then be cooked by adding the pastes of *mṛṇāla, padma, bisa, kiñjalka,* flower of *mālatī, hrībera, madhuka, sārivā, padma keśara, medā, punarnavā, drākṣā, mañjiṣṭhā, bṛhatī, kaṇṭakārī, tvak, elā, harītakī, bibhītaka, āmalakī, patra, mustā, candana* and *padmaka.* This medicated recipe cures aggravated *vāyu* in *raktāśaya* (spleen and liver), *raktapitta* (a disease characterised by bleeding from different parts of the body) and menorrhagia. It promotes nourishment and strength.

It promotes *māṃsa* (muscle tissue) of emaciated persons. It cures diseases of the female genital tract and those caused by the aggravated *vāyu.* It corrects the ailments caused by ulcers. It promotes the virility of even impotent persons. It is used in the form of *pāna* (taking internally), *abhyaṅga* (massage) and *avagāhana* (oil-bath).

"कुष्ठं मुस्तं हरिद्रे द्वे पिप्पली कटुरोहिणी ।
काकोली क्षीरकाकोली विडङ्गं त्रिफला वचा ॥३४॥
मेदा रास्ना विडङ्गानि[२७] देवदारु सहिंगुकम् ।
द्वे सारिवे शताह्वा च वचा[२८] यष्टी प्रियङ्गुकाम्[२९] ॥३५॥
अजमोदा महामेदा चन्दनं रक्तचन्दनम् ॥३६॥
जातिफलं[३०] तुगाक्षीरी कट्फलं सितशर्करा[३१] ।
एतैरक्षसमैः कल्कैर्घृतप्रस्थं भिषक्तमः ॥३७॥
चतुर्गुणेन पयसा विपचेद् गोमयाग्निना ।
सुदिने[३२] पुष्यसंयुक्ते भाण्डे ताम्रमये दृढे ॥३८॥
कलशे हेमकल्याणे[३३] कृतकौतुकमंगलम्[३४] ।
सर्पिरेतन्नरः पीत्वा स्त्रीषु नित्यं वृषायते ॥३९॥
या च वन्ध्या भवेन्नारी या च कन्याप्रजायिनी ।
या चैवास्थिरगर्भा[३५] स्याद्या च सूता पुनः स्थिता ॥४०॥
अल्पायुष[३६] वा जनयेद्या च जनयते मृतम् ।
तादृशं[३७] जनयेत्पुत्रं वेदवेदांगपारङ्गम् ॥४१॥
रूपलावण्यसम्पन्नं शतायुर्विगतरुजा ।
नाम्ना फलघृतं ह्येतद्भारद्वाजेन निर्मितम् ॥४२॥
॥ बृहत्फलघृतम् ॥
(भारतभैषज्यरत्नाकर : तृतीयभाग : पृष्ठ ५४३-५४४)

***Bṛhat Phala Ghṛta***

One *prastha* of ghee and four *prasthas* of milk should be cooked by adding the pastes of one *akṣa* of each of *kuṣṭha, mustā, haridrā, dāruharidrā, pippalī, kaṭurohiṇī, kākolī, kṣīrakākolī, viḍaṅga, harītakī, bibhītaka, āmalakī, vacā, medā, rāsnā, viḍaṅga, devadāru, hiṅgu, sārivā, kṛṣṇasārivā, śatāhvā, vacā* (?), *yaṣṭimadhu*, *priyaṅgu*, *ajamodā*, *mahāmedā*, *candana*, *raktacandana*, *jātiphala*, *tugākṣīrī*, *kaṭphala* and *sita śarkarā*. The cooking should be performed with the help of the fire of cowdung cakes on an auspicious day during *puṣya* constellation in a strong vessel prepared of copper. This medicated ghee should be stored in an auspicious jar made of gold after performing benedictory rituals. Intake of this medicated ghee promotes virility in men as a result of which they indulge in sex with ladies everyday. It is useful for women who suffer from sterility, who give birth to female progeny, who get habitual abortion, who fail to conceive after first delivery, who give birth to short-lived progeny and who give birth to dead-foetus. It helps a woman to get a son who will be well versed in the Vedas and Vedāṅgas, who are endowed with beauty and good complexion and who live for one hundred years free from diseases. This recipe is called *Phala ghṛta* and it was propounded by the sage Bharadvaja.

"नीलोत्पलोशीरमधूकयष्टी-
द्राक्षाविदारीकुशपञ्चमूलैः ।
स्याज्जीवनीयैश्च घृतं विपक्वं
शतावरीकारसदुग्धमिश्रम् ॥४३॥
तच्छर्करापादयुतं प्रशस्त-
मसृग्दरे मारुतरक्तपित्ते ।
क्षीणे बले रेतसि च प्रणष्टे
कृच्छ्रे च पित्तप्रभवे च गुल्मे" ॥४४॥
॥ नीलोत्पलादि घृतम् ॥

(भारतभैषज्यरत्नाकर : तृतीयभाग : पृष्ठ १९२)

**Nīlotpalādi Ghṛta**

Ghee (one part), juice of *śatāvarī* (one part), milk (one part) and sugar (1/4th part) should be cooked by adding the pastes of *nīlotpala*, *uśīra*, *madhūka*, *yaṣṭimadhu*, *drākṣā*, *vidārī*, roots of *kuśa*, *kāśa*, *śara*, *darbha* and *ikṣu* and of drugs belonging to the *Jīvanīya* group. It is useful in the treatment of menorrhagia, *vātika* type diseases, *raktapitta* (a disease characterised by bleeding from different parts of the body), emaciation, seminal disorders, dysuria and *gulma* (phantom tumour) caused by the aggravated *pitta*.

"सिद्धार्थकं वचा ब्राह्मी शङ्खपुष्पी पुनर्नवा ।
पयस्याभयायष्ट्याह्वकटुका[३८] च फलत्रयम् ॥४५॥
सारिवे रजनी पाठा भृङ्गदारुसुवर्चला: ।
मञ्जिष्ठा त्रिफला श्यामा वृषपुष्पं सगैरिकम् ॥४६॥
इमान्[३९] पक्त्वा घृतप्रस्थं सम्यक् मन्त्राभिमन्त्रितम् ।
द्विमासगर्भिणी नारी षण्मासानुपयोजयेत्[४०] ॥४७॥
सर्वज्ञं जनयेत्पुत्रं सर्वामयविवर्जितम् ।
अस्य प्रयोगात् कुक्षिस्थः स्फुटवाग्व्याहरत्यपि ॥४८॥
योनिदुष्टाश्च या नार्यो रेतोदुष्टाश्च ये नराः ।
वन्ध्यापि लभते पुत्रं शूरं पण्डितमानिनम् ॥४९॥
जडगद्गदमूकत्वं पानादेवापकर्षति ।
सप्तरात्रप्रयोगेण नरः श्रुतिधरो भवेत् ॥५०॥
नाग्निर्दहति तद्वेश्म न वज्रमुपहन्ति च ।
न तत्र म्रियते बालो यत्रास्ते सोमसंज्ञितम्' ॥५१॥
॥ सोमघृतम्[४१] ॥

(भैषज्यरत्नावली : स्त्रीरोगाधिकार : १७४-१८०)

*Soma Ghṛta*

One *prastha* of ghee should be cooked by adding *siddhārthaka*, *vacā*, *brāhmī*, *śaṅkhapuṣpī*, *punarnavā*, *payasyā*, *abhayā*, *yaṣtimadhu*, *kaṭukā*, *harītakī*, *bibhītaka*, *āmalakī*, *sārivā*, *kṛṣṇa sārivā*, *haridrā*, *pāṭhā*, *bhṛṅgarāja*, *devadāru*, *suvarcalā*, *mañjiṣṭhā*, *harītakī*, *bibhītaka*, *āmalakī*, *śyāmā*, flowers of *vāsaka* and *gairika*. This medicated ghee should be given to a woman who is in the second month of pregnancy for six months. This recipe helps her to get an intelligent son who is free from all diseases. Her child, even while in laps (early infancy) starts talking clearly. A woman having faults in her genital tract, a man having ailments of semen and even a sterile woman conceive and get a brave as well as intelligent son by the intake of this recipe. Its intake cures a *jaḍa* (dumb), *gadgada* (stammering) and *mūka* (mute). Its use for seven nights makes a person *śrutidhara* (a who can retain in memory whatever he hears). His house does not get burnt by fire nor does it get destroyed by thunderbolt. In the house, where this recipe called "*Soma ghṛta*" is used, there will be no infantile death.

**इति श्रीमहाराजाधिराजश्रीटोडरमल्लविरचिते टोडरानन्दे आयुर्वेदसौख्ये स्त्रीरोगनिदानचिकित्साकथनं नाम षड्सप्ततितमो हर्षः ॥**

Thus, ends the 76th chapter dealing with the diagnosis and treatment of female diseases in the *Āyurveda saukhya* of *Ṭoḍarānanda* composed by the great king Ṭoḍaramalla.

## NOTES AND REFERENCES

१. प्रदूषितः इति प्रथमपुस्तके पाठः ।

२. स्त्रीरोगनिदानम् पाठोऽयं पंचमपुस्तके अधिकमुपलभ्यते ।

३. 'अष्टौ दोषश्च नारीणां नवमः पुरुषस्य च ।
रक्तं पित्तं तथा वातः श्लेष्मा च सन्निपाततः ।
ग्रहदोषविकारश्च पुरुषस्य च रेतसः ।
काकवन्ध्या मृतापत्या गर्भस्रावा तथैव च ।
जातांते चापि वन्ध्या च दोषैरेभिर्न्न चान्यथा ।
मासि मासि रजः स्त्रीणां ऋतौ च स्रवति त्र्यहम् ।
वत्सराद्द्वादशादूर्द्ध्वं याति पंचाशतं क्षयम् ।
॥ स्त्रीरोगनिदानम् ॥' पाठोऽयं चतुर्थपुस्तके अधिकमुपलभ्यते ।

४. 'हरिद्रादिं ..... विशुद्धये' पाठोऽयं चतुर्थपुस्तके अधिकमुपलभ्यते ।

५. त्र्यहं इति आकरे पाठः ।

६. शिफाकुक्करमर्द्दस्य दंतक्षुणा घृता मुखे ।
स्तन्यवृद्धिकरो स्त्रीणां स्तनकीलकनाशनाः ।
पाठोऽयं चतुर्थपुस्तके अधिकमुपलभ्यते ।

७. 'अथवा त्रिफला मुस्तं निम्बं कटुकरोहिणीं'
पाठोऽयं चतुर्थपुस्तके अधिकमुपलभ्यते ।

८. .स्तीक्ष्णैर्धात्रीं च वामयेत् इति चतुर्थषष्ठपुस्तकयोः पाठः ।

९. क्रुष्टिको इति आकरे पाठः ।

१०. हिंगुपत्रिका कासमर्दकम् इति आकरे पाठः ।

११. तथाऽन्यच्च इति षष्ठपुस्तके पाठः ।

१२. कसेल्लकं इति आदर्शपुस्तकेषु पाठः ।

१३. कुष्ठं दीप्यकमेव च इति आकरे पाठः ।

१४. गुडस्य च शतं इति आकरे पाठः ।

१५. 'शीती ..... क्षिपेत्' पाठोऽयं आकरे नोपलभ्यते ।

१६. ज्वरं क्षयम् इति आकरे पाठः ।

१७. घ्नन्ति पीनोन्नतकुचाः इति आकरे पाठः ।

१८. स्त्रियो नित्यमलक्ष्मीमलवर्जिताः इति आकरे पाठः ।

१९. पञ्चजीरकगुडः इति आकरे पाठः ।

२०. 'मंजिष्ठा ..... दीयते' पाठोऽयं प्रथमपंचमपुस्तकयोः नोपलभ्यते ।

२१. (क) फलकल्याणघृतम् इति आकरे पाठः ।
(ख) मध्यमफलघृतम् इति चतुर्थषष्ठपुस्तकयोः पाठः ।

२२. कल्कैर्मृणालशालुकबिस. इति आकरे पाठः ।

२३. एलैलवालुत्रिफलामुस्तचन्दनपद्मकैः इति आकरे पाठः ।

२४. रेतोयोनि. इति आकरे पाठः ।

२५. पानाभ्यङ्गानुवासनैः इति आकरे पाठः ।

२६. अश्वगन्धातैलम् इति आकरे पाठः ।

२७. विशाला च देवदारु प्रियङ्गुका इति आकरे पाठः ।

२८. दन्ती मधुकमुत्पलम् इति आकरे पाठः ।

२९. 'मेदापयस्या काकोली मूलं चैत्राश्वगन्धकम्' पाठोऽयं षष्ठपुस्तके अधिकमुपलभ्यते ।

३०. जातिपुष्पं इति आकरे पाठः ।

३१. हिंगु इति आकरे पाठः ।

३२. पुष्पनक्षत्रसम्पन्नं भाण्डे हेमादिजे स्थितम् इति आकरे पाठः ।

३३. कल्याणो इति चतुर्थपुस्तके पाठः ।

३४. मंगलः इति षष्ठपुस्तके पाठः ।

३५. पीत्वैतत्स्थिरगर्भा इति आकरे पाठः ।

३६. अनायुषं या इति आकरे पाठः ।

३७. सा च सञ्जनयेत्पुत्रं दीर्घायुषमरोगिणम् ।
वेदवेदाङ्गशास्त्रज्ञं सर्वावयवसुन्दरम् ।
नानेन सदृशं किञ्चिदौषधं चान्यदुत्तमम् ।

वर्तते मर्त्यलोकेऽत्र योषितां पुत्रदं परम् ।
नाम्ना फलघृतं ह्येतद्भारद्वाजेन निर्मितम् ।
अनुक्तं लक्ष्मणामूलं क्षिप्यन्त्यत्र चिकित्सकाः ।
जीवद्वत्सैकवर्णाया घृतमस्मिन् प्रशस्यते ।
आरण्यगोमयेनात्र वह्निज्वालाविधिः स्मृतः ।
इति आकरे पाठः ।

३८. मधुयष्ठ्याह्वाकटुकैल्लानिष्कण्टकम् इति आदर्शपुस्तकेषु पाठः ।

३९. एभिः इति आदर्शपुस्तकेषु पाठः ।

४०. .मासान्स्तत्प्रत्ययोजयेत् इति आदर्शपुस्तकेषु पाठः ।

४१. 'छर्दिरम्लेच्छता प्रातः ष्ठीवनं राजिरञ्जनम् ।
अरुचिः स्तनयोः कार्श्न्यं ग्लानिः रायेपनिस्तरः ।
कुक्षौ अक्ष्णोश्च संसित्वं गर्भिण्याः स्फुटलक्षणम्' ।
इति षष्ठपुस्तके अधिको पाठः ।

# CHAPTER VII

## ॥ बालरोगनिदानं चिकित्सा च ॥

*(Diagnosis and Treatment of Children's Diseases)*

त्रिविधः कथितो बालः क्षीरान्नोभयवर्त्तनः ।
स्वस्थ्यः तेषामदुष्टायां दुष्टायां रोगसंभवः ॥१॥

***Three Stages of Infancy***

*Bāla* (infancy) has the following three stages :

(1) *Kṣīrāda* (when the child depends exclusively upon milk for nourishment);

(2) *Kṣīrānnāda* (when the child depends upon both milk and cereals for nourishment); and

(3) *Annāda* (when the child depends upon cereals for nourishment).

If the milk and cereals are not polluted then the child remains healthy. If, however, the child is given polluted milk and cereals then he suffers from diseases.

दन्तोद्भेदश्च रोगाणां सर्वेषामपि कारणम् ।
विशेषाद् ज्वरविड्भेदकासच्छर्दिशिरोरुजाम् ।

अभिष्यन्दश्च पोथक्यो विसर्पोऽस्य च जायते ॥२॥
(योगरत्नाकर : बालरोगाधिकार : पृष्ठ ४३६)

### *Teething Time*

Teething time in a child is the cause of all diseases. During this period, he specially suffers from fever, diarrhoea, cough, vomiting, headache, conjuctivitis, *pothaki* (an eye-disease characterised by the appearance of hard papules of the size of mustard seed inside the eyelids accompanied with purulent discharge, itching and pain) and erysipelas.

षृष्ठभंगे[1] विडालानां बर्हिणां च शिखोद्गमे ।
दंतोद्भेदे च बालानां न हि किंचिन्न दूयते ॥३॥

### *Significance of Teething Time*

During the period of *pṛṣṭha bhaṅga* (breaking or bending of the back or vertibral column) in kitten, *śikhodgama* (appearance of crest or comb) in peacock and teething of children, there is no disease which do not afflict them.

"वातदुष्टं स्तन्यं पिबन् बालः वातगदातुरः ।
क्षामस्वरः कृशाङ्गः स्याद्बद्धविण्मूत्रमारुतः ॥४॥

### *Milk Vitiated by Vāyu*

If the child takes milk vitiated by *vāyu* then he suffers from *vātarogas* (diseases caused by aggravated *vāyu*); his voice becomes hoarse, his body becomes emaciated and there will be obstruction to his passage of stool, urine as well as flatus.

स्विन्नो भिन्नमलो बालः कामलापित्तरोगवान् ।
'तृष्णालुरुष्णसर्वाङ्गः[2] पित्तदुष्टं पयः पिबन् ॥५॥

### *Milk Vitiated by Pitta*

If the child takes milk vitiated by *pitta*, then he perspires and suffers from diarrhoea, jaundice, diseases caused by aggravated *pitta*, thirst and excessive heat in the body.

कफदुष्टं पिबन् क्षीरं लालालुः श्लेष्मरोगवान् ।
निद्रान्वितो जडः शूनवक्त्राक्षश्छर्दनः शिशुः' ॥६॥

(माधवनिदान : बालरोग : ६८ : १-३)

*Milk Vitiated by Kapha*

If the child takes milk vitiated by *kapha* then he suffers from excessive salivation and diseases caused by aggravated *kapha*. He gets excessive sleep and remains inactive. His face and eyes get swollen and he suffers from vomiting.

"शिशोस्तीव्रामतीव्रां च रोदनाल्लक्षयेद्रुजम्" ॥

(माधवनिदान : बालरोग : ६८ : ४)

"स्रोतांस्यङ्गानि सर्वांश्च[3] पश्येद्यत्नान्मुहुर्मुहुः ॥७॥

*Diagnosis of Pain in a Child*

Acuteness or otherwise of the pain in a child is to be determined from the nature of his cries. The physician should carefully examine the orifices (ears, eyes, nose, etc.) and limbs frequently.

कुकूणकः क्षीरदोषाच्छिशूनामेव वर्त्मनि ।
जायते तेन तन्नेत्रं कण्डूरं च स्रवेन्मुहुः ॥८॥
शिशु कुर्याल्ललाटाक्षिकूटनासावघर्षणम् ।
शक्तो नार्कप्रभां द्रष्टुं न वर्त्मोन्मीलनक्षमः ॥९॥

*Kukūṇaka (Ophthalmia)*

A disease called *kukūṇaka* appears in the eyelids of the child because of the intake of polluted milk. As a result of this, there will be itching in eyes and frequent lachrymation. The child rubs his forehead, eyes and nose. He becomes incapable of looking at the sun-rays. It becomes even difficult for him to open the eyelids.

मातुः कुमारो गर्भिण्याः स्तन्यं प्रायः पिबन्नापि।
कासाग्निसादवमथुतन्द्राकार्श्यारुचिभ्रमैः ॥१०॥

युज्यते कोष्ठवृद्ध्या च तमाहुः पारिगर्भिकम् ।
रोगं परिभवाख्यं च युञ्ज्यात्तत्राग्निदीपनम् ॥११॥

*Pārigarbhika*

Generally, by the intake of the milk of a pregnant mother the child suffers from cough, suppression of the power of digestion, vomiting, drowsiness, emaciation, anorexia, giddiness and protruted abdomen. This condition is called *Pārigarbhika*. It is also called *Paribhava* and in such a condition, the child should be given digestive stimulants.

तालुमांसे[४] कफः क्रुद्धः कुरुते तालुकण्टकम् ।
तेन तालुप्रदेशस्य निम्नता मूर्ध्नि जायते ॥१२॥
तालुपातः[५] स्तनद्वेषः[६] कृच्छ्रात् पानं शकृद्द्रवम् ।
तृडक्षिकण्ठास्यरुजा ग्रीवादुर्धरता वमिः ॥१३॥

*Tālukaṇṭaka*

Aggravation of *kapha* in the palatal muscles of the child produces a disease called *Tālukaṇṭaka*. As a result of this, the *mūrdhā* (anterior fontanel) above the region of the palate gets depressed. The palate of the child hangs down (*tālu pāta*) and he dislikes sucking the breasts. He takes milk with difficulty, passes loose motions, becomes thirsty and gets pain in the eyes, throat and mouth. He becomes incapable of holding the neck (head) straight and gets vomiting.

विसर्पस्तु शिशोः प्राणनाशनो बस्तिशीर्षजः ।
पद्मवर्णो महापद्मो[७] रोगो दोषत्रयोद्भवः ।
शङ्खाभ्यां हृदयं यो वा हृदयाद्वा गुदं व्रजेत् ॥१४॥

*Visarpa (Erysipelas)*

Erysipelas in the child, which is fatal, is of two types, viz., one which appears in the head and the other which appears in the region of urinary bladder. It is red like the colour of the lotus, and therefore, it is called *Mahāpadma*. It is caused by the simultaneous vitiation of all the three *doṣas*. The first variety travels from the regions of two temples to the cardic region and the second variety travels from the cardiac region towards the anal region.

क्षुद्ररोगे[९] च कथिते अजगल्यहिपूतने ॥१५॥

*Ajagallikā and Ahiputanā*

These two diseases, viz., *ajagallikā* and *ahiputanā* are already described in the chapter on the diagnosis and treatment of *kṣudrarogas* (diseases of minor importance).

ज्वराद्या व्याधयः सर्वे महतां ये पुरेरिताः ।
बालदेहेऽपि[१०] ते तद्वद्विज्ञेयाः कुशलैः सदा ॥१६॥

*Other Diseases of the Child*

Fever, etc., which are already described earlier, (which generally occurs in adults) also appear in the children. Their diagnosis and treatment as described earlier should be followed in the case of children also.

क्षणादुद्विजते बालः क्षणात् त्रस्यति रोदिति ।
नखैर्दन्तैर्दारयति धात्रीमात्मानमेव वा ॥१७॥
'ऊर्ध्वं'[११] निरीक्षते दन्तान् खादेत् कूजति जृम्भते ।
भ्रुवौ क्षिपति दन्तौष्ठं फेनं वमति चासकृत् ॥१८॥
क्षामोऽति निशि जागर्ति शूनाक्षो भिन्नविट्स्वरः ।
मत्स्यशोणितगन्धिश्च[१२] न चाश्नाति यथा पुरा ।
सामान्यं ग्रहजुष्टानां लक्षणं समुदाहृतम् ॥१९॥

*Signs and Symptoms in General of Grahāveśa*

If the child is possessed by *grahas* (evil spirits), the following signs and symptoms in general, appear in the child :

(1) The child gets irritated and terrified suddenly and he starts crying suddenly;

(2) he scratches himself and the wet-nurse with help of teeth & nails;

(3) he looks upwards and bites (gnaws) teeth;
(4) he produces coojing (murmuring) sound and yawns;
(5) he draws down the eyebrows;
(6) he bites lips with the help of teeth;
(7) he frequently vomits frothy material;
(8) he becomes prostrated and remains excessively awake at night;
(9) his eyes become swollen, he gets diarrhoea and his voice becomes hoarse;
(10) smell of fish and blood comes out of his body; and
(11) he does not take feed as before.

एकनेत्रस्य गात्रस्य स्रावः स्पन्दनकम्पनम् ।
उध्वं दृष्ट्या निरीक्षेत वक्रास्यो रक्तगन्धिकः ॥२०॥
दंतान् खादति वित्रस्त[१३] स्तन्यं नैवाभिनन्दति ।
स्कन्दग्रहगृहीतानां रोदनं चाल्पमेव च ॥२१॥
नष्टसंज्ञो वमेत्फेनं त्रस्तो[१४] हसति रोदिति ।
पूयशोणितगन्धित्वं स्कन्दापस्मारलक्षणम् ॥२२॥

### *Seizure by Skanda-graha*

If the child is possessed by the evil spirit called Skanda, then the following signs and symptoms are manifested :

(1) There is lachrymation from one eye;
(2) there is perspiration, throbbing and trembling of the body;
(3) the child looks upwards;
(4) smell of blood comes out from his face and mouth;
(5) he gnaws teeth and appears terrified;
(6) he does not like to suck breasts (take milk); and
(7) he cries less.

### *Skandāpasmāra (Epileptic Fit Because of Seizure by Skanda)*

If the child gets epileptic fits because of seizure by the evil spirit called Skanda (*Skandāpasmāra*), then the following signs and symptoms are manifested :

(1) He becomes unconscious and vomits frothy material;
(2) he becomes fearful, he laughs and cries; and
(3) smell of pus and blood comes out from his body.

स्रस्ताङ्गो भयचकितो विहङ्गगन्धिः
साम्रावव्रणपरिपीडितः समन्तात् ।
स्फोटैश्चोपचिततनुः[१५] सदाहपाकै[१६]-
र्विज्ञेयो भवति शिशुः क्षतः शकुन्या ॥२३॥

*Seizure by Śakunī*

The following signs and symptoms are indicative of the seizure by the evil spirit called Śakunī:

(1) Prostrated body;
(2) getting up with fearfulness;
(3) smell of birds coming out of the body;
(4) affliction by exudating ulcers all over the body; and
(5) affliction of the entire body by pustular eruptions associated with burning sensation and putrification.

व्रणैः स्फोटैश्चितं गात्रं पङ्कगन्धं स्रवेदसृक् ।
भिन्नवर्चो ज्वरो दाहो रेवतीग्रहलक्षणम् ॥२४॥

*Seizure by Revatī*

If the child is possessed by the evil spirit called Revatī then the following signs and symptoms are manifested :

(1) The body of the child becomes surrounded with ulcers and pustular eruptions;
(2) smell of mud comes out of the body of the child;
(3) exudation of blood from different parts of the body; and
(4) diarrhoea, fever and burning sensation.

अतीसारो ज्वरस्तृष्णा[१८] स्रस्ताङ्गं चातिरोदनम् ।
नष्टनिद्रस्तथोद्विग्नो ग्रस्तः पूतनया शिशुः ॥२५॥

*Seizure by Pūtanā*

The following signs and symptoms appear if the child is possessed by the evil spirit called Pūtanā :

(1) Diarrhoea, fever, thirst and prostration;
(2) excessive cry; and
(3) lack of sleep and irritability.

'छर्दिः[१९] श्वासो[२०] ज्वरस्तृष्णा वसागन्धोऽतिरोदनम् ।
स्तन्यद्वेषोऽतिसारश्च अन्धपूतनया[२१] भवेत् ॥२६॥

*Seizure by Andha Pūtanā*

Seizure of the child by the evil spirit called Andha Pūtanā gives rise to the following signs and symptoms :

(1) Vomiting, asthma, fever and thirst;
(2) the body emits the smell of *vasā* (muscle fat);
(3) excessive cry;
(4) dislike for taking milk; and
(5) diarrhoea.

वेपते कासते क्षीणो नेत्ररोगो विगन्धिता ।
छर्द्यतीसारयुक्तश्च शीतपूतनया शिशुः ॥२७॥

*Seizure by Śīta Pūtanā*

The following signs and symptoms appear in the child possessed by the evil spirit called Śīta Pūtanā :

(1) Trembling, cough and emaciation;
(2) appearance of eye diseases;
(3) foul smell coming out of the body; and
(4) vomiting as well as diarrhoea.

प्रसन्नवर्णवदनः सिराभिरभिसंवृतः ।
मूत्रगन्धी च बह्वाशी मुखमण्डिकया[२२] भवेत् ॥२८॥
छर्दीस्पन्दनकण्ठास्यशोषो[२३] मूर्च्छा विगन्धिता ।
उर्ध्वं पश्येद्दंशेद्दन्तान् नैगमेषग्रहं वदेत् ॥२९॥

॥ बालरोगनिदानम् ॥

(माधवनिदान : बालरोग : ६८ : ७-२९)

*Seizure by Mukha Maṇḍikā*

Seizure of the child by the evil spirit called Mukha Maṇḍikā gives rise to the following signs and symptoms :

(1) Bright complexion of the child's body;

(2) appearance of veins prominently all over the body of the child;
(3) the body emits foul smell like that of the urine; and
(4) desire for eating more.

*Seizure by Naigameṣa*

If the child is possessed by the evil spirit called Naigameṣa, then the following signs and symptoms are manifested :

(1) Vomiting, trembling, dryness of the throat and the mouth and fainting;
(2) foul smell coming out of his body; and
(3) looking upwards.

Thus, ends the diagnosis of children diseases.

"कुष्ठं वचाभयाब्राह्मीकनकं क्षौद्रसर्पिषा ।
वर्णायुःकान्तिजननं लेहं बालस्य दापयेत् ॥३०॥

*Recipe*

Intake of the powder of *kuṣṭha, vacā, abhayā, brāhmī* and *svarṇa bhasma* along with honey and ghee promotes the complexion, longevity and complexion of the child.

स्तन्याभावे पयश्छागं गव्यं वा तद्गुणं पिबेत् ॥३१॥

***Substitutes of Mother's Milk***

In the case of the non-availability of mother's milk (or the milk of the wet-nurse), the child should be given goat's milk or cow's milk because of their similarity in property with that of the former (mother's milk).

'तर्क्वधो गुडिकां तप्तां निर्वाप्य कटुतैलके ।
तत्तैलं पानतो हन्ति बालानां कफमुद्धतम्[२४] ॥३२॥

(भैषज्यरत्नावली : बालरोगाधिकार : ५-७)

The iron ball placed at the bottom of a *tarkū* (spinning spindle) should be made hot and immersed in mustard oil.

Administration of this medicated oil cures the aggravated *kapha* located in the throat of the child.

व्योषशिवोग्ररजनीकल्कं वा पीतमथ पयसौं[२५] ।
तत्तुनिसेव्य कुरुते पटुतां बालस्य चाभ्यस्तात् ॥३३॥

The paste of *śuṇṭhī, pippalī, marica, harītakī, vacā* and *haridrā* should be mixed with milk and given to the child every day for its good health. [There seems to be errors in this verse].

"बालो[२६] योऽचिरजातः[२७] स्तन्यं गृह्णाति नो तदा तस्य[२८]।
सैन्धवधात्रीमधुघृतपथ्याकल्केन घर्षयेज्जिह्वाम्" ॥३४॥
(योगरत्नाकर : बालरोगचिकित्सा : पृष्ठ ४४०)

*Feed of Child Immediately After Birth*

If a child who is recently born, do not take feed, his tongue should be rubbed with the paste of *saindhava, āmalakī*, honey, ghee and *harītakī*. This will enable to child to take feed.

मयूरचूलिकामूलमादित्यग्रहणोद्धृतम् ।
बालकस्य करे बद्धं समस्तग्रहदोषहृत् ॥३५॥

The root of *mayūra candrikā* should be collected (uprooted) during solar eclipse. Tying this root (in the form of a talisman) in the arm of the child cures all types of afflictions by evil spirits.

"मृत्पिण्डेनाग्नितप्तेन क्षीरसिक्तेन सोष्मणा ।
स्वेदयेदुत्थितां नाभिं शोथस्तेन प्रशाम्यति[२९] ॥३६॥

*Swelling in Umbilicus*

A bolus of mud should be made hot by exposing to the flame of the fire. Over it, milk should be poured. With the help of this bolus, when it is lukewarm, fomentation should be applied over the umbilicus which cures its swelling.

नाभिपाके निशालोध्रप्रियङ्गुमधुकैः शृतम् ।
तैलमभ्यञ्जने शस्तमेभिर्वाप्यवचूर्णयेत्[३०] ॥३७॥

### Inflammation of Umbilicus

Oil cooked with *niśā, lodhra, priyangu* and *madhuka* should be gently rubbed over the umbilicus which cures its inflammation. For this purpose, the powder of the above mentioned drugs should also be dusted over the umbilicus.

सोमग्रहणे विधिवत् केकिशिखामूलमुद्धृतं बद्धम् ।
जघनेऽथ कन्धरायां क्षपयत्यहिण्डिका[31] नियतम् ॥३८॥

### Recipe for Marasmus

The root of *mayūra śikhā* should be collected during lunar eclipse. Tying this root either in the thigh or in the arm certainly cures *ahiṇḍikā bāla śoṣa*=marasmus) in the child.

सप्तदलपुष्पमरिचं पिष्टं गोरोचनासहितम् ।
पीतं तद्वत्तण्डुलभक्तकृतो दग्धपिष्टकप्रायः ॥३९॥

Flowers of *sapta parṇa, marica* and *gorocanā* should be made to a paste. This should be given to drink which cures marasmus in the infant. Similarly, administration of burnt pastry prepared of rice-flour cures marasmus in the child.

जम्बूकनासा वायसजिह्वा नाभिर्वराहसम्भूता ।
कांस्यं रसोऽथ मिलितं विधृतं ग्रीवादि कटिदेशे ।
आहिण्डिकाप्रशमनमत्यर्थं[32] नाभिपाके विधिः ॥४०॥

Nose of jackal, tongue of crow, umbilicus of wild boar, *kāṃsya bhasma* and mercury (in *bhasma* form) should be triturated together and made to a paste. Application of this paste in the neck and lumber region cures *ahiṇḍikā* (marasmus). This paste may also be applied over the umbilicus which cures its inflammation.

अनामके घुर्घुरिका[33] मृद्वीकामरिचरोचनाः ।
नवनीतञ्च सम्मिश्र्य खादेत्तद्रोगनाशनम्"[34] ॥४१॥

(भैषज्यरत्नावली : बालरोगाधिकार : ८-१४)

***Recipe for Anāmaka***

If the child is suffering from *anāmaka* (ulceration of the anus), then he should be given the paste of *ghurghurikā* (a type of insect), *mṛdvīkā*, *marica* and *gorocanā* mixed with butter.

'पटोलत्रिफलारिष्ट'[३५] हरिद्रा त्रिफला पिबेत् ।
तत्तत् विस्फोटविसर्पज्वराणां शान्तये शिशुः' ॥४२॥

***Recipe***

The dedoction of *paṭola, harītakī, bibhītaka, āmalakī* and *ariṣṭa* or the decoction of *haridrā, harītakī, bibhītaka* and *āmalakī* should be administered to the child for the cure of *visphoṭa* (pustural eruption), erysipelas and fever.

"तैलाक्तशिरसस्तालुनि सप्तदलार्कस्नुहीक्षीरम्'[३६] ।
दत्त्वा रजनीचूर्णे दत्ते न स्यादनामाख्यः ॥४३॥

***Recipe for Prevention of Anāmaka***

The head and *tālu* (anterior fontanel) of the child should be smeared with oil. Thereafter, he should be administered the milky-latex of *saptaparṇa, arka* and *snuhī* mixed with the powder of *haridrā*. This prevents *anāmaka* (ulceration of the anus) of the child.

लेहयेच्च शुना बालं नवनीतेन लेपितम् ।
स्फुटकपत्रजरसेनोद्वर्त्तनञ्च तद्धितम् ॥४४॥

***Recipe for Anāmaka***

The body of the child should be smeared with butter and a dog should be allowed to lick the child thereafter. This cures *anāmaka* (anal ulcer). Similarly, rubbing the juice of the leaf of *sphuṭaka* cures *anāmaka*.

तैलस्य भागमेकं मूत्रस्य द्वौ द्वौ च शिम्बीदलरसस्य च।
गव्यं पयश्चतुर्गुणमेवं दत्त्वा पचेत्तैलम् ।
तेनाभ्यङ्गः सततं रोगमनामाख्यमपहरति ॥४५॥

*Medicated Oil*

One part of oil, two parts of cow's urine, two parts of the juice of the leaves of *śimbī* and four parts of cow's milk should be cooked together. It's constant application cures *anāmaka* (anal ulcer) in the child.

अर्कतूलकमाविकरोमाण्यादाय[३७] केशराजस्य ।
स्वरसेनाक्ते वस्त्रे कृत्वा वर्त्तिञ्च तैलाक्ताम् ॥४६॥
तज्जातकज्जलाञ्जितलोचनयुगलोऽप्यलङ्कृतो बालः ।
कष्टमनामकरोगं क्षपयति भूतादिकञ्चापि ॥४७॥

*Collyrium*

The cotton collected from the ripe fruits of *arka* and hair of sheep should be soaked in the juice of *bhṛṅgarāja*. It should then be rolled in a piece of cloth which should be smeared with oil. This should then be ignited. The collyrium, thus prepared, should be applied over the eye-lids of the child. It cures *anāmaka* (anal ulcer) and seizures by evil spirits.

चालमिकांतःस्थितपोत[३८] सम्प्लाव्य गव्यमूत्रेण ।
आकोदशालिकायां रजकक्षारोदकस्नानम् ॥४८॥

*Recipe for Bath*

In a bathroom, the child should be made to sit inside a sieve over which cow's urine should be poured so that the child gets fully bathed in it. Thereafter, he should be bathed with alkali water collected from the house of a washerman. This cures *anāmaka* (anal ulcer).

दासक्रयणश्रावणवटिका रसेन्द्रपूरिता धृता कण्ठे ।
नलिनीदले च शयनं दुष्टमनामाख्यरोगहरम् ॥४९॥

(भैषज्यरत्नावली : बालरोगाधिकार : १५-२१)

*Talisman*

Through the servant one should buy a cowri shell from a charlatan. It should be filled with mercury, sealed and tied to the neck of the child. He should be made to sleep over the lotus leaves. This is found to cure the disease called *anāmaka* (anal ulcer) of the child.

"भैषज्य[३९] पूर्वमुद्दिष्टं नराणां यज्ज्वरादिषु ।
कार्यं तदेव बालानां मात्रा त्वस्य[४०] कनीयसी" ॥५०॥
(भैषज्यरत्नावली : बालरोगाधिकार : ३६)

*Dose of Medicines for Child*

Earlier, various recipes have been described for the treatment of diseases like fever of human beings. Same recipes should be used for the treatment of fever, etc., of the child. These recipes should, however, be administered in a smaller dose.

'प्रथमे मासि जातस्य[४१] शिशोर्भेषजरक्तिका ।
अवलेह्या तु कर्त्तव्या मधुक्षीरसिताघृतैः ॥५१॥
एकैकां वर्धयेत्तावद्यावत्संवत्सरो भवेत् ।
तदूर्ध्वं माषवृद्धिः स्याद्यावत्षोडशवत्सराः'[४२] ॥५२॥
(योगरत्नाकर : बालरोगचिकित्सा : पृष्ठ ४३९)

During the first month of the new-born child, medicines should be administered in a dose of one *ratti*. These medicines should be mixed with honey, milk and sugar, made to a linctus-form and given to the child to lick. Thereafter, every month, the dose should be increased by one *ratti* per month till he becomes one year old. Thereafter, the dose should be increased by one *māṣa* (per year) till he becomes 16 years of age.

"हरिद्राद्वययष्ट्याह्वसिंहीशक्रयवैः कृतः ।
शिशोर्ज्वरातिसारघ्नः[४३] कषायः स्तन्यदोषजित्" ॥५३॥
(भैषज्यरत्नावली : बालरोगाधिकार : ३७)

*Recipe*

The decoction of *haridrā, dāru haridrā, yaṣṭimadhu, siṃhī* and *indrayava* cures fever and diarrhoea in a child. It also cures diseases caused by the intake of polluted milk.

लाजांजनसितावांशीमधुकैः सूक्ष्मचूर्णितैः ।
बालस्य देयो मधुना लेहः[४४] सर्वज्वरापहः ॥५४॥

*Recipe for Fever*

Intake of the fine powder of *lājā, añjana*, sugar, *vaṃśalocana* and *yaṣṭimadhu* mixed with honey (in the form of a linctus) cures all types of fever in the child.

शर्करा क्षौद्रसंयुक्ता तिक्ता लीढा ज्वरं जयेत् ॥५५॥

Powder of *tiktā* should be mixed with sugar and honey. In the form of a linctus, this potion should be given to the child which cures fever.

"घनकृष्णारुणाशृङ्गीचूर्णं क्षौद्रेण संयुतम् ।
शिशोर्ज्वरातिसारघ्नं कासश्वासवमीहरम्" ॥५६॥
॥ बालचातुर्भद्रिका[४५] ॥
(भैषज्यरत्नावली : बालरोगाधिकार : ४०)

***Bāla Cāturbhadrikā***

Administration of the powder of *mustā, pippalī, aruṇā* (*ativiṣā*) and *śṛṅgī* mixed with honey cures fever, diarrhoea, cough, asthma and vomiting of the child.

"मुस्तकूष्माण्डबीजानि[४६] भद्रदारुकलिङ्गकान् ।
पिष्ट्वा तोयेन लेपोयं[४७] शोफघ्नः परमः शिशोः" ॥५७॥
(योगरत्नाकर : बालरोगचिकित्सा : पृष्ठ ४४५)

*Recipe for Oedema*

*Mustā*, seeds of *kuṣmāṇḍa, bhadradāru* and *kaliṅgaka* should be made to a paste by triturating with water. Its external use cures oedema of the child.

"धातकीबिल्वधान्यकलोध्रेन्द्रयवबालकैः[४८] ।
लेहः क्षौद्रेण बालानां ज्वरातीसारवान्तिजित् ॥५८॥
॥ धातक्यादिचूर्णम् ॥

***Dhātakyādi Cūrṇa***

The powder of *dhātakī, bilva, dhānyaka, lodhra, indrayava* and *hrībera* should be made to a linctus by mixing with honey and given to the child which cures his fever, diarrhoea and vomiting.

रजनी दारु सरलं श्रेयसी बृहतीद्वयम् ।
पृश्निपर्णी शताह्वा च लीढं माक्षिकसर्पिषा ॥५९॥
ग्रहणीदीपनं हन्ति मारुतार्त्तिं सकामलाम् ।
ज्वरातिसारपाण्डुघ्नं बालानां सर्वकासनुत्[४९] ।
(भैषज्यरत्नावली : बालरोगधिकार : ४१-४३)
बालस्य सर्वरोगेषु पूजितं बलवर्णदम् ॥६०॥

***Recipes***

*Haridrā, devadāru, sarala, śreyasī, bṛhatī, kaṇṭakārī, pṛśniparṇī* and *śatāhvā* should be made to a linctus by adding honey and ghee. Administration of this potion stimulates the functioning of *grahaṇī* (duodenum) and it cures diseases caused by *vāyu*, jaundice, fever, diarrhoea, anemia and all types of cough of children. It is useful in all the children-diseases and it promotes strength as well as complexion.

'हिंगुशुण्ठी[५०] कणा पथ्या निशा पंचामृतामृतम् ।
सर्वबालामयान् हन्ति पाचनं दीपनं परम्' ॥६१॥

Intake of *hiṅgu, śuṇṭhī, pippalī, harītakī, haridrā, pañcāmṛta* (cow's ghee, curd prepared of cow's milk, cow's milk, honey and sugar taken together) and *amṛta* (*drākṣā*) cures all children diseases. It is carminative and digestive stimulant.

"मिसीकृष्णाञ्जनं लाजा शृङ्गीमरिचमाक्षिकैः ।
लेहः शिशोर्विधातव्यश्छर्दिकासज्वरापहः ॥६२॥

Powder of *misī, pippalī, añjana* (*dārvī rasāñjana*), *lājā, śṛṅgī* and *marica* should be mixed with honey and made to a linctus. Administration of this potion cures vomiting, cough and fever in a child.

शृङ्गीं समुस्तातिविषां विचूर्ण्य
लेहं विदध्यात् मधुना शिशूनाम्।
कासज्वरछर्दिभिरर्दितानां
समाक्षिकां चातिविषामथैकाम् ॥६३॥

Powder of *śṛṅgī, mustā* and *ativiṣā* should be mixed with honey and made to a linctus. It cures cough, fever and vomiting of the child. Even *ativiṣā* alone taken along with honey cures these ailments.

पीतं पीतं वमेद्यस्तु स्तन्यं तं मधुसर्पिषा ।
द्विवार्त्ताकीफलरसं पञ्चकोलञ्च लेहयेत् ॥६४॥

*Recipes for Vomiting*

If the child gets vomiting while taking breast-milk, he should be given the fruit juice of *bṛhatī* and *kaṇṭakārī* or the powders of *pippalī, pippalīmūla, cavya, citraka* and *śuṇṭhī* along with honey and ghee.

आम्रास्थिलाजसिन्धूत्थैर्लेहः क्षौद्रेण च्छर्दिनुत् ॥६५॥

Intake of the powder of *āmrāsthi* (pulp inside the seed of mango), *lājā* and *saindhava* along with honey cures vomiting of the child.

पिप्पलीमरिचानां तु चूर्णं समधुशर्करम्"[१] ।
रसेन मातुलुङ्गस्य हिक्काच्छर्दिनिवारणम्" ॥६६॥
(भैषज्यरत्नावली : बालरोगाधिकार : ४४-४८)

Powder of *pippalī* and *marica* should be mixed with honey and sugar. Intake of this potion along with the juice of *mātuluṅga* cures hiccup, and vomiting of the child.

"व्याघ्रीकुसुमसंजातकेसरैरवलेहिका ।
पञ्चापि"[२] चिरसंजातः शिशोः कासान् व्यपोहति ॥६७॥

***Recipes for Cough***

Stamens of the flowers of *kaṇṭakārī* should be made to a paste (by triturating with honey). Intake of this cures five varieties of cough of a child even if these ailments have become chronic.

मुस्तकातिविषावासाकणाशृङ्गीरसं लिहन् ।
मुच्यते मधुना बालः कासैः पंचभिरेव"[13] च"[14]" ॥६८॥

(योगरत्नाकर : बालरोगचिकित्सा : पृष्ठ ४४२)

The decoction of *mustā, ativiṣā, vāsā, pippalī* and *śṛṅgī* should be added with honey and made to a linctus form. Intake of this cures five varieties of cough in the child.

"तुगा च क्षौद्रसंयुक्ता"[15] कासश्वासहरा शिशोः" ॥६९॥

(योगरत्नाकर : बालरोगचिकित्सा : पृष्ठ ४४३)

Intake of *vaṃśa locana* mixed with honey cures cough and asthma of the child.

"पेटीपाठामूलाज्जम्ब्वाः सहकारवल्कलकल्कः ।
इत्येकशश्च पिण्डो विधृतो हृन्नाभिताल्वादौ ।
छर्द्यतिसारजं वेगं प्रबलं धत्ते तदेव च नियमेन" ॥७०॥

(भैषज्यरत्नावली : बालरोगाधिकार : ४९)

Roots of *peṭi* (?) and *pāṭhā*, and barks of *jambū* and *āmra* should be made to a paste and tied in a cloth into a bolus form. Placing this on the cardiac region, umbilicus and *tālu* (anterior fontanel) cures the acute attacks of vomiting and diarrhoea of the child.

"बिल्वञ्च पुष्पाणि च धातकीनां
जलं सलोध्रं गजपिप्पली च ।
क्वाथावलेहौ मधुना विमिश्रौ
बालेषु योज्यावतिसारितेषु" ॥७१॥

(भैषज्यरत्नावली : बालरोगाधिकार : ५६)

***Recipes for Diarrhoea***

The decoction or linctus of *bilva, dhātakī* flower, *hrībera, lodhra* and *gaja pippalī* should be mixed with honey and given to the child which cures diarrhoea.

"समङ्गाधातकीलोध्रशारिवाभिः शृतं जलम् ।
दुर्द्धरेऽपि शिशोर्देयमतीसारे समाक्षिकम् ॥७२॥

The decoction of *samaṅgā, dhātakī, lodhra* and *śārivā* should be mixed with honey and given to the child which cures even acute form of diarrhoea.

'नागरातिविषामुस्तबालकेन्द्रयवैः[५६] शृतम् ।
कुमारं पाययेत्प्रातः सर्वातीसारनाशनम्" ॥७३॥
(भैषज्यरत्नावली : बालरोगाधिकार : ५९-६०)

Intake of the decoction of *śuṇṭhī, ativiṣā, mustā, hrībera* and *indrayava* in the morning cures all types of diarrhoea in the child.

"समङ्गाधातकी[५७] पद्मवयस्थाकच्छुरा तथा ।
पिष्टैरेतैयवागूः स्याद्रक्तातीसारनाशिनी"[५८] ॥७४॥
(भैषज्यरत्नावली : बालरोगाधिकार : ६३)

Gruel prepared with the paste of *samaṅgā, dhātakī, padma, vayasthā* and *kacchurā* cures *raktātisāra* (diarrhoea with blood in the stool) of the child.

सितासर्जरसं[५९] सर्पिर्लेहोऽतीसारनाशनः ।
धात्रीमरिचबिल्वं वा सदध्ना सह मिश्रितम् ॥७५॥

Intake of the linctus prepared of sugar, *sarja rasa* and ghee cures diarrhoea of the child.

Intake of *dhātrī, marica* and *bilva* along with curd cures diarrhoea of a child.

क्षीरादस्य शिशोः कासं शुष्कं दृष्ट्वा सदारुणम् ।
माषयूषं पिबेद्धात्रीपिप्पलीघृतभर्जितम् ॥७६॥

*Recipe for Dry Cough*

If the child, who is *kṣīrāda* (who exclusively depends upon breast milk for nourishment), suffers from dry cough, then the mother (or wet nurse) should be given the soup of *māṣa*. She should also be given *pippalī* fried by adding ghee.

रामठाघ्राणतो हन्ति सर्वहिक्कां सदुस्तराम् ॥७७॥

*Recipe for Hiccup*

Inhalation of the powder of *rāmaṭha* (*hiṅgu*) cures serious type of hiccup of the child.

मूत्रग्रहे तु बलानां चटकस्य च विट् ध्रुवम् ॥७८॥

*Recipe for Anuria*

If there is suppression of urination in a child, then the stool of *caṭaka* (sparrow) should be made to a paste and applied over the region of urinary bladder. It certainly causes urination.

तत्रस्थामभयां त्रिषु पुनः शुष्कां विचूर्णयेत् ।
विश्वं जातीफलं दीप्यं सिंधुं क्षिप्त्वा वटीकृता ॥७९॥
बदरास्थिनिभा भुक्ता चातीसारं निवारयेत् ।
भुक्तं च पाचयत्येव शिशूनां च न संशयः ॥८०॥

[The meaning of these verses is not clear].

बिल्वमूलकषायेण लाजाश्चैव सशर्कराः ।
आलोढ्य पाययेद्बालं छर्द्यतीसारनाशनम् ॥८१॥

*Recipes for Vomiting*

*Lājā* and sugar should be cooked with the decoction of the root of *bilva*. This should be given to child. It cures vomiting and diarrhoea.

"कल्कः प्रियङ्गुकोलास्थिमज्जमुस्तरसाञ्जनैः ।
क्षौद्रलीढः कुमारस्यच्छर्दितृष्णातिसारनुत् ॥८२॥

The paste of *priyangu*, seed pulp of *kola, mustā* and *rasāñjana* should be mixed with honey and given to the child. It cures vomiting, morbid thirst and diarrhoea.

मोचरसः समङ्गा च धातकी पद्मकेशरम् ।
पिष्टैरेतैर्यवागुः स्याद्रक्तातीसारनाशिनी ॥८३॥

Gruel prepared with the paste of *mocarasa, samangā, dhātakī* and stamens of lotus cures *raktātisāra* (diarrhoea associated with bleeding) of the child.

लेहस्तैलसिताक्षौद्रतिलयष्ट्याह्वकल्कितः ।
बालस्य रुंध्यान्नियतं[६०] रक्तस्रावं प्रवाहिकाम् ॥८४॥

*Recipes for Dysentery and Sprue*

Sessame seeds and *yaṣṭimadhu* should be made to a paste, and to this oil, sugar and honey should be added. Administration of this linctus certainly cures dysentery associated with bleeding.

लाजाः[६१] सयष्टीमधुकं शर्कराक्षौद्रमेव च ।
तण्डुलोदकसंमिश्रं क्षिप्रं हन्ति प्रवाहिकाम् ॥८५॥

*Lājā, yaṣṭimadhu*, sugar and honey should be mixed with rice-wash (*taṇḍulodaka*) and given to the child. It instantaneously cures dysentery.

अंकोठमूलमथवा तण्डुलसलिलेन कुटजमूलं वा ।
पीतं हन्त्यतिसारं ग्रहणीरोगञ्च[६२] दुर्वारम्" ॥८६॥

(भैषज्यरत्नावली : बालरोगाधिकार : ६२-६६)

Root of *ankoṭha* or *kuṭaja* should be triturated by adding rice-wash and given to child. It cures obstinate type of diarrhoea and *grahaṇī* (sprue).

"सितजीरकसर्जचूर्णं बिल्वदलोत्थाद्विमिश्रितं[६३] पीतम् ।
हन्त्याशु[६४] रक्तशूलं गुडसहितं श्वेतसर्जो वा" ॥८७॥

(भैषज्यरत्नावली : बालरोगाधिकार : ५८)

Intake of *śveta jīraka* and *sarja* powder along with the juice of *bilva* leaf instantaneously cures dysentery associated with bleeding and colic pain. In this condition, the powder of the white variety of *sarja rasa* along with jaggery is also useful.

"मरिचमहौषधकुटजं द्विगुणीकृतमुत्तरोत्तरं क्रमशः ।
गुडतक्रयुक्तमेतद् ग्रहणीरोगं निहन्त्याशु[६५] ॥८८॥

One part of *marica*, two parts of *śuṇṭhī* and four parts of *kuṭaja* should be added with jaggery and butter-milk. Intake of this cures *grahaṇī* (sprue).

बिल्वशक्राम्बुमोचाब्दसिद्धमाजं पयः शिशोः[६६] ।
सामां[६७] सरक्तां ग्रहणीं पीतं[६८] हन्यात् त्रिरात्रतः ।
तद्वदजाक्षीरसमो जम्बुत्वगुद्भवो रसः" ॥८९॥

(भैषज्यरत्नावली : बालरोगाधिकार : ६७-६९)

*Bilva, indrayava, hrībera, mocarasa* and *mustā* should be cooked in goat's milk. Intake of this medicated milk cures *grahaṇī* (sprue) associated with mucus and blood in three nights.

Similarly, goat's milk boiled with the bark of *jambū* cures sprue.

"गुदपाके तु बालानां पित्तघ्नीं कारयेत् क्रियाम् ।
रसाञ्जनं विशेषेण पानालेपनयोर्हितम्" ॥९०॥

(भैषज्यरत्नावली : बालरोगाधिकार : ७२)

***Recipe for Inflammed Anus***

In the anal inflammation of the child, the physician should administer therapies for the alleviation of *pitta*. *Rasāñjana* is specially useful for internal as well as external use.

(मूत्रग्रहे कणादिलेहः)

"कणोषणसिताक्षौद्रसूक्ष्मैलासैन्धवैः कृतः ।
मूत्रग्रहे प्रयोक्तव्यः शिशूनां लेह उत्तमः ॥९१॥

*Kaṇādi Leha for Anuria*

A linctus should be prepared of *pippalī, marica*, sugar, honey, *sūkṣmailā* and *saindhava* and administered to the child for curing strangury (obstruction) to the passage of urine. It is an excellent recipe.

(आनाहशूलचिकित्सा)

घृतेन सिन्धुविश्वैलाहिङ्गुभार्ङ्गीरजो लिहन् ।
आनाहं वातिकं शूलं जयेत्तोयेन वा शिशुः ॥९२॥

*Recipe for Flatulence*

Intake of the powder of *saindhava, śuṇṭhī, elā, hiṅgu* and *bhārṅgī* along with either ghee or water cures flatulence and colic pain caused by aggravated *vāyu* in a child.

(तालुपातचिकित्सा)

हरीतकीवचाकुष्ठकल्कं माक्षिकसंयुतम् ।
पीत्वा कुमारः स्तन्येन मुच्यते तालुपातनात् ॥९३॥

*Recipe for Tālupāta*

If the child takes the paste of *harītakī, vacā, kuṣṭha* and honey along with breast-milk, then he becomes free from *tālupāta* (depression of the palate and the anterior fontanel).

(मुखपाकचिकित्सा)

मुखपाके तु बालानां साम्रसारमयोरजः ।
गैरिकं क्षौद्रसंयुक्तं भेषजं सरसाञ्जनम् ॥९४॥

***Recipe for Stomatitis***

Application of the paste of *āmrasāra* (pulp of the mango-seed), *lauha bhasma, gairika bhasma,* honey and *rasāñjana* cures stomatitis of children.

अश्वत्थत्वग्दलक्षौद्रैर्मुखपाके प्रलेपनम् ।
दार्वीयष्ट्यभयाजातीपत्रक्षौद्रैस्तथाऽपरम्[६९] ॥९५॥

The powder of the leaves and bark of *aśvattha* should be made to a paste by adding honey. Application of this paste in the mouth cures stomatitis. Similarly, the application of the paste of *dārvī, yaṣṭimadhu, abhayā* and the leaf of *jātī* cures stomatitis in the child.

सह जम्बीररसेन स्नुग्दलरसघर्षणं सद्यः ।
कृतमुपहन्ति हि पाकं मुखजं बालस्य वाश्वेव ॥९६॥

Paste should be prepared of the leaves of *snuhī* by triturating with the juice of *jambīra*. Rubbing this paste in the mouth of the child instantaneously cures stomatitis.

लावतित्तिरिवल्लूररजः पुष्परसान्वितम् ।
द्रुतं करोति बालानां दन्तं केशरवन्मुखम् ॥९७॥

***Recipes for Teething Trouble***

Dried meat of *lāva* and *tittiri* should be made to a powder. To this, honey should be added and made to a paste. Its application helps in teething and promotes the complexion of the face.

दन्तोद्भवोत्थरोगेषु[७०] न बालमभिमन्त्रयेत् ।
स्वयमेवोपशाम्यन्ति जातदन्तस्य ते गदाः" ।

(भैषज्यरत्नावली : बालरोगाधिकार : ७७-८४)

For teething trouble of children, one should avoid drugging the child (in excess) because when teeth are out, those diseases automatically subside.

सदन्तो यस्तु जायेत दन्तो वा प्रथमोत्तराः ।
कुर्युस्तस्य कृते शान्ति बालस्याऽपि द्विजातयः ।
दद्यात्सदक्षिणां बाल[७१] नैगमेषं प्रपूजयेत् ॥९९॥

If a child is born with teeth and when the first tooth appears, benedictory rituals should be performed, offerings should be made to the brahmins and prayer should be offered to the evil spirit Naigameṣa.

"पञ्चमूलीकषायेण सघृतेन पयः शृतम् ।
सशृङ्गवेरं सगुडं शीतं 'हिक्कार्दितः[७२] पिबेत् ॥१००॥

*Recipe for Hiccup*

Intake of the milk boiled with the decoction of the roots of *bilva, śyonāka, gambhārī, pāṭalī* and *gaṇikārikā*, and ghee cures hiccup in the child. It should be added with the juice of *ārdraka* and jaggery, and cooled before administration.

सुवर्णगैरिकस्यापि चूर्णानि मधुना सह ।
लीढ्वा सुखमवाप्नोति क्षिप्रं' हिक्कार्दितः शिशुः ॥१०१॥

Paste should be prepared of *suvarṇa bhasma* and *gairika* by adding honey. Intake of this paste gives relief to the child suffering from hiccup instantaneously.

चित्रकं शृङ्गवेरं च तथा[७३] दन्ती गवाक्ष्यपि ।
चूर्णं कृत्वा तु सर्वेषां सुखोष्णेनाम्बुना पिबेत् ।
श्वासं कासमथो हिक्कां कुमाराणां प्रणाशयेत्[७४] ॥१०२॥

*Citraka, śuṇṭhī, dantī* and *gavākṣī* should be made to a powder. Intake of this powder along with warm water cures asthma, cough and hiccup of a child.

(कासश्वासचिकित्सा)

द्राक्षायासाभयाकृष्णाचूर्णं सक्षौद्रसर्पिषा ।
लीढं श्वासं निहन्त्याशु कासञ्च तमकं तथा ॥१०३॥

*Recipes for Cough and Asthma*

*Drākṣā, yavāsā, harītakī* and *pippalī* should be made to a powder. To this, honey and ghee should be added and made to a paste. Administration of this portion instantaneously cures cough and *tamaka* type of asthma in a child.

(पुष्करादिचूर्णम)

'पुष्करातिं'[७५] विषाशृङ्गीमागधीधन्वयासकैः[७६] ।
चूर्णं तु मधुना लीढं शिशुनां पञ्चकासनुत्' ॥१०४॥

*Puṣkarādi Cūrṇa*

The powder of *puṣkara mūla, ativiṣā, śṛṅgi, pippalī* and *dhanvayāsaka* should be added with honey and given to the child. It cures five varieties of *kāsa* (bronchitis).

(तृष्णायां दाडिमादिचूर्णम्)

दाडिमस्य च बीजानि जीरकं नागकेशरम् ।
चूर्णितं शर्कराक्षौद्रलीढं तृष्णाविनाशनम् ॥१०५॥

*Recipes for Morbid Thirst*

*Dāḍimādi Cūrṇa*

Seeds of *dāḍima, jīrā* and *nāgakeśara* should be made to a powder and added with sugar and honey. Administration of this paste cures morbid thirst in a child.

मायूरपक्षभस्मव्युषितजल[७७] तेन[७८] भावितं पेयम् ।
तृष्णाघ्नं वटकाष्ठभस्मजल[७९] वक्त्रशोषहृद्वक्त्रे[८०] ॥१०६॥

Ash of peacock-feather should be diluted with water. Intake of this cures morbid thirst in a child. Similarly, the ash of the burnt banyan wood should be mixed with water and given to the child for curing morbid thirst.

(नेत्ररोगचिकित्सा)

पिष्टैश्छागेन पयसा दार्वीमुस्तकगैरिकैः ।
बहिरालेपनं शस्तं शिशोर्नेत्रामयापहम्[81] ॥१०७॥

*Recipes for Eye Diseases*

*Dārvī, mustā* and *gairika* should be made to a paste by triturating with goat's milk. Its external application cures eye diseases of the child.

मनःशिला शङ्खनाभिः पिप्पल्योऽथ रसाञ्जनम् ।
वर्त्तिः क्षौद्रेण संयुक्ता बाले सर्वाक्षिरोगनुत् ॥१०८॥

A *varti* (elongated pill) should be prepared of *manaḥśilā, śaṅkha nābhi, pippalī* and *rasāñjana*. This *varti* should be rubbed with honey and the paste, thus prepared, should be applied over the eyelids as collyrium. It cures all eye diseases of the child.

मातृस्तन्यकटुस्नेहकाञ्जिकैर्भावितो जयेत् ।
स्वेदाद्दीपशिखातप्तो नेत्रामयमलक्तकः ॥१०९॥

*Alaktaka* (cotton smeared with lac) should be soaked in mother's milk, mustard oil and *kāñjī* (vinegar) and made warm by exposing to the flame of an oil lamp. Fomentation with this cures eye diseases of a child.

(कुकूणके आश्च्योतनम्)

शुण्ठीभृङ्गनिशाकल्कः पुटपाकः[82] ससैन्धवः ।
कुकूणकेऽक्षिरोगेषु भद्रमाश्च्योतनं[83] हितम् ॥११०॥

The paste of *śuṇṭhī, bhṛṅgarāja* and *haridrā* should be cooked by *puṭapāka* method. The juice of this paste should then be sprinkled over the eyes. It cures *kukūṇaka* (ophthalmia) and other eye diseases of the child.

कृमिघ्नालशिलादार्वीलाक्षाचन्दनगैरिकैः[८५] ।
चूर्णाञ्जनं कुकूणाक्षे[८५] शिशूनां पोतकीषु च ॥१११॥

The powder of *viḍaṅga, haritāla, manaḥśilā, dārvī, lākṣā, candana* and *gairika* should be used as collyrium which cures *kukūṇaka* (ophthalmia) and *potakī* (trachoma) in a child.

सुदर्शनामूलचूर्णादञ्जनं स्यात्कुकूणके ॥११२॥

Application of the collyrium with the help of the powder of the root of *sudarśanā* cures *kukūṇaka* (ophthalmia) in the child.

(सिध्मादिचिकित्सा)
गृहधूमनिशाकुष्ठराजिकेन्द्रयवैः शिशोः ।
लेपस्तक्रेण हन्त्याशु सिध्मपामाविचर्चिकाः ॥११३॥

### Recipe for Leucoderma, etc.

*Gṛha dhūma* (house-shoot), *haridrā, kuṣṭha, rājikā* and *indrayava* should be made to a paste by triturating with butter-milk. Its external application cures leucoderma, scabies and eczema in the child.

पादकल्केऽश्वगन्धायाः क्षीरे दशगुणे पचेत् ।
घृतं पेयं कुमाराणां पुष्टिकृद् बलवर्धनम् ॥११४॥
॥ अश्वगन्धाघृतम् ॥

### Aśvagandhā Ghṛta

Ghee (one part) should be cooked with the paste of *aśvagandhā* ($^1/_4$th part) and milk (10 parts). Intake of this medicated ghee promotes nourishment and strength of the child.

चाङ्गेरीस्वरसे सर्पिश्छागक्षीरसमें[६] पचेत् ।
कपित्थव्योषसिन्धूत्थसमङ्गोत्पलबालकैः ॥११५॥
सबिल्वधातकीमोचैः सिद्धं सर्वातिसारनुत् ।
ग्रहणीं दुस्तरां हन्ति बालानान्तु विशेषतः ॥११६॥
॥ बालचाङ्गेरीघृतम् ॥

*Bāla Cāngerī Ghṛta*

Ghee (one part), juice of *cāngerī* (one part) and goat's milk (one part) should be cooked by adding the paste of *kapittha, śuṇṭhī, pippalī, marica, saindhava, samangā, utpala, hrībera, bilva, dhātakī* and *mocarasa*. This medicated ghee cures all types of diarrhoea and serious type of *grahaṇī* (sprue) specially of children.

शंखपुष्पी वचा ब्राह्मी कुष्ठं त्रिफलया सह ।
द्राक्षा सशर्करा शुण्ठी जीवन्ती जीवकं[८७] बला ॥११७॥
शटी दुरालभा बिल्वं दाडिमः सुरसः स्थिरा ।
मुस्तं पुष्करमूलञ्च सूक्ष्मैला गजपिप्पली ॥११८॥
एषां कर्षसमैर्भागैर्घृतंप्रस्थं विपाचयेत् ।
कषाये कण्टकार्याश्च क्षीरे तस्माच्चतुर्गुणे ॥११९॥
एतत्कुमारकल्याणं घृतरत्नं सुखप्रदम् ।
बलवर्णकरं धन्यं पुष्ट्यग्निबलवर्द्धनम् ॥१२०॥
छायासर्वग्रहालक्ष्मीकृमिदन्तगदापहम् ।
सर्वबालामयहरं दन्तोद्भेदं विशेषतः ॥१२१॥
॥ कुमारकल्याणघृतम्[८८] ॥

*Kumāra Kalyāṇa Ghṛta*

One *prastha* of ghee should be cooked by adding four *prasthas* of the decoction of *kaṇṭakārī*, four *prasthas* of milk, the paste of one *karṣa* of the each of *śankhapuṣpī, vacā, brāhmī, kuṣṭha, harītakī, bibhītaka, āmalakī, drākṣā*, sugar, *śuṇṭhī, jīvantī, jīvaka, balā, śaṭī, durālabhā, bilva, dāḍima, surasa, sthirā, mustā, puṣkaramūla, sūkṣmailā* and *gaja pippalī*. This excellent recipe of medicated ghee is called *Kumāra kalyāṇa ghṛta*. It promotes strength, complexion, nourishment and the power of digestion. It cures seizures by evil spirits, inauspiciousness, *kṛmidanta* (carries teeth) and all the children diseases, specially those appearing during the teething period.

वचा कुष्ठं तथा ब्राह्मी सिद्धार्थकमथापि च ।
शारिवा सैन्धवञ्चैव पिप्पली घृतमष्टकम्[८९] ॥१२२॥
मेध्यं घृतमिदं सिद्धं पातव्यञ्च दिने दिने ।
दृढस्मृतिः क्षिप्रमेधाः कुमारो बुद्धिमान् भवेत् ॥१२३॥
'न[९०] पिशाचा न यक्षांसि[९१] न भूता न च मातरः ।
प्रभवन्ति कुमाराणां पिबतामष्टमङ्गलम्' ॥१२४॥
॥ अष्टमङ्गलघृतम्[९२]" ॥
(भैषज्यरत्नावली : बालरोगाधिकार : ८६-११०)

*Aṣṭamaṅgala Ghṛta*

Ghee cooked with *vacā, kuṣṭha, brāhmī, sarṣapa, sārivā, saindhava* and *pippalī* promotes strong memory, sharp intellect and wisdom of the child. This medicated ghee should be used everyday. The child using this medicated ghee does not get afflicted by *piśācas, yakṣas*, evil spirits and evil goddesses (*mātṛ*). This recipe is called *Aṣṭamaṅgala*.

"लाक्षारससमं सिद्धं तैलं मस्तु चतुर्गुणम् ।
रास्नाचन्दनकुष्ठाब्दवाजिगन्धानिशायुगैः[९३-९४] ॥१२५॥
शताह्वादारुयष्ट्याह्वमूर्वातिक्ताहरेणुभिः ।
बालानां ज्वररक्षोघ्नमभ्यङ्गाद्बलवर्णकृत् ॥१२६॥
॥ लाक्षादि[९५] तैलम्' ॥
(भैषज्यरत्नावली : बालरोगाधिकार : १२१-१२२)

*Lākṣādi Taila*

Oil (one part), one part of *lākṣā rasa* (aqueous extract of lac) and four parts of *mastu* (a type of butter-milk) should be cooked with the paste of *rāsnā, candana, kuṣṭha, mustā, aśvagandhā, haridrā, dāru haridrā, śatāhvā, devadāru, yaṣṭimadhu, mūrvā, tiktā* and *hareṇu*. This medicated oil cures fever and seizures by evil spirits. It should be used for massage. This promotes strength and complexion of the child.

भैषज्यं[१६] पूर्वमुद्दिष्टं महतां यज्ज्वरादिषु ।
कार्यं गदेषु बालानां तेषु दाहादिकं विना ॥१२७॥
त एव दोषा दूष्याश्च ज्वराद्याः व्याधयश्च ते ।
अतस्तदेव भैषज्यं मात्रा त्वस्य कनीयसी ॥१२८॥

*Line of Treatment of Other Diseases*

Recipes for fever, etc., of adults have already been described before. The same therapies should be used for the treatment of fever, etc., of children. But *dāha* (cauterisation) therapy etc., (earlier prescribed for adults) should not be administered to children.

In the fever, etc., of both the adults and children, the same *doṣas* and *dhātus* (tissue elements) get afflicted in the process of pathogenesis. Therefore, similar therapies are to be given to both the adults and children. However, in the case of children, these recipes should be administered in a smaller dose.

'विडङ्गफलमात्रं[१७] तु जातमात्रस्य भेषजम् ।
मासि मासि प्रयोक्तव्यं विडङ्गानां प्रवर्द्धनम् ॥१२९॥
अब्दादूर्ध्वं कुमारस्य दद्यात् कोलास्थिमात्रकम् ।
क्षीरान्नादशिशौ कोलमात्रा स्याद्बदरोपमा' ॥१३०॥

*Dosage for Children*

For children immediately after birth, the dose of medicines should be of the weight of a seed of *viḍaṅga*. As the child grows, every month, the dose should be increased by one *viḍaṅga* every month. After one year of age, the child should be given medicines in a dose of one *kolāsthi* (seed of jujube). In the *kṣīrānnāda* stage (when the child is given both milk and cereals for nourishment), the dose should be of the weight of the seed of *badara* (big size jujube).

"सह मुण्डितिकोदीच्यक्वाथस्नानं[९८] ग्रहापहम् ।
सप्तच्छदनिशाकुष्ठचन्दनश्चानुलेपनम्[९९] ॥१३१॥

***Bath and Unguentum***

Bath with the decoction of *muṇḍitikā* and *udīcya* cures seizures by evil spirits. Similarly, the unguentum of the paste of *saptacchada, haridrā, kuṣṭha* and *candana* cures these ailments.

सर्पत्वग्लशुनं मूर्वासर्षपारिष्टपल्लवाः ।
विडालविडजालोममेषशृङ्गं वचा मधु ।
धूपः शिशोर्ज्वरघ्नोऽयमशेषग्रहनाशनः" ॥१३२॥
(भैषज्यरत्नावली : बालरोगाधिकार : १२३-१२४)

***Recipes for Fumigation***

Fumigation with the slough of snake, garlic, *mūrvā*, mustard, leaves of *nimba*, cat-stool, goat-hair, sheep-horn, *vacā* and honey cures fever and all the ailments caused by the seizure of evil spirits in the child.

धूपश्चन्दनकुंकुमागुरुनखश्रीवासलाक्षारसैः ।
कुष्ठत्वग्वचसर्जमुस्तसरलैर्युक्तं रुक्फेण च[१००] ॥१३३॥
कर्पूरेण सहिङ्गुना मृगमदेनैकीकृतः[१०१] सर्पिषा ।
देयो निम्बरसोनसर्षपयवैर्भूतादिदोषापहः[१०२] ॥१३४॥

Fumigation with *candana, kuṅkuma, aguru, nakha, śrīvāsa, lākṣā, kuṣṭha, tvak, vacā, sarjarasa, mustā, sarala, samudra phena, karpūra, hiṅgu* and *kastūrī* mixed with ghee, *nimba, rasona, sarṣapa* and *yava* cures ailments caused by the seizure of evil spirits of the child.

बलिशान्तीष्टकर्माणि[१०३] कार्याणि ग्रहशान्तये ।
मन्त्रश्चायं प्रयोक्तव्यस्तत्रादौ सार्वकार्मिकः ॥१३५॥
ॐ[१०४] नमो भगवते गरुडाय त्र्यम्बकाय स्वस्त्यस्तु स्वाहा ॥१३६॥

ॐ फट्[१०५] वैनतेयाय नमः । ॐ ह्रौं ह्रीं क्षः ॥१३७॥

(भैषज्यरत्नावली : बालरोगाधिकार : १९२-१९३)

ॐ कारिणि[१०६] सुवर्णयक्षिणि रक्ष रक्ष बालकं स्वाहा ॥१३८॥

*Mantras for Propitiation of Grahas*

For the propitiation of *grahas* (evil spirits), one should make offerings (*bali*) and perform benedictory as well as auspicious rituals with the help of the *mantras* (sacred incantations) described in the line nos. 136-138 above.

बालदेहप्रमाणेन पुष्पमालान्तु सर्वतः ।
प्रगृह्य मुष्टिकाभक्तं[१०७] बलिर्देयस्तु शान्तिकः ॥१३९॥

(भैषज्यरत्नावली : बालरोगाधिकार : १९४-१९५)

A garland should be prepared of the size of the child. Inside an earthen plate, cooked rice should be kept surrounded by this garland. This should then be offered to the gods for endowing peace over the child.

(अथ रावणकृतं कुमारतन्त्रम्)

Text on Paediatrics by Rāvaṇa.

ॐ नारायणाय नमः ॥१४०॥

*Invocation*

*Oṃ namo Nārāyaṇāya.*

प्रथमे दिवसे मासे वर्षे वा गृह्णाति नन्दा नाम मातृका ।
तथा गृहीतमात्रेण[१०९] प्रथमं भवति ज्वरः । अशुभं शब्दं
मुञ्चति । सीत्काराश्च[११०] भवन्ति, स्तन्यं न गृह्णाति ॥१४१॥
बलिं तस्य प्रवक्ष्यामि येन सम्पद्यते शुभम् ॥१४२॥
नद्युभयतटमृत्तिकां गृहीत्वा पुत्तलिकां कृत्वा शुक्लौदनं,

शुक्लपुष्पं, शुक्लसप्तध्वजाः, सप्त प्रदीपाः, सप्त वटकाः, सप्त स्वस्तिकाः, सप्तशष्कुलिकाः, सप्त जम्बूलिकाः[१११], स्विन्नमाषाः, गंधं, ताम्बूलं, मत्स्यं, मांसं, सुराग्रभक्तञ्च—पूर्वस्यां दिशि चतुष्पथे मध्याह्ने बलिर्दातव्यः । ततोऽश्वत्थपत्रं[११२] कुम्भे[११३] निक्षिप्य[११४] शान्त्युदकेन स्नापयेत् । रसोन-सिद्धार्थकमेषशृङ्गनिम्बपत्रशिवनिर्माल्यैर्बालकं धूपयेत् । ॐ नमो रावणाय अमुकस्य[११५] व्याधिं हन हन मुञ्च मुञ्च ह्रीं फट् स्वाहा । 'एवं[११६] दिनत्रयं कारयेत् ततश्चतुर्थे दिवसे ब्राह्मणं भोजयेत् ॥१४३॥
ततः सम्पद्यते शुभम् ॥१४४॥

*Seizure by Nandā*

During the first day, first month or the first year, the child gets possessed by the *mātṛkā* (evil goddess) called Nanda. Immediately after the seizure the child suffers from fever, produces inauspicious sounds including whistling sound and does not take breast-milk.

Now the offerings (*bali*) to be sacrificed for curing the child and bestowing auspiciousness will be described.

A small idol should be prepared out of the mud collected from both the banks of a river. Along with this, white rice, white flower, seven white flags, seven oil lamps, seven *vaṭakas* (a type of food preparation), steamed *māṣa*, perfume (incense), betel leaf, fish and meat beginning with alcohol should be given as offering in the eastern side during mid-day in a cross-road. Then leaves of *aśvattha* should be immersed in a jar filled with water and with this, the child should be given bath. Then the child should be fumigated with the help of garlic, mustard, sheep-horn, leaves of *nimba* and *śiva nirmālya*. Then the sacred incantation (described in the text) should be recited. This ritual should be performed for three days. On the fourth day, brahmins should be fed with meals. Thus, the child becomes free from the seizure of Nandā.

द्वितीये दिवसे मासे वर्षे वा गृह्णाति सुनन्दा नाम मातृका । तया गृहीतमात्रेण प्रथमं भवति ज्वरः ।

चक्षुरुन्मीलयति, गात्रमुद्वेजयति, न शेते, क्रन्दति, स्तन्यं न गृह्णाति, आत्कारश्च भवति ॥१४५॥
बलिं तस्य प्रवक्ष्यामि येन सम्पद्यते शुभम् ॥१४६॥
तण्डुलहस्तमुष्टैकं गृहीत्वा दधिगुडघृतमिश्रितं शरावैकं, गन्धता[११७]म्बूलं, पीतपुष्पं पीतसप्तध्वजाश्चत्वारः प्रदीपाः दश- स्वस्तिकाः मत्स्यमांसं[११८] सुरातिलचूर्णं च पश्चिमायां[११९] दिशि चतुष्पथे बलिर्दातव्यः । दिनानि त्रीणि संध्यायां, ततः शान्त्युदकेन स्नापयेत् । शिवनिर्माल्यसिद्धार्थकमार्जाररोमोशीरबालकघृतैः धूपं दद्यात् । 'ॐ नमोनारायणाय[१२०] अमुकस्य व्याधिं हन[१२१] मुञ्च हूँ फट् स्वाहा ।' चतुर्थे दिवसे ब्राह्मणं भोजयेत् ॥१४७॥
ततः सम्पद्यते शुभम् ॥१४८॥

### *Seizure by Sunandā*

On the second day, second month or second year, the child gets possessed by the *mātṛkā* (evil goddess) called Sunandā. Immediately after the seizure, the child suffers from fever, keeps eyes opened, gets irritation of the body, does not get sleep, weeps, does not take milk and produces *ā* sound while crying.

Now the offerings (*bali*) to be sacrificed for curing the child and bestowing auspiciousness will be described.

Along with one fistful of rice, an earthen plate containing curd, jaggery and ghee, incense, betel leaf, yellow flower, seven flags prepared of yellow cloth, four oil-lamps, ten *svastikas* (a type of *yantra*), fish, meat, alcohol and sessame powder should be given as offering (*bali*) in a cross-road in the western direction for three days in the evening. Thereafter, the child should be bathed with *śāntyudaka* (peace-betowing water). Then he should be fumigated with *śiva nirmālya*, mustard, cat-hair, *uśīra, hrībera* and ghee. This offering should performed by reciting the sacred incantation "*Oṃ, namo Nārāyaṇāya, amukasya* (the name of the child is to be inserted here) *vyādhiṃ hana muñca huṃ phaṭ svāhā.*" On the fourth day, meals should be served to the *brāhmaṇas*. Thereafter, the child becomes free from the seizure.

तृतीये दिवसे मासे वर्षे वा गृह्णाति पूतना नाम मातृका, तया गृहीतमात्रेण प्रथमं भवति ज्वरः, गात्रमुद्वेजयति, स्तन्यं न गृह्णाति मुष्टिं बध्नाति क्रन्दति ऊर्ध्वं निरीक्षते ॥१४९॥ बलिं तस्य प्रवक्ष्यामि येन सम्पद्यते शुभम् ॥१५०॥ नद्युभयतटमृत्तिकां गृहीत्वा पुत्तलिकां कृत्वा रक्तचन्दनं, गंधं, ताम्बूलं, रक्तसप्तध्वजाः, सप्त प्रदीपाः, सप्त स्वस्तिकाः, पक्षिमांससुराग्रभक्तञ्च दक्षिणस्यां दिशि अपराह्ने चतुष्पथे बलिर्दातव्यः । शिवनिर्माल्यगुग्गुलुसर्षपनिम्बपत्रमेषशृङ्गैर्दिनत्रयं धूपयेत् । "ॐ नमो नारायणाय नमः । बालस्य व्याधिं हन मुञ्च त्रासं च स्वाहा" । चतुर्थे दिवसे ब्राह्मणं भोजयेत् ॥१५१॥ ततः सम्पद्यते शुभम् ॥१५२॥

*Seizure by Pūtanā*

On the third day, third month or third year, the child gets possessed by the *mātṛkā* (evil goddess) called Pūtana. Immediately after the seizure, the child gets fever, irritation in the body, does not take milk, clinches the fists, cries and looks upwards.

Now, the offerings (*bali*) to be sacrificed for curing the child and bestowing auspiciousness will be described.

An earthen statue should be prepared out of the mud collected from both the banks of a river. Along with this, red sandal-wood-paste, incense, betel leaf, seven red flags, seven oil lamps, seven *svastikas* (a type of *yantra*) and bird-meat beginning with alcohol should be offered in the southern direction, in a cross-road during the afternoon. The child should be fumigated with *śiva nirmālya, guggulu, sarṣapa,* leaf of *nimba* and sheep-horn for three days. This offering should be performed with the sacred incantation "*Oṃ namo Nārāyaṇāya namaḥ, bālasya vyādhiṃ hana muñca trāsañca svāhā*". On the fourth day, meals should be served to the *brāhmaṇas.* Thereafter, the child becomes free from the seizure.

चतुर्थे दिवसे मासे वर्षे वा यदा[२३] गृह्णाति मुखमुण्डिका नाम मातृका । तया गृहीतमात्रेण प्रथमं भवति ज्वरः ।

ग्रीवां नमयति चक्षुरुन्मीलयति,[१२४] स्तन्यं न गृह्णाति, रोदिति, स्वपिति, मुष्टिं बध्नाति ॥१५३॥
बलिं तस्य प्रवक्ष्यामि येन सम्पद्यते शुभम् ॥१५४॥
नद्युभयतटमृत्तिकां गृहीत्वा पुत्तलिकां निर्माय उत्पलपुष्पं, गन्धं, ताम्बूलं, शुक्लदशध्वजाः, चत्वारः प्रदीपाः, त्रयोदश स्वस्तिकाः, मत्स्यमांससुराग्रभक्तञ्च उत्तरस्यां दिशि अपराह्णे चतुष्पथे बलिर्दातव्यः । "ॐ नमो रावणाय हन२[१२५] मथ२ स्वाहा" । चतुर्थे दिवसे ब्राह्मणान् भोजयेत् ॥१५५॥
ततः सम्पद्यते शुभम् ॥१५६॥

*Seizure by Mukha Muṇḍikā*

On the fourth day, fourth month or fourth year, the child gets possessed by the *mātṛkā* (evil goddess) called Mukha muṇḍikā. Immediately after the seizure, the child gets fever, his neck gets bent, eyes remain opened, he does not take milk, cries, sleeps in excess and clinches his fists.

Now the offerings (*bali*) to be sacrificed for curing the child and bestowing auspiciousness will be described.

An earthen statue should be prepared out of the mud collected from both the banks of a river. Along with this, lotus flower, incense, betel leaf, ten white flags, four oil lamps, thirteen *svastikas* (a type of *yantra*), fish and meat beginning with alcohol should be offered in the northern direction, in a cross-road during the afternoon. This offering should be performed with the sacred incantation "*Oṃ namo Rāvaṇāya hana hana matha matha svāhā*". On the fourth day, meals should be served to the *brāhmaṇas*. Thereafter, the child becomes free from the seizure.

पञ्चमे दिवसे मासे वर्षे वा यदा गृह्णाति कटपूतना नाम मातृका । तया गृहीतमात्रेण प्रथमं भवति ज्वरः; गात्रमुद्वेजयति, स्तन्यं न गृह्णाति, मुष्टिं बध्नाति ॥१५७॥
बलिं तस्य प्रवक्ष्यामि येन सम्पद्यते शुभम् ॥१५८॥
कुम्भकारचक्रस्य मृत्तिकां गृहीत्वा पुत्तलिकां निर्माय[१२६]

गन्धं, ताम्बूलं, शुक्लौदनं, शुक्लपुष्पं, पञ्चध्वजाः, पंचप्रदीपाः[१२७], पञ्चवटकाः, ऐशान्यां दिशि बलिर्दातव्यः । शान्त्युदकेन स्नापयेत् । शिवनिर्माल्यसर्पनिर्मोकगुग्गुलुनिम्बपत्रबालकधृतैर्धूपं दद्यात् । "ॐ नमो नारायणाय[१२८] चूर्णय स्वाहा । चतुर्थे दिवसे ब्राह्मणान्[१२९] भोजयेत् ॥१५९॥
ततः सम्पद्यते शुभम् ॥१६०॥

*Seizure by Kaṭa Pūtanā*

On the fifth day, fifth month or fifth year, the child gets possessed by the *mātṛkā* (evil goddess) called Kaṭapūtanā. Immediately after the seizure, the child suffers from fever, gets irritation in the body, does not take milk and clinches fists.

Now the offerings (*bali*) to be sacrificed for curing the child and bestowing auspiciousness will be described.

An earthen statue should be made out of the mud from the potmakers wheel. Along with this, incense, betel-leaf, white rice, white flower, five flags, five oil-lamps, five *vaṭakas* (a type of food preparation) should be offered in the *aiśānya* (north-eastern) direction. The child should be given bath with *śāntyudaka* (auspicious water which bestows peace). Then he should be fumigated with *śivanirmālya*, slough of snake, *guggulu*, leaves of *nimba, hrībera* and ghee. This offering should be performed with the sacred incantation, "*Oṃ namo Nārāyaṇāya cūrṇaya svāhā.*" On the fourth day, meals should be served to the *brāhmaṇas*. Thereafter, the child becomes free from the seizure.

षष्ठे दिवसे मासे वर्षे वा गृह्णाति शुकनिका नाम मातृका । तया गृहीतमात्रेण प्रथमं भवति ज्वरः । गात्रभेदञ्च दर्शयति । दिवारात्रौ[१३०] उत्तानं भवति, उर्ध्वं निरीक्षते ॥१६१॥
बलिं तस्य प्रवक्ष्यामि येन सम्पद्यते शुभम् ॥१६२॥
पिष्टकेन पुत्तलिकां कृत्वा शुक्लपुष्पं[१३१], रक्तपुष्पं, पीतपुष्पं, गन्धताम्बूलं दशप्रदीपं[१३२], दशस्वस्तिकाः, दशवटकाः, क्षीरजम्बूतिलपिष्टकाः,[१३३] मस्त्यमांससुराः—आग्नेय्यां दिशि

ग्राम निष्क्रान्ते मध्याह्ने बलिर्दातव्यः । शान्त्युदकेन स्नापयेत् । शिवनिर्माल्यरसोनगुग्गुलुसर्पनिर्मोक-निम्बपत्रघृतैर्धूपं दद्यात् । "ॐ नमो नारायणाय[134] चूर्णय ३ हन ३ स्वाहा । चतुर्थे दिवसे ब्राह्मणं[135] भोजयेत् ॥१६३॥
ततः सम्पद्यते शुभम् ॥१६४॥

*Seizure by Śukanikā*

On the sixth day, sixth month or sixth year, the child gets possessed by the *matṛkā* (evil goddess) called Śakunikā. Immediately after the seizure, the child gets fever, his body appears cracked, he remains on the back all the day and night and he looks upwards.

Now the offerings (*bali*) to be sacrificed for curing the child and bestowing auspiciousness will be described.

A statue should be prepared with the paste of corn-flour. Along with this, white flower, red flower, yellow flower, incense, betel-leaf, ten oil-lamps, ten *svastikas* (a type of *yantra*), ten *vaṭakas* (a type of food preparation), milk, jamun, sessame paste, fish, meat and alcohol should be offered in the *āgneya* (south-east) direction at the end of the village and during the mid day. The child should be given bath in *śantyudaka* (auspicious water). The child should be fumigated with *śiva nirmālya*, garlic, *guggulu*, slough of the snake, leaf of *nimba* and ghee. This offering should be performed with the sacred incantation, "*Oṃ namo Nārāyaṇāya cūrṇaya cūrṇaya cūrṇaya, hana hana hana svāhā*". On the fourth day, meals should be offered to the *brāhmaṇas*. Thus, the child becomes free from seizure.

सप्तमे दिवसे मासे वर्षे वा यदा गृह्णाति शुष्करेवती नाम मातृका । तया गृहीतमात्रेण प्रथमं भवति ज्वरः । गात्रमुद्वेजयति, मुष्टिं बध्नाति, रोदिति ॥१६५॥
बलिं तस्य प्रवक्ष्यामि येन सम्पद्यते शुभम् ॥१६६॥
रक्तं पुष्पं, शुक्लपुष्पं, गन्धं, ताम्बूलं, रक्तौदनं, कृशराः त्रयोदशस्वस्तिकाः, (त्रयोदश शष्कुलिकाः[136]), जम्बुडिका[137], मत्स्यमांससुराः, त्रयोदशध्वजाः, पञ्चप्रदीपाः

पश्चिमदिग्भागे[१३८] ग्रामनिष्क्रामेऽपराह्ने[१३९] वृक्षमाश्रित्य[१४०] बलिं दद्यात्[१४१] । शान्त्युदकेन स्नानम्[१४२] । गुग्गुलुमेषशृङ्गसर्षपोशीरबालकघृतैर्धूपयेत्[१४३] । "ॐ नमो नारायणाय[१४४] दीप्ततेजसे हन २ मुञ्च २ स्वाहा" ।
चतुर्थदिवसे ब्राह्मणं[१४५] भोजयेत् ॥१६७॥
ततः सम्पद्यते शुभम् ॥१६८॥

*Seizure by Śuṣka Revatī*

On the seventh day, seventh month or seventh year, the child gets possessed by the *mātṛkā* (evil goddess) called Śuṣka Revatī. Immediately after the seizure, the child suffers from fever, his body gets irritated, he clinches fists and cries.

Now, the offerings (*bali*) to be sacrificed for curing the child and bestowing auspiciousness is being described.

Red flower, white flower, incense, betel-leaf, red rice, *kṛśarā* (a type of gruel), thirteen *svastikas* (a type of *yantra*), thirteen *śaṣkulikās* (a type of food preparation), jamun fruits, fish, meat, alcohol, thirteen flags and five oil lamps should be offered in the western direction at the exit of the village below a tree during the afternoon. The child should be given bath in the *śāntyudaka* (auspicious water). Thereafter, the child should be fumigated with *guggulu*, sheep-horn, mustard, *uśīra*, *hrībera* and ghee. The offering should be performed with the sacred incantation, *"Oṃ namo Nārāyaṇāya dīptatejase hana hana muñca muñca svāhā"*. On the fourth day, meals should be offered to the *brāhmaṇas*. Thereafter, the child becomes free from the seizure.

अष्टमे दिवसे मासे वर्षे वा यदा गृह्णाति गृहीनाम[१४६] मातृका । तया गृहीतमात्रेण प्रथमं भवति ज्वरः । गृध्रगन्धः पूतिगन्धश्च जायते, आहारं न गृह्णाति, उद्वेजयति गात्राणि ॥१६९॥
बलिं तस्य प्रवक्ष्यामि येन[१४७] सम्पद्यते शुभम् ॥१७०॥
रक्तपीतध्वजाश्चन्दनं, पुष्पं[१४८], शष्कुल्यः, पर्पटिकाः, मत्स्यमांसजम्बूडिकाः[१४९] सुराः प्रत्यूषे बलिर्देयः[१५०] प्रातरेव ।

"ॐ नमो रावणाय त्रैलोक्य-विद्रावणाय चतुर्दिशमोक्षणाय व्याधिं[१५१] हन हन मुञ्च[१५२] ३ ज्वल ३ हल ३ दह ३ ॐ हुं फट् स्वाहा ।" चतुर्थे दिवसे ब्राह्मण[१५३] भोजयेत् ॥१७४॥ ततः सम्पद्यते शुभम् ॥१७२॥

*Seizure by Gṛhī*

On the eighth day, eighth month or eighth year, the child gets possessed by the *mātṛkā* (evil goddess) called Gṛhī. Immediately after the seizure, the child suffers from fever, smell of the vulture and putrid smell emits from his body, the child does not take food and his body gets irritated.

Now, the offerings (*bali*) to be sacrificed for curing the child and bestowing auspiciousness will be described.

Flags of red and yellow colour, sandal-wood paste, flower, *śaṣkulīs* (a type of food preparation), *parpaṭikā* (another type of food preparation), fish, meat, *jambūḍikā* (fruit of jamun) and alcohol should be offered during early or late in the morning. This offering should be performed with the sacred incantation, "*Oṃ namo Rāvaṇāya, trailokyavidravaṇāya caturdiśamokṣaṇāya vyādhiṃ hana hana muñca muñca muñca jvala jvala jvala hala hala hala daha daha daha oṃ huṃ phaṭ svāhā*". On the fourth day, meals should be served to the *brāhmaṇas*. Thereafter, the child becomes free from the seizure.

नवमे दिवसे मासे वर्षे वा गृह्णति सूतिका नाम मातृका । तया गृहीतमात्रस्य[१५४] प्रथमं भवति ज्वरः । नित्यं छर्दिर्भवति,[१५५] गात्रभेदं दर्शयति मुष्टिं बध्नाति स्वापो[१५६] भवति ॥१७३॥

बलिं तस्य प्रवक्ष्यामि येन सम्पद्यते शुभम् ॥१७४॥

नद्युभयतटमृत्तिकां गृहीत्वा पुत्तलिकां कृत्वा[१५७] शुक्लवस्त्रेण वेष्टयेत् । शुक्लपुष्प[१५८], गन्धताम्बूलं, शुक्लत्रयोदशध्वजाः, त्रयोदश प्रदीपाः, त्रयोदशस्वस्तिकाः, त्रयोदशपुपलिकाः[१५९], मत्स्यमांससुराः, उत्तरदिग्विभागे ग्रामनिष्क्रामे[१६०] बलिं दापयेत् । शान्त्युदकेन स्नानम्[१६१] ।

गुग्गुलुनिम्बपत्रगोशृङ्गश्वेतसर्षपघृतैर्धूपं[१६२] दद्यात् । "ॐ नमो नारायणाय[१६३] चतुर्भुजाय हन हन मुञ्च ३ स्वाहा" ।
चतुर्थे दिवसे ब्राह्मणं भोजयेत् ॥१७५॥
ततः सम्पद्यते शुभम् ॥१७६॥

*Seizure by Sūtikā*

On the ninth day, ninth month or ninth year, the child gets possessed by the *mātṛkā* (evil goddess) called Sūtikā. Immediately after the seizure, the child suffers from fever. He vomits everyday, exhibits pain in the body, clinches the fists and always sleeps.

Now the offering (*bali*) to be sacrificed for curing the child and bestowing auspiciousness will be described.

A statue should be prepared of the mud collected from both the banks of a river. This should be wrapped with a white cloth. Along with this, white flower, incense, betel-leaf, thirteen white flags, thirteen oil-lamps, thirteen *svastikas* (a type of *yantra*), thirteen *pupalikās* (a type of food preparation), fish, meat and alcohol should be offered in the northern direction at the exit of the village. The child should be given bath with *śāntyudaka* (auspicious water). Then he should be fumigated with *guggulu*, leaf of *nimba*, cow's horn, white variety of mustard and ghee. The offering should be performed with the sacred incantation, "*Oṃ namo Nārāyaṇāya caturbhujāya, hana hana muñca muñca muñca svāhā*." On the fourth day, meals should be served to the *brāhmaṇas*. Then the child becomes free from the seizure.

दशमे दिवसे मासे वर्षे वा गृह्णाति नैर्ऋता[१६४] नाम मातृका । तया गृहीतमात्रेण प्रथमं भवति ज्वरः । गात्रमुद्वेजयति, रोदिति[१६५], मूत्रपुरीषं भवति ॥१७७॥
बलिं तस्य प्रवक्ष्यामि येन सम्पद्यते शुभम् ॥१७८॥
पारावारमृत्तिकां गृहीत्वा पुत्तलिकां निर्माय[१६६] गन्धताम्बूलं, रक्तपुष्पं, रक्तचन्दनं, पञ्चवर्णध्वजाः, पञ्चप्रदीपाः, पञ्चस्वस्तिकाः, पञ्चपूपलिका,[१६७] मत्स्यमांससुराः वायव्यां दिशि बलिं दद्यात् । काकविष्टागोमांसगोशृङ्गरसोनमार्जारलोमनिम्बपत्रघृतैर्धूपयेत् ।

"ॐ नमो नारायणाय[१६८] चूर्णित-हस्ताय मुञ्च २
स्वाहा । चतुर्थे दिवसे ब्राह्मणं[१६९] भोजयेत् ॥१७९॥
ततः सम्पद्यते[१७०] शुभम् ॥१७९॥

*Seizure by Nairṛtā*

On the tenth day, tenth month and tenth year, the child becomes possessed by the *mātṛkā* (evil goddess) called Nairṛtā. Immediately after the seizure, the child suffers from fever, gets irritation in the body, cries and voids urine and stool in excess.

Now the offering (*bali*) to be sacrificed for curing the child and bestowing auspiciousness will be described.

A statue should be prepared of the mud collected from a lake. Along with this, incense, betel-leaf, red flower, paste of red sandal wood, five red flags, five oil-lamps, five *svastikas* (a type of *yantra*), five *pūpalikās* (a type of food preparation), fish, meat and alcohol should be offered in the *vāyavya* (north-west) direction. The child should be fumigated with the crow-stool, beef, cow-horn, garlic, cat-hair, leaf of *nimba* and ghee. The offering should be performed with the sacred incantation, "*Oṃ namo Nārāyaṇāya cūrṇitahastāya muñca muñca svāha.*" On the fourth day, meals should be served to *brāhmaṇas*. Thereafter, the child gets cured of the seizure.

एकादशे दिवसे मासे वर्षे वा यदा[१७१] गृह्णाति
पिलिपिच्छिका[१७२] नाम मातृका, तया गृहीतमात्रेण
प्रथमं भवति ज्वरः, आहारं न गृह्णाति, उदध्र्वदृष्टिर्भवति,
आत्कारश्च गात्रभंगो भवति ॥१८०॥
बलिं तस्य प्रवक्ष्यामि येन सम्पद्यते शुभम् ॥१८१॥
पिष्टकपुत्तलिकां,[१७३] रक्तचन्दनाक्तां तस्या मुखं दुग्धेन
सिञ्चयेत् । पीतं पुष्पं, गन्धताम्बूलं, सप्तपीतध्वजाः,
सप्तप्रदीपाः, अष्टौ वटकाः, (अष्टौ शष्कुलिकाः[१७४]), अष्टौ
पूपिकाः, मस्त्यमांससुराः पूर्वस्यां दिशि बलिं दद्यात्[१७५] ।
शान्त्युदकेन स्नानम्[१७६] ।

शिवनिर्माल्यगुग्गुलुगोशृङ्गसर्पनिर्मोकघृतैर्धूपयेत् । "ॐ नमो नारायणाय[१७७] मुञ्च मुञ्च स्वाहा ।" चतुर्थे दिवसे ब्राह्मणं भोजयेत् । ततः स्वस्थो[१७८] भवति बालकः ॥१८२॥

(तेन सम्पद्यते शुभम्[१७९]) ॥१८३॥

*Seizure by Pilipicchikā*

On the eleventh day, eleventh month or eleventh year, the child gets possessed by the *mātṛkā* (evil goddess) called Pilipicchikā. Immediately after the seizure, the child suffers from fever, he does not take food, he looks upwards, he cries with the sound *'ā'* and gets pain in the body.

Now the offerings (*bali*) to be sacrificed for curing the child and bestowing auspiciousness will be described.

A statue prepared of the paste of rice should be smeared with the paste of red sandal-wood. Its face should be sprinkled with milk. Along with this, yellow flower, incense, betel-leaf, seven yellow flags, seven oil-lamps, eight *vaṭakas* (a type of food preparation), eight *śaṣkulikās* (another type of food preparation), eight cakes, fish, meat and alcohol should be offered in the eastern direction. The child should be given bath with *śāntyudaka* (auspicious water). Thereafter; he should be fumigated with *śiva nirmālya*, *guggulu*, cow's horn, slough of the snake and ghee. The offering should be performed with the sacred incantation, "*Oṃ namo Nārāyaṇāya muñca muñca svāhā.*" On the fourth day, meals should be served to the *brāhmaṇas*. Thereafter, the child becomes free from the seizure.

द्वादशे दिवसे मासे वर्षे वा यदा[१८०] गृह्णाति कामुका नाम मातृका, तया गृहीतमात्रेण प्रथमं भवति ज्वरः । विहस्याकारणं[१८१] वादयति, तर्जयति, गृह्णाति, क्रमति, निःश्वसिति, मुहुर्मुहुः छर्दयति, आहारं न करोति, कृशता भवति ॥१८४॥

बलिं तस्य प्रवक्ष्यामि येन[१८२] सम्पद्यते शुभम्[१८३] ॥१८५॥

क्षीरेण पुत्तलिकां कृत्वा गन्धताम्बूलं, शुक्लपुष्पं, शुक्लसप्तध्वजाः, (सप्तशष्कुलिका[१८४]), सप्तप्रदीपाः,

करम्भकेण[१८५] सर्वं[१८६] कर्मबलिं दद्यात् । शान्त्युदकेन स्नापयेत् शिवनिर्माल्यगुग्गुलुसर्षपघृतैर्धूपं[१८७] दद्यात्[१८८] । "ॐ नमो नारायणाय[१८९] मुञ्च मुञ्च हन हन स्वाहा" । चतुर्थे दिवसे ब्राह्मणं[१९०] भोजयेत् । ततः स्वस्थो भवति बालकः" ॥१८७॥

(भैषज्यरत्नावली : बालरोगाधिकार : १९७-२०८)

*Seizure by Kāmukā*

On the twelfth day, twelfth month or twelfth year, the child gets possessed by the *mātṛkā* (evil goddess) called Kāmukā. Immediately after the seizure, the child gets fever, he smiles without any cause, beats, makes fearful posture, clinches, moves, deeply breaths, frequently vomits, does not take food and becomes emaciated.

Now, the offerings (*bali*) to be sacrificed for curing the child and bestowing auspiciousness will be described.

A statue should be prepared of rice-paste and milk. Along with this, incense, betel-leaf, white flower, seven white flags, seven *śaṣkulikās*, seven oil-lamps and *karambha* (a type of food preparation, curd-rice) should be offered. The child should be given bath with *śāntyudaka* (auspicious water). He should be fumigated with *śiva nirmālya, guggulu, sarṣapa* and ghee. The offering should be performed with the sacred incantation, "*Oṃ namo Nārāyaṇāya muñca muñca hana hana svahā.*" On the fourth day, meals should be served to the *brāhmaṇas*. Thereafter, the child becomes cured of the seizure.

अथ भूतनिवारणमन्त्रानुच्यते ॥१८८॥

कंकणं वामहस्तेन शंखमन्येन धारयेत् ।
आत्मरक्षां ततः कृत्वा पूर्वद्वारे बलिं क्षिपेत् ।
विधायैवं ततो मंत्रान्[१९१] कुर्यान्निग्रहनुन्ग्रहम् ॥१८९॥
सुग्रीवप्रमुखैर्मंत्रैः सर्वभूतभयंकरम् ॥१९०॥

ॐ नमो भगवते रुद्राय चिलि[१९२] २ मिलि पशुपतिराज्ञापयति स्वाहा ॥१९१॥

एष बलिनिवेदनमंत्रः[१९३] ॥१९२॥

***Incantation for Dispelling Evil Spirits***

Now the sacred incantation for dispelling evil-spirits will be described.

In the left hand, one should wear *kankaṇa* (metallic bangle) and in the right hand he should carry *śankha* (conch-shell). After protecting himself (by sacred incantations), one should throw *bali* (sacred offerings) in the eastern gate. While doing so, he should recite sacred incantations to alleviate the effects of evil spirits. In this connection *sugrīva mantra*, etc., should be recited. All the evil spirits are afraid of these incantations. Offerings should be sacrificed with the sacred incantation, "*Oṃ namo bhagavate Rudrāya cili cili mili paśupatirājñāpayati svāhā.*"

ॐ नमश्चन्द्ररुद्राय कुरु २ मुरु २ भूत समये विष्वतर[१९४] स्वाहा । भूतगृहीतस्य शिर[१९५] आबंधः ॥१९३॥

The head of child seized with the evil spirit should be tied with the sacred incantation, "*Oṃ namaścandrarudrāya kuru kuru muru muru bhūtasamaye viṣvatara svāhā*".

ॐ नमः पशुपतये नानाभूताधिपतये ॐ नमो रुद्राय खट्वांगघंटाकपालमालाधराय व्याघ्रचर्मपरीधानाय शशाङ्ककृतशेखराय कृष्णसर्पयज्ञोपवीतिने चल[१९६] चल चल[१९७] अनिवर्त्तकपालमालिने हन ह्रीं ह्रीं ह्रीं सर्वभूतान् त्रासय त्रासय मंडलमध्ये कट्ट २ रुद्रांकुशेन समय[१९८] प्रवेशय[१९९] २ आवाहय २ चंद्रासि धाराधिपति रुद्रो ज्ञापयति हूँ फट् स्वाहा खड्गरावणः सर्वभूतज्वरान्नाशयति[२००] ॥१९४॥

***Khaḍga Rāvaṇa Mantra***

The following *khaḍgarāvaṇa mantra* cures all types of fever caused by the seizure of evil-spirits :

*Oṃ namaḥ paśupataye nānābhūtādhipataye oṃ namo Rudrāya khaṭvāngaghaṇṭākapālamālādharāya vyāghracarmaparidhānāya śaśānkakṛtaśekharāya kṛṣṇasarpayajñopavītine cala cala cala anivartakapālamāline hana hrīṃ hrīṃ hrīṃ sarvabhūtān trāsaya trāsaya maṇḍalamadhye katta katta rudrāṅkuśena samayaṃ praveśaya praveśaya āvāhaya āvāhaya huṃ phaṭ svāhā.*

॥ इति रावणकृतं कुमारतन्त्रं समाप्तम् ॥१९५॥

Thus, ends the *Kumāratantra* (text on paediatrics) composed by Rāvaṇa.

इति श्रीमहाराजाधिराजश्रीटोडरमल्लविरचिते टोडरानन्दे आयुर्वेदसौख्ये बालरोगनिदानचिकित्साकथनं नाम पंचसप्ततितमो हर्षः ॥

Thus, ends the 75th chapter *Āyurveda saukhya* dealing with the diagnosis and treatment of children-diseases in of *Ṭoḍarānanda* composed by the great king Ṭoḍaramalla.

## NOTES AND REFERENCES

१. दृष्टिभंगे इति षष्ठपुस्तके पाठः ।

२. 'तृष्णालु. ...... श्लेष्मरोगवान्' पाठोऽयं प्रथमपुस्तके नोपलभ्यते ।

३. सन्धींश्च इति आकरे पाठः ।

४. तालुमध्ये कफं शुद्धः इति षष्ठपुस्तके पाठः ।

५. (क) तालुपाके इति प्रथमपुस्तके पाठः ।
(ख) तालुपाते इति पंचमपुस्तके पाठः ।

६. स्तनद्वेषी इति षष्ठपुस्तके पाठः ।

७. महापद्मनामा इति आकरे पाठः ।

८. याति इति आकरे पाठः ।

९. क्षुद्ररोगेन इति आदर्शपुस्तकेषु पाठः ।

१०. बालदेहोऽपि इति प्रथमपुस्तके पाठः ।

११. 'उर्ध्वं ...... चासकृत्' पाठोऽयं प्रथमपुस्तके नोपलभ्यते ।

१२. मांसशोणित. इति आकरे पाठः ।

१३. वित्रस्तः इति आकरे पाठः ।

१४. संज्ञावानतिरोदिति इति आकरे पाठः ।

१५. प्रचिततनुः इति आकरे पाठः ।

१६. सदाहपाकौ. इति प्रथमपुस्तके पाठः ।

१७. भिन्नवर्चा ज्वरी दाही इति आकरे पाठः ।

१८. तिर्यक्प्रेक्षणरोदनम् इति आकरे पाठः ।

१९. 'छर्दिः ...... शिशुः' पाठोऽयं प्रथमपुस्तके नोपलभ्यते ।

२०. कासो इति आकरे पाठः ।

२१. गन्धपूतनया इति चतुर्थपुस्तके पाठः ।

२२. मुखमण्डितिकाग्रहे इति प्रथमपुस्तके पाठः ।

२३. .शोष. इति आकरे पाठः ।

२४. बालानामुल्वणम् इति आकरे पाठः ।

२५. पद्मशानतुति सेव्य कुरु पटुतां इति षष्ठपुस्तके पाठः ।

२६. "बालो ..... घर्षयेज्जिह्वाम्" पाठोऽयं प्रथमपुस्तके नोपलभ्यते ।

२७. यश्चिर(रे)जातः इति चतुर्थषष्ठपुस्तकयोः पाठः ।

२८. तस्य सह इति चतुर्थपुस्तके पाठः ।

२९. शोथस्तेनोपशाम्यति इति आकरे पाठः ।

३०. .चूर्णनम् इति आकरे पाठः ।

३१. क्षपयति शिशोरहं त्रिकायां इति चतुर्थपुस्तके पाठः ।

३२. .प्रशमनमभ्यङ्गो नातिपथ्यविधिः इति आकरे पाठः ।

३३. घुर्घुरिकाबुक्कामरिचरोचनाः इति आकरे पाठः ।

३४. खादेत्तत्कोपनाशनम् इति आकरे पाठः ।

३५. 'पटोल. ..... शिशु' पाठोऽयं प्रथमपुस्तके नोपलभ्यते ।

३६. .स्नुहीभवं क्षीरम् इति आदर्शपुस्तकेषु पाठः ।

३७. आर्कं इति आकरे पाठः ।

३८. चालनिकातलसंस्थिबालं इति आकरे पाठः ।

३९. 'सुवर्णगैरिकस्यापि चूर्णं तु मधुना सह ।
लीढात्सुखमवाप्नोतिप्रवाहिकार्दितः शिशुः ।
यथारोगं यथादोषं यथोद्रेकं यथाबलम् ।
विभज्य देशकालादीन् यथा योग्यं भिषज्जितम् ।' पाठोऽयं षष्ठपुस्तके अधिकमुपलभ्यते ।

४०. मात्रा चात्र इति आकरे पाठः ।

४१. बालाय देया भैषज्यरक्तिका इति आकरे पाठः ।

४२. स्याद्यावदाषोडशब्दिकः इति प्रथमपुस्तके पाठः ।

४३. 'शिशो. ...... क्षौद्रेण संयुतम्' पाठोऽयं प्रथमपुस्तके नोपलभ्यते ।

४४. देयः इति षष्ठपुस्तके पाठः ।

४५. बालानां चातुर्भद्रिका इति चतुर्थपुस्तके पाठः ।

४६. (क) "मुस्त. ...... शिशोः" पाठोऽयं प्रथमपुस्तके नोपलभ्यते ।
(ख) मुस्ताकूष्माण्डवातारि भद्रदारुकलिङ्गकैः इति आदर्शपुस्तकेषु पाठः ।

४७. संलिम्पेल्लेपोऽयं शोथहृच्छिशोः इति आकरे पाठः ।

४८. .धान्याक. इति आकरे पाठः ।

४९. सर्वरोगजित् इति आकरे पाठः ।

५०. 'हिंगु ...... दीपनं परम्' पाठोऽयं षष्ठपुस्तके अधिकमुपलभ्यते ।

५१. मधुरशर्करैः इति प्रथमपुस्तके पाठः ।

५२. मधुना चिरसंजातशिशोः इति आकरे पाठः ।

५३. पञ्चभिरुच्छ्रितैः इति आकरे पाठः ।

५४. "व्याघ्री ...... पंचभिरेव च" पाठोऽयं प्रथमपुस्तके नोपलभ्यते ।

५५. क्षौद्रसंलीढा कासश्वासौ शिशोर्जयेत् इति आकरे पाठः ।

५६. 'नागराति. ...... सर्वातीसारनाशनम्' पाठोऽयं चतुर्थषष्ठपुस्तकयोः नोपलभ्यते ।

५७. मोचरसः समङ्गा च धातकी पद्मकेशरम् इति आकरे पाठः ।

५८. .तीसारविनाशनी इति चतुर्थषष्ठपुस्तकयोः पाठः ।

५९. 'सितासर्जरस ...... छर्दतीसारनाशनम्' पाठोऽयं प्रथमपंचमपुस्तकयोः नोपलभ्यते ।

६०. रक्षेयान्नियतं इति षष्ठपुस्तके पाठः ।

६१. धान्यं इति चतुर्थषष्ठपुस्तकयोः पाठः ।

६२. ग्रहणीरोगं सुदुर्वारम् इति प्रथमपुस्तके पाठः ।

६३. बिल्वदलोत्थाम्बुमिश्रितं इति आकरे पाठः ।

६५. 'छुछुन्दरीमलोमांसीहरिद्राबिल्वपत्रकम् ।
इन्द्रशिरीषपत्रं च धूपे नित्यं प्रयोजयेत् ।
निहन्ति रोदनं रात्रौ बालस्याशु न संशयः ।
कर्कटाघ्रिं क्षीरपक्वं घृताभ्यङ्गेन नश्यति ।
दंतशकृत्कक्यंध्रिलेपाद्धौ दंतयोजितः ।'
पाठोऽयं चतुर्थषष्ठपुस्तकयोः अधिकमुपलभ्यतें ।

६६. पिबेत् इति चतुर्थषष्ठपुस्तकयोः पाठः ।

६७. (क) सामानुबन्धां इति चतुर्थपुस्तके पाठः ।
(ख) पाठोऽयं षष्ठपुस्तके नोपलभ्यते ।

६८. 'पीतं.....जम्बूत्व.' पाठोऽयं चतुर्थषष्ठपुस्तकयोः नोपलभ्यते ।

६९. 'पिष्ट्वा भूम्यामली लेपं कुर्यात्पाणिपदौः शिशोः ।
मुखपाकं हरत्याशु दृष्टप्रत्ययमौषधम् ।'
पाठोऽयं चतुर्थषष्ठपुस्तकयोः अधिकमुपलभ्यते ।

७०. दन्तोद्भेदोत्थरोगेषु इति आकरे पाठः ।

७१. (क) गावं नैगमेषं प्रपूजयेत् इति चतुर्थपुस्तके पाठः ।
(ख) गावै नैगमयं प्रपूजयेत् इति षष्ठपुस्तके पाठः ।

७२. 'हिक्कार्दित ...... क्षिप्रं' पाठोऽयं चतुर्थषष्ठपुस्तकयोः नोपलभ्यते ।

७३. वज्रदन्ती इति चतुर्थषष्ठपुस्तकयोः पाठः ।

७४. विनाशयेत् इति चतुर्थषष्ठपुस्तकयोः पाठः ।

७५. 'पुष्करातिविषा. ...... पंचकासनुत्' पाठोऽयं प्रथमपुस्तके नोपलभ्यते ।

७६. मागधी त्वचपययाचकैः इति चतुर्थपुस्तके पाठः ।

७७. भस्मयुषितजलं इति प्रथमपुस्तके पाठः ।

७८. तैलेन इति षष्ठपुस्तके पाठः ।

७९. वटकास्थितं जलं इति षष्ठपुस्तके पाठः ।

८०. वक्त्रशोषहृद्वक्रे इति षष्ठपुस्तके पाठः ।

८१. शिशोर्नेत्रामयार्त्तिजित् इति आकरे पाठः ।

८२. पुटपक्वः इति आकरे पाठः ।

८३. तद्रसाश्च्योतनं इति आकरे पाठः ।

८४. लाक्षाकाञ्जिकगैरिकैः इति षष्ठपुस्तके पाठः ।

८५. कुकूणे स्यात् शिशुना पोथकीषु च इति आकरे पाठः ।

८६. .समं इति आकरे पाठः ।

८७. जीरकं इति पंचमपुस्तके पाठः ।

८८. कुमारकल्याणकं घृतम् इति प्रथमपुस्तके पाठः ।

८९. घृतमष्टमम् इति आकरे पाठः ।

९०. 'न ..... पिबतामष्टमङ्गलम्' पाठोऽयं चतुर्थषष्ठपुस्तकयोः नोपलभ्यते ।

९१. रक्षांसि इति आकरे पाठः ।

९२. अष्टमङ्गलकं घृतम् इति प्रथमपुस्तके पाठः ।

९३. कृष्णाब्द. इति प्रथमपुस्तके पाठः ।

९४. युतैः इति षष्ठपुस्तके पाठः ।

९५. लाक्षाद्यं घृतम् इति चतुर्थषष्ठपुस्तकयोः पाठः ।

९६. भैषज्यं सर्वमुद्दिष्टं बालनां इति चतुर्थषष्ठपुस्तकयोः पाठः ।

९७. 'विडङ्गपलमात्रं ...... .द्वदरोपमा' पाठोऽयं प्रथमपुस्तके नोपलभ्यते ।
९८. स्नुहीमुण्डितिकोदीच्यक्वाथै स्नानं इति प्रथमपुस्तके पाठः ।
९९. सप्तछदामयानिशाचन्दनैश्चानुलेपनम् इति प्रथमपुस्तके पाठः ।
१००. पाठोऽयं चतुर्थषष्ठपुस्तकयोः नोपलभ्यते ।
१०१. कृतं चूर्णितम् इति चतुर्थषष्ठपुस्तकयोः पाठः ।
१०२. 'देयो.....दोषापहः' पाठोऽयं चतुर्थषष्ठपुस्तकयोः नोपलभ्यते ।
१०३. शान्तीष्टिकर्म्मणि इति प्रथमपुस्तके पाठः ।
१०४. पाठसंलग्ना टिप्पणी द्रष्टव्या ।
१०५. कं टं यं शं वैनतेयाय इति आकरे पाठः ।
१०६. ॐ कारि सुवर्णपक्षीश इति आकरे पाठः ।
१०७. मृच्छिकाभक्तबलिर्देयस्तु शान्तिकः इति आकरे पाठः ।
१०८. पाठोऽयं आदर्शपुस्तकेषु नोपलभ्यते ।
१०९. गृहीतमात्रस्य इति आकरे पाठः ।
११०. आत्कारञ्च करोति इति आकरे पाठः ।
१११. जम्बुडिका, सप्तमुस्तकाः, गंध, पुष्पं, ताम्बूलं इति आकरे पाठः ।
११२. अश्वत्थपत्रं इति प्रथमपुस्तके पाठः ।
११३. जलकुम्भे इति आकरे पाठः ।
११४. प्रक्षिप्य इति प्रथमपुस्तके पाठः ।
११५. य इति आदर्शपुस्तकेषु पाठः ।
११६. (क) 'एवं.......ततश्च' पाठोऽयं प्रथमपुस्तके नोपलभ्यते ।
(ख) सर्व इति चतुर्थपुस्तके पाठः ।
११७. कृत्वा गन्धताम्बूलं इति पंचमपुस्तके पाठः ।
११८. मत्स्यमांससुराग्रभक्ततिलचूर्णानि इति आकरे पाठः ।
११९. पश्चिमस्यां इति प्रथमपुस्तके पाठः ।
१२०. रावणाय इति आकरे पाठः ।
१२१. हन हन मुञ्च मुञ्च ह्रीं फट् स्वाहा इति आकरे पाठः ।
१२२. रावणाय अमुकस्य व्याधिं हन हन मुञ्च मुञ्च हासय हासय स्वाहा इति आकरे पाठः ।
१२३. गृहणति नाम मातृका इति आदर्शपुस्तकेषु पाठः ।
१२४. अक्षिउन्मीलयति इति प्रथमपुस्तके पाठः ।
१२५. अमुकस्य व्याधिं हन हन मुञ्च मुञ्च स्वाहा इति आकरे पाठः ।
१२६. विधाय इति आकरे पाठः ।

१२७. सप्त इति आकरे पाठः ।

१२८. रावणाय अमुकस्य व्याधिं चूर्णय चूर्णय हन हन स्वाहा इति आकरे पाठः ।

१२९. ब्राह्मणान् इति आकरे पाठः ।

१३०. मुष्टिं बध्नाति, दिवारात्रावुत्थानं इति आकरे पाठः ।

१३१. शुक्लौदनं इति आकरे पाठः ।

१३२. दीपाः दशपीतध्वजाः इति आकरे पाठः ।

१३३. क्षीरजम्बूतिलपिष्टिकाः इति आदर्शपुस्तकेषु पाठः ।

१३४. रावणाय अमुकस्य व्याधिं चूर्णय चूर्णय हन हन स्वाहा इति आकरे पाठः ।

१३५. ब्राह्मणान् इति आकरे पाठः ।

१३६. पाठोऽयं आदर्शपुस्तकेषु नोपलभ्यते ।

१३७. जम्बुलिका इति आकरे पाठः ।

१३८. पश्चिमायां दिशि इति आकरे पाठः ।

१३९. ग्रामनिष्काशे इति आकरे पाठः ।

१४०. वक्षमाश्रित्य इति आदर्शपुस्तकेषु पाठः ।

१४१. बलिर्दातव्यः इति आकरे पाठः ।

१४२. स्नापयेत् इति आकरे पाठः ।

१४३. बालकघृतैर्धूपं दद्यात् इति आकरे पाठः ।

१४४. रावणाय दीप्ततेजसे हन हन मुञ्च मुञ्च इति आकरे पाठः ।

१४५. ब्राह्मणान् इति आकरे पाठः ।

१४६. आर्य्यका नाम इति आकरे पाठः ।

१४७. यतः इति आकरे पाठः ।

१४८. पीतपुष्पं इति आकरे पाठः ।

१४९. जम्बूलिका इति आकरे पाठः ।

१५०. बलि दद्यात् इति आकरे पाठः ।

१५१. अमुकस्य व्याधिं इति आकरे पाठः ।

१५२. मुञ्च मुञ्च दह दह ॐ ह्री फट् स्वाहा इति आकरे पाठः ।

१५३. ब्राह्मणान् इति आकरे पाठः ।

१५४. गृहीत मांत्रेण इति आकरे पाठः ।

१५५. छर्दयति इति आकरे पाठः ।

१५६. निद्रातितरां स्यात् इति आकरे पाठः ।

१५७. निर्माय इति आकरे पाठः ।

१५८. शुक्लौदनं इति आकरे पाठः ।

१५९. पूपिकाः इति आदर्शपुस्तकेषु पाठः ।

१६०. ग्राम निष्काशे इति आकरे पाठः ।

१६१. स्नापयेत् इति आकरे पाठः ।

१६२. गोधूम इति आकरे अधिकः पाठः ।

१६३. रावणाय इति आकरे पाठः ।

१६४. निर्हृता इति आकरे पाठः ।

१६५. आत्कारं करोति, रोदिति मुष्टिं बध्नाति, मूत्रं पुरीषञ्च भवति इति आकरे पाठः ।

१६६. कृत्वा इति आकरे पाठः ।

१६७. पञ्चपुत्तलिकाः इति आकरे पाठः ।

१६८. रावणाय चूर्णित हस्ताय हन हन मुञ्च मुञ्च स्वाहा इति आकरे पाठः ।

१६९. ब्राह्मणान् इति आकरे पाठः ।

१७०. स्वस्थो भवति बालकः इति प्रथमपुस्तके पाठः ।

१७१. यदि इति प्रथमपुस्तके पाठः ।

१७२. पिप्लिपिञ्जिका इति प्रथमपुस्तके पाठः ।

१७३. पिष्टकेन पुत्तलिका कृत्वा रक्तचन्दनं, रक्तपुष्पं इति आकरे पाठः ।

१७४. पाठोऽयं आदर्शपुस्तकेषु नोपलभ्यते ।

१७५. बलिर्दातव्यः इति आकरे पाठः ।

१७६. स्नापयेत् इति आकरे पाठः ।

१७७. रावणाय इति आकरे पाठः ।

१७८. सुस्थो इति आकरे पाठः ।

१७९. पाठोऽयं आदर्शपुस्तकेषु नोपलभ्यते ।

१८०. यदि इति प्रथमपुस्तके पाठः ।

१८१. वादयति करेण तर्जयति इति आकरे पाठः ।

१८२. तेन इति आकरे पाठः ।

१८३. सुखम् इति पंचमपुस्तके पाठः ।

१८४. पाठोऽयं आदर्शपुस्तकेषु नोपलभ्यतें ।

१८५. करम्भभक्तेन इति आदर्शपुस्तकेषु पाठः ।

१८६. गर्वकर्मबलिं इति आकरे पाठः ।

१८७. श्वेतसर्षप इति आकरे पाठः ।

१८८. धूपयेत् इति आकरे पाठः ।

१८९. रावणाय इति आकरे पाठः ।

१९०. विप्रान् इति आकरे पाठः ।

१९१. यंत्रनिग्रहनुन्ग्रहक्षमान इति षष्ठपुस्तके पाठः ।

१९२. मिलि चतुर्थषष्ठपुस्तकयोः पाठः ।

१९३. वेदेन मंत्रः इति षष्ठपुस्तके पाठः ।

१९४. तिष्टातर इति षष्ठपुस्तके पाठः ।

१९५. शिखाबंधः इति षष्ठपुस्तके पाठः ।

१९६. वल इति षष्ठपुस्तके पाठः ।

१९७. वला इति षष्ठपुस्तके पाठः ।

१९८. शमय अवेशय आवादय २ इति षष्ठपुस्तके पाठः ।

१९९. आवाह २ इति चतुर्थपुस्तके पाठः ।

२००. नाशयेत् इति षष्ठपुस्तके पाठः ।

# CHAPTER VIII

## ।। अथ विषनिदानं चिकित्सा च ।।

*(Diagnosis and Treatment of Diseases Caused by Poisons)*

"स्थावरं जङ्गमं चैव द्विविधं विषमुच्यते ।
मूलाद्यात्मकमाद्यं स्यात् परं सर्पादिसम्भवम् ।।१।।

***Classification of Poisons***

Poisons are of two categories, viz., *sthāvara* (derived from inanimate objects) consisting of roots of plants, etc., and *jaṅgama* (derived from animals) comprising snake poison, etc.

निद्रां तन्द्रां क्लमं दाहं संतापं रोमहर्षणम् ।
शोथं चैवातिसारं च कुरुते जङ्गमं विषम् ।।२।।

***Jaṅgama Type of Poison***

*Jaṅgama* (derived from animals) type of poison causes excessive sleep, drowsiness, exhaustion, burning sensation, rise in body temperature, horripilation, oedema and diarrhoea.

'स्थावरं[1] तु ज्वरं हिक्कां दन्तहर्षं गलग्रहम् ।
फेनच्छर्द्यरुचिश्वासं मूर्च्छां च कुरुते विषम्' ॥३॥

### *Sthāvara Type of Poison*

*Sthāvara* (derived from inanimate objects) type of poison produces fever, hiccup, tingling sensation in teeth, obstruction in the throat, vomiting of frothy material, anorexia, asthma and fainting.

'इङ्गितज्ञो मनुष्याणां वाक्चेष्टामुखवैकृतैः ।
जानीयाद्विषदातारमेभिर्लिङ्गैश्च बुद्धिमान् ॥४॥
न ददात्युत्तरं पृष्टो विवक्षुर्मोहमेति च ।
अपार्थं बहुसंकीर्णं भाषते चापि मूढवत् ॥५॥
हसत्यकस्मात्स्फोटत्यङ्गुलीर्विलिखेन्महीम् ।
वेपथुश्चास्य भवति त्रस्तश्चान्योन्यमीक्षते[1] ॥६॥
विवर्णवक्त्रो ध्यामश्च नखैः किञ्चिच्छिनत्त्यपि ।
आलभेतासनं दीनः करेण च शिरोरुहम् ॥
वर्त्तते विपरीतं च विषदाता विचेतनः" ॥७॥

(सुश्रुत : कल्पस्थान : १ : १८-२३)

### *A Person Who has Administered Poison*

The person who has administered poison can be ascertained by a wise physician from the hints (activities) like the perversion in speech, activities and facial features of that person. Details of such hints (perverted activities) are as follows :

(1) The person who has administered poison does not answer when questioned;
(2) he faints while trying to speak (give answers);
(3) like a fool, he gives irrelevant and clumsy replies;
(4) he suddently starts laughing;
(5) he crackles his finger joints and scratches the ground;
(6) he trembles, and with fear, looks here and there (lit. each other);
(7) his face becomes discoloured and distorted;
(8) when asked to sit, he does it with humility;

(9) he pulls his hair;
(10) he behaves in an erratic manner; and
(11) he loses his consciousness.

उद्वेष्टनं मूलविषे प्रलापो मोहं एव च ।
जृम्भणं वेपनं श्वासो ज्ञेयं पत्रविषेण तु ॥८॥

*Root and Leaf-Poisons*

If a person is administered a poisonous root, then he suffers from cramps, delirium and delusion. Leaf-poison makes a person to yawn frequently, tremble and breathless.

मुष्कशोथः फलविषैर्दाहोऽन्नद्वेषं एव च ।
भवेत् पुष्पविषैश्छर्दिराध्मानं श्वास एव च ॥९॥

*Fruit and Flower-Poison*

If a person is administered a poisonous fruit, then he gets swelling in the scrotum, burning sensation and aversion for the intake of food. A poisonous flower gives rise to vomiting, flatulence and dyspnoea.

"त्वक्सारनिर्यासविषैरुपयुक्तैर्भवन्ति" च ।
आस्यदौर्गन्ध्यपारुष्यशिरोरुक्कफसंस्रवाः ॥१०॥

*Bark-Poison, etc.*

Administration of poisonous barks, *sāra* (heart wood) and *niryāsa* (gum resin) causes foul smell coming out of the mouth, roughness of the face, headache and excessive salivation.

फेनागमः क्षीरविषैर्विड्भेदो गुरुजिह्वता ।
हृत्पीडनं धातुविषैर्मूर्च्छा दाहश्च तालुनि ॥११॥

*Latex and Mineral Poisons*

Administration of poisonous *kṣīra* (milky latex) causes froth coming out of the mouth, diarrhoea and heaviness of the tongue. Mineral poisons cause pain in the cardiac region, fainting and burning sensation in palates.

प्रायेण कालघातीनि विषाण्येतानि निर्दिशेत्' ॥१२॥
(सुश्रुत : कल्पस्थान : २ : ९-२२)

*Time of Death*

Because of the administration of these varieties of poisons, the patient generally succumbs to death after some time (*kālaghāti*).

सद्यः क्षतं पच्यते यस्य जन्तोः
स्रवेद्रक्तं पच्यते चाप्यभीक्ष्णम् ।
कृष्णीभूतं क्लिन्नमत्यर्थपूति
क्षतान्मांसं शीर्यते चापि यस्य ॥
तृष्णा मूर्च्छा ज्वरदाहौ च यस्य
दिग्धाहतं तं पुरुषं व्यवस्येत् ॥१३॥

*Injury by Poisonous Weapon*

Following signs appear in a person who is wounded by a weapon smeared with poisonous substance :

(1) The fresh wound gets suppurated;
(2) bleeding and suppuration take place very frequently;
(3) the wound becomes black, sticky and excessively putrified;
(4) the flesh from the wound gets shrivelled; and
(5) he suffers from morbid thirst, fainting, fever and burning sensation.

लिङ्गान्येतान्येव कुर्यादमित्रैः[१]-
र्व्रणे विषं यस्य दत्तं प्रमादात् ॥१४॥

*Smearing Wounds with Poisons*

At times, enemies smear the wound of a person with poisons. In such cases also, the above signs will be manifested.

सवात[10] गृहधूमाभं पुरीषं 'योऽतिसार्यते[11] ।
फेनमुद्वमते चापि विषपीतं तमादिशेत् ॥१५॥

*Suicide by Poisons*

If a person voids very frequent loose motions having the colour of house-shoot along with flatus and vomits frothy material, then it should be ascertained that he has taken poison [to commit suicide].

वातपित्तकफात्मानो भोगिमण्डलिराजिलाः ।
यथाक्रमं समाख्याता[12] इतरा द्वन्द्वरूपिणः' ॥१६॥

*Nature of Snakes*

Snakes of *bhogi* type (those having hoods), *maṇḍali* type (those having circular patches in their bodies) and *rājila* (those having coloured strips in their bodies) are dominated by *vāyu, pitta* and *kapha* respectively. Other varieites are dominated by two of these *doṣas.*

दंशो भोगिकृतः कृष्णः सर्ववातविकारकृत्[13] ।
पीतो मण्डलिजः[14] शोथो मृदुः पित्तविकारवान्[15] ॥१७॥

*Bhogi and Maṇḍali Types of Snakes*

If a person gets bitten by a *bhogi* (hooded) type of snake, then the place of bite becomes black in colour and he suffers from all symptoms caused by the aggravated *vāyu.* If a person is bitten by a *maṇḍali* (having circular patches) type of snake, the site of bite which is swollen and soft becomes yellow in colour and he suffers from all the symptoms caused by the aggravated *pitta.*

राजिलोत्थो भवेद्दंशः स्थिरशोथश्च पिच्छिलः ।
पाण्डुः स्निग्धाऽतिसान्द्रासृक्[16] सर्वश्लेष्मविकारकृत् ॥१८॥

*Rājila Type of Snake*

If a person is bitten by a *rājila* (having coloured strips) type of snake, then the swelling at the site of bite becomes stable and slimy. It is pale-yellow in colour and unctuous containing thick blood. It produces all the signs and symptoms caused by the aggravated *kapha* in the patient.

अश्वत्थदेवायतनश्मशान-
बल्मीकसंध्यासु चतुष्पथेषु ।
याम्ये च पैत्रे[१७] परिवर्जनीया
ऋक्षे सिरामर्मसु[१८] ये च दष्टाः ॥१९॥

*Prognosis*

If a person is bitten by a snake near an *aśvattha* tree, in a temple, in a crematorium, near an ant-hill, during evening, in a cross-road, during *pitṛpakṣa* (during the fortnight when oblations are offered to manes) or during the constellation of *bharaṇī* and if he is bitten in a site of *śirāmarma* (vital spot in the body having the predominance of vessels), then such a patient is incurable.

दर्वीकराणां विषमाशु घाति सर्वाणि चोष्णे द्विगुणीभवन्ति ।
अजीर्णपित्तश्रमपीडितेषु[१९] वृद्धेषु बालेषु बुभुक्षितेषु ॥
क्षीणक्षते मेहिनि कुष्ठयुक्ते[२०] रूक्षेऽबले गर्भवतीषु चापि ॥२०॥

Bite by the *darvīkara* or *bhogi* type of snake (ones having hood) kills the person instantaneously. During summer season, the effects of poisons become doubled. Similarly, these effects become doubly powerful in a person suffering from indigestion, aggravated *pitta* and exhaustion, in an old person, in the children, in hungry persons, in persons suffering from consumption, *prameha* (obstinate urinary disorders including diabetes), *kuṣṭha* (obstinate skin diseases including leprosy), in ununctuous and weak persons and in pregnant women.

"शस्त्रक्षते यस्य न रक्तमस्ति[२१]
'राज्यो[२२] लताभिश्च न संभवन्ति ।
शीताभिरद्भिश्च न रोमहर्षो
विषाभिभूतं परिवर्जयेत्तम् ॥२१॥

If a person does get bleeding from a cut by a weapon, if no spot appears on the skin when thrashed by a rope or creeper and if there is no horripilation when sprinkled with cold water such a person afflicted with poison should not be treated.

जिह्मं मुखं यस्य च केशशातो
नासावसादश्च सकण्ठभङ्गः ॥
कृष्णः सरक्तः श्वयथुश्च दंशे
हन्वोः स्थिरत्वं च विवर्जनीयः ॥२२॥

If there is deformity in the face, if the hairs get depilated by slight pulling, if the nose becomes depressed, if the patient is unable to support his head with the help of his neck, if the site of bite becomes swollen with black or red coloration and if the jaws get locked then such a patient should not be treated.

वर्तिर्घना[23] यस्य निरेति वक्त्राद्
रक्तं स्रवेदूर्ध्वमधश्च यस्य ।
दंष्ट्रानिपाताश्चतुरश्च[24] यस्य
तं चापि वैद्यः परिवर्जयेत्तु ॥२३॥

If from the mouth of the patient, thick phlegm comes out in the form of a wick, if bleeding takes place from the upward and downward tracts of his body, if in his skin there are spots indicating biting by four teeth of the snake [the term '*daṃṣṭrānipātaścaturaśca*' has been interpreted differently by different authors], such a patient should not be entertained for treatment by the physician.

उन्मत्तमत्यर्थमुपद्रुतं वा
हीनस्वरं वाऽप्यथवा विवर्णम् ।
सारिष्टमत्यर्थमवेगिनं च
जह्यान्नरं कर्म तत्र न कुर्यात्" ॥२४॥

(सुश्रुत : कल्पस्थान : ३ : ४०-४४)

If the patient has gone mad, if he is afflicted by complications in excess, if his voice has become thin, if he has become discolored, if bad prognostic signs have already appeared in the patient and if he becomes incapable of passing stool and urine, then such a patient should not be treated.

"जीर्णं विषघ्नौषधिभिर्हतं वा
दावाग्निवातातपशोषितं वा ।
स्वभावतो वा गुणविप्रहीनं
विषं हि दूषीविषतामुपैति ॥
वीर्याल्पभावान्न निपातयेत्तत्
कफान्वितं[१५] वर्षगणानुबन्धि ॥२५॥

*Dūṣīviṣa*

If the poison has become old, if the poison is treated by anti-poison drugs and if the poison is dried up because of exposure to forest-fire or air or sunrays, then it gets reduced in potency. This type of poison is called *duṣīviṣa* and it does not cause death of the person. In association with *kapha* [it does not get digested] and remains in the body for years together producing adverse effects.

तेनार्दितो भिन्नपुरीषवर्णो
विगन्धवैरस्ययुतः[१६] पिपासी ।
मूर्च्छां[१७] भ्रमं गद्गदवाग्वमिश्च
विचेष्टमानोऽरतिमाप्नुयाद्वा ॥२६॥

*Signs and Symptoms of Dūṣīviṣa*

A person who has consumed *dūṣīviṣa* suffers from diarrhoea discoloration of the skin, foul smell coming out of the body, bad taste in the mouth, morbid thirst, fainting, giddiness, stammering speech, vomiting, perverted activities and disliking for doing any work.

आमाशयस्थे कफवातरोगी
पक्वाशयस्थेऽनिलपित्तरोगी ।
भवेत्समुद्ध्वस्तशिरोरुहाङ्गो
विलूनपक्षस्तु यथा विहङ्गः ॥२७॥

*Location in Stomach and Colon*

If this *dūṣīviṣa* gets lodged in the stomach including small intestine, then the person suffers from diseases caused by aggravated *kapha* and *vāyu.* If, however, it gets lodged in the colon, then the person suffers from diseases caused by the aggravated *vāyu* and *pitta* and hairs from his head and body get depilated. Thus, he looks like a bird whose feathers have been pulled out.

स्थितं रसादिष्वथवा यथोक्तान्
करोति धातुप्रभवान् विकारान् ॥२८॥

*Location in Tissues*

If this *dūṣīviṣa* gets lodged in the tissue elements like *rasa* (plasma), etc., then it produces ailments involving those tissues.

कोपं च शीतानिलदुर्दिनेषु
यात्याशु, पूर्वं शृणु तस्य[२८] रूपम् ॥
निद्रा गुरुत्वं च विजृम्भणं च
विश्लेषहर्षावथवाऽङ्गमर्दः ॥२९॥
ततः करोत्यन्नमदाविपाकान्
विरोचकं मण्डलकोठजन्म[२९] ।
मांसक्षय[३०] पादकरास्यशोथं
मूर्च्छां तथा छर्दिमथातिसारम् ।
दूषीविष[३१] श्वासतृषज्वरांश्च
कुर्यात्सवृद्धिं[३२] जठरस्य चापि ॥३०॥

उन्मादमन्यज्जनयेत्तथाऽन्यदानाहमन्यत् क्षपयेच्च शुक्रम् ।
गाद्गद्यमन्यज्जनयेच्च कुष्ठं तांस्तान् विकारांश्च बहुप्रकारम् ॥३१॥

*Other Signs and Symptoms*

Effects of *dūṣīviṣa* get enhanced by exposure to cold, strong wind and during rainy season. Other signs and symptoms caused by the intake of *dūṣīviṣa* are excessive sleep, heaviness, yawning, looseness of joints, horripilation and malaise. Thereafter, it causes *annamada* (feeling of intoxication after the intake of food), indigestion, anorexia, *maṇḍala koṭha* (urticuria), wasting of muscles, oedema in the feet, legs and face, fainting, vomiting, diarrhoea, asthma, morbid thirst, fever and swelling of the abdomen.

In addition, different types of *dūṣīviṣa* produce different specific types of symptoms, for example, some of these poisons cause insanity, some others cause flatulence, some cause reduction in semen, some cause stammering and some of them cause *kuṣṭha* (obstinate skin diseases including leprosy). Similarly, several other ailments are manifested because of *dūṣīviṣa.*

दूषितं देशकालान्नदिवास्वप्नैरभीक्ष्णशः ।
यस्मात्संदूषयेद्धातून् तस्मादूषीविषं स्मृतम्" ॥३२॥
(सुश्रुत : कल्पस्थान : २ : २५-३३)

*Another Definition of Dūṣīviṣa*

A substance which is produced because of the pollution of the place of habitation, temporal including seasonal perversions, improper food, sleep of the individual during the daytime and which causes vitiation of tissue elements, is called *dūṣīviṣa.*

"साध्यमात्मवतः सद्यो याप्यं संवत्सरोषितम्[३३] ।
दूषीविषमसाध्यं स्यात् क्षीणस्याहितसेविनः" ॥३३॥
(सुश्रुत : कल्पस्थान : २ : ५५)

*Prognosis*

In a person with a strong will power, the ailments caused by *dūṣīviṣa* get easily cured. If these are afflicting the patient continuously for one year, then the condition becomes palliable (*yāpya*). If the patient is emaciated and if he indulges in the unwholesome food, then his ailments become incurable.

सौभाग्यार्थं स्त्रियः स्वेदं रजो नानाङ्गजान् मलान्।
शत्रुप्रयुक्तांश्च गरान् प्रयच्छन्त्यन्नमिश्रितान् ॥३४॥

*Gara Poison*

Ladies for getting bestowed with auspiciousness, and enemies to cause harm to their foes administer sweat, menstrual blood and excreta from different parts of the body mixed with food. This is called *gara* type of poison.

तैः स्यात् पाण्डुः कृशोऽल्पाग्निर्ज्वरश्चास्योपजायते[३४]।
मर्मप्रधमनाध्मान[३५] हस्तयोः शोथलक्षणम् ॥३५॥
जठरं ग्रहणीदोषो यक्ष्मा गुल्मः क्षयो ज्वरः ।
एवंविधस्य चान्यस्य व्याधेर्लिङ्गानि दर्शयेत् ॥३६॥

*Signs and Symptoms of Gara Poison*

Because of *gara* type of poison, a person suffers from anemia, emaciation, less power of digestion, *marma pradhamana* (pain in the vital parts of the body), flatulence, oedema in hands, *jathara* (obstinate abdominal disorders including ascites), *grahaṇī doṣa* (sprue syndrome), tuberculosis, *gulma* (phantom tumour), consumption, fever and several such other ailments.

"यस्माल्लून[३६] तृणं प्राप्ता मुनेः प्रस्वेदविन्दवः ।
तस्माल्लूताश्च भाष्यन्ते संख्यया ताश्च षोडश" ॥३७॥

(सुश्रुत : कल्पस्थान : ८ : ९३)

*Lūtā (Spider) Poison*

Since sweat-drops from the forehead of the sage Vaśiṣṭha fell on cut pieces (*lūna*) of grass and gave rise to poisonous spiders, these are called *lūtā.* [This gives the mythological origin of spiders. Once the sage Viśvāmitra wanted to forcibly take away the *Kāmadhenu* (Wish-fulfilling Cow) of the sage *Vaśiṣṭha.* This attempt enraged the latter as a result of which sweat drops came out of his forehead]. These are of sixteen varieties.

"ताभिर्दष्टे दंशकोथः प्रवृत्तिः क्षतजस्य च ।
ज्वरो दाहोऽतिसारश्च गदाः स्युश्च त्रिदोषजाः ॥३८॥
पिडका विविधाकारा मण्डलानि महान्ति च ।
शोथा महान्तो मृदवो रक्ताः श्यावाश्चलास्तथा ॥
सामान्यं सर्वलूतानामेतत् दंशस्य लक्षणम्" ॥३९॥

(सुश्रुत : कल्पस्थान : ८ : ९६-१००)

॥ लूतादंशनिदानम् ॥

*Signs of Lūtā Poison*

When bitten by a poisonous spider, the following signs and symptoms appear in general :

(1) Putrification at the site of the bite;
(2) profuse bleeding;
(3) fever, burning sensation, diarrhoea, and other diseases caused by the simultaneous vitiation of all the three *doṣas*;
(4) different types of carbuncles and big circular patches over the body; and
(5) excessive swelling which is soft, red, grayish black and shifting.

दंशमध्य[३७] तु यत् कृष्णं श्यावं वा जालकाचितम्[३८] ।
दग्धाकृति[३९] भृंशपाकं क्लेदकोथज्वराधिकम्[४०] ।
दूषीविषाभिर्लूताभिर्भूताभिर्दष्टमादिशेत्[४१] ॥४०॥

If the spot where the person is bitten is black or grayish black, if it is surrounded by net work of vessels, if it appears as if burnt, if it is excessively putrified and if there is excessive sticky material, sloughing and fever, he is to be diagnosed as a case bitten by the venomous spider. This is a form of *dūṣīviṣa.*

शोथः[४२] श्वेताः सिता रक्ताः पीता वा पिडका ज्वरः ।
प्राणान्तिको[४३] भवेद्दाहः श्वासहिक्काशिरोरुजः[४४] ॥४१॥

*Prognosis*

If there is excess of oedema, if papules of white, whitish red or yellow colour appear in the skin and if there is fever accompanied with burning sensation, dyspnoea, hiccup and headache, then the patient is destined to death.

आदंशाच्छोणितं पाण्डुमण्डलानि ज्वरोऽरुचिः ।
लोमहर्षश्च दाहश्चाप्याखुदूषीविषार्दिते[४५] ॥४२॥

*Rat-Poison*

If a person is afflicted by rat-poison, then bleeding takes place from the site of bite, circular patches having yellowish white colour appear over the skin, there is fever, anorexia, horripilation and burning sensation.

मूर्च्छाङ्गशोथवैवर्ण्यक्लेदमंत्रस्रुतिज्वराः[४६] ।
शिरोगुरुत्वं लालासृक्छर्दिश्चासाध्यमूषकैः[४७] ॥४३॥

*Prognosis*

If the person bitten by a poisonous rat suffers from fainting, swelling in the limbs, discoloration of the skin, stickiness, exudation from the intestine (through the anus), fever, heaviness of the head and vomiting of sticky saliva and blood, then he is incurable.

कार्ष्ण्यं[४८] शोथत्वमथवा[४९] नानावर्णत्वमेव च[५०] ।
मोहोऽथ वर्चसो भेदो[५१] दष्टे स्यात् कृकलासकैः ॥४४॥

*Chameleon-Poison*

Because of the poison of chemeleon-bite, the swollen skin becomes black or of different colours and the patient suffers from unconsciousness as well as diarrhoea.

दहत्यग्निरिवादौ च[५२] भिनत्तीवोर्ध्वमाशु च ।
वृश्चिकस्य विषं याति दंशे पश्चाच्च[५३] तिष्ठति ॥४५॥

*Scorpion-Poison*

Because of scorpion-bite, the patient gets excruciating burning sensation as if the site is touched by fire. Thereafter, the burning sensation enters to deeper part of the body and spreads upwards. This burning sensation persists for some time and thereafter subsides.

दष्टोऽसाध्यश्च[५४] हृद्घ्राणरसनोपहतो नरः ।
मांसैः पतद्भिरत्यर्थं[५५] वेदनार्तो जहात्यसून् ॥४६॥

*Prognosis*

If in the patient of scorpion-bite, there is affliction of heart, power of smelling and the gustatory sensation, if there is excessive sloughing out of the muscle tissue and if there is excessive pain, then he succumbs to death.

विसर्पः श्वयथुः शूलं ज्वरश्छर्दिरथापि च[५६] ।
लक्षणं कणभैर्दष्टे[५७] दंशश्चैवावसीदति ॥४७॥

*Wasp-Poison*

If a person is stung by a *kaṇabha* (wasp), then the swelling at the site of bite spreads like erysipelas, there will be colic pain, fever, vomiting and depression at the site of the bite.

हृष्टलोमोच्चिटिङ्गेन स्तब्धलिङ्गो भृशार्तिमान् ।
दष्टः शीतोदकेनेव सिक्तान्यङ्गानि मन्यते ॥४८॥

*Poisonous Crab*

If a person is bitten by a *uccițiṅga* (poisonous crab), then there will be horripilation, stiffness and excruciating pain and the patient will feel as if his body is smeared with cold water.

एकदंष्ट्रार्दितः शूनः सरुजः पीतकः सतृट्[५८] ।
छर्दिर्निद्रा च सविषैर्मण्डूकैर्दष्टलक्षणम् ॥४९॥

*Poisonous Frog*

If a person is bitten by one tooth of a poisonous frog, then there will be swelling associated with yellow coloration and pain, morbid thirst and excessive sleep.

मत्स्यास्तु सविषाः कुर्युर्दाहं शोथं रुजं तथा ।
कण्डूं शोथं ज्वरं मूर्च्छां सविषास्तु[९] जलौकसः ॥५०॥

*Poisonous Fish and Leeches*

If stung by a poisonous fish, the person suffers from burning sensation, oedema and pain.

If a person is bitten by a poisonous leech, then he suffers from itching, oedema, fever and fainting.

विदाहं श्वयथुं तोदं स्वेदं च गृहगोधिका ।
दंशे स्वेदं रुजं[१०] दाहं कुर्याच्छतपदीविषम् ॥५१॥

*Poison of House Lizard and Centipede*

Bite of house lizard produces burning sensation, oedema, pricking pain and sweating.

If bitten by a centipede, the person gets perspiration, pain and burning sensation.

कण्डूमान् मशकैरीषच्छोथः स्यान्मन्दवेदनः ।
असाध्यकीटसदृशमसाध्यं मशकक्षतम् ॥५२॥

*Mosquito-Bite*

If bitten by mosquito, a person gets itching, slight swelling and dull pain. If the mosquito is of excessively poisonous type, the bitten person develops those incurable signs and symptoms which are similar to the bite of excessively poisonous insects.

सद्यः प्रस्राविणी श्यावा दाहमूर्च्छाज्वरान्विता ।
पिडका मक्षिकादंशे तासां तु स्थगिकाऽसुहृत्[११] ॥५३॥

### *Bee-Poison*

If a person is stung by bee, then immediately there will be bleeding from the site of the bite, the skin will be grayish black in colour, there will be burning sensation, fainting, fever and papular eruptions. If the bee is of *sthagikā* type, then bitten person succums to death.

चतुष्पद्भिर्द्विपद्भिश्च नखदन्तविषं च यत् ।
शूयते[६२] पच्यते वापि स्रवति ज्वरयत्यपि" ॥५४॥
(माधवनिदान : विषरोग : ६९ : १-५६)

### *Other Poisonous Bites*

Attacks by the claws (nails) and teeth of quadruped and biped animals cause swelling, putrifiction, exudation and fever.

प्रसन्नदोषं[६३] प्रकृतिस्थधातुमन्नाभिकामं[६४] सममूत्रविट्कम्।
प्रसन्नवर्णेन्द्रियचित्तचेष्टं वैद्योऽवगच्छेदविषं मनुष्यम् ॥५५॥
॥ विषनिदानम् ॥

### *Signs of Poison-Free State*

If in the person (who was earlier afflicted by poison) *doṣas* return back to the state of equilibrium, *dhātus* (tissues) become normal, there is desire for food, the person voids urine and stool in normal quantity, the complexion becomes clear, the sensory organs work appropriately, there is happiness of the mind and other physical activities become normal, then the physician should diagnose him as free from poison.

Thus, ends the diagnosis of poisoning.

"स्थावरं[६५] जङ्गमं चैव द्विविधं विषमुच्यते" ।
(सुश्रुत : कल्पस्थान : २ : ३)

"तत्र, क्लीतकाश्वमारगुञ्जासुगन्धगर्गरककरघाट- विद्यु-च्छिखाविजयानीत्यष्टौ मूलविषाणि; विषपत्रिकाल-म्बावरदारुकरम्भमहाकरम्भाणि पञ्चपत्रविषाणि; कुमुद्वतीवेणुकाकरम्भमहाकरम्भ'कर्कोटकरेणुकख

द्योतकचर्मरीभगन्धासर्पघातिनन्दनसारपाकानीति द्वादशफल-
विषाणि; वेत्रकादम्बवल्लीजकरम्भमहाकरम्भाणि पञ्चपुष्पविषाणि;
अन्त्रपाचककर्त्तरीथसौरीयककरघाटकरम्भनन्दननाराचकानि
सप्त त्वक्सारनिर्यासविषाणि; कुमुदघ्नीस्नुहीजालक्षीरीणि
त्रीणि क्षीरविषाणि; फेनाश्मभस्महरितालं च द्वे धातुविषे;
कालकूटवत्सनाभसर्षपकपालककर्दमकवैराटकमुस्तक-
शृङ्गीविषप्रपुण्डरीकमूलकहालाहलमहाविषकर्कटकानीति
त्रयोदश कन्दविषाणि; इत्येवं पञ्चपञ्चाशत् स्थावरविषाणि
भवन्ति ॥५७॥

चत्वारि वत्सनाभानि मुस्तके द्वे प्रकीर्तिते ।
षट् चैव सर्षपाण्याहुः शेषाण्येकैकमेव च" ॥५८॥

(सुश्रुत : कल्पस्थान : २ : ५-६)

"दशाधिष्ठानमाद्यं स्यात् द्वितीयं षोडशाश्रयम् ।
मूलं पत्रं फलं पुष्पं त्वक् क्षीरं सार एव च ।
निर्यासो धातवश्चैव कन्दश्च दशमः स्मृतः" ॥५९॥

(सुश्रुत : कल्पस्थान : २ : ३-४)

॥ इति विषभेदाः ॥

### Enumeration of Sthāvara Poison

Poisons are of two categories, viz., *sthāvara* (derived from inanimate objects) and *jaṅgama* (derived from animals). [This is a repetition of the first line in verse no. 1.]

The former category is further classified into the following groups :

*Mūlaviṣa (Plants whose Roots are Poisonous)*

*Klītaka, aśvamāra, guñjā, sugandha, gargaraka, karaghāṭa, vidyucchikhā* and *vijayā.*

*Patraviṣa (Plants whose Leaves are Poisonous)*

*Viṣapatrikā, lambā, varadāru, karambha* and *mahākarambha.*

*Phalaviṣa (Plants whose Fruits are Poisonous)*

*Kumudvatī, veṇukā, karambha, mahākarambha, karkoṭaka, reṇuka, khadyotaka, carmarī, ibhagandhā, sarpaghātī, nandana* and *sārapāka.*

*Puṣpaviṣa (Plants whose Flowers are Poisonous)*

*Vetra, kādambha, vallīja, karambha* and *mahākarambha.*

*Tvaksāraniryāsaviṣa (Plants whose Barks, Heartwood and Resins are Poisonous)*

*Antrapācaka, karttarītha, saurīyaka, karaghāṭa, karambha, nandana* and *nārācaka.*

*Kṣīraviṣa (Plants whose Latex are Poisonous)*

*Kumudaghnī, snuhī* and *jālakṣīrī.*

*Dhātuviṣa (Poisonous Minerals)*

*Phenāśma* and *haratāla.*

*Kandaviṣa (Plants whose Rhizomes and Tubers are Poisonous)*

*Kālakūṭa, vatsanābha, sarṣapaka, pālaka, karddamaka, vairāṭaka, mustaka, śṛṅgīviṣa, prapuṇḍarīka, mūlaka, hālāhala, mahāviṣa* and *karkaṭaka.*

The above 55 varieties constitute *sthāvaraviṣa* (inanimate substances having poisonous effects).

In the above four varieties of *vatsanābha*, two varieties of *mustaka* and six varieties of *sarṣapa* are described. Others are of one variety each.

*Sthāvaraviṣa* (inanimate substances having poisonous effects) are of ten types as described above, viz., those derived from roots, leaves, fruits, flowers, barks, *kṣīra* (milky-latex), *sāra* (heart-wood), *niryāsa* (resinous exudates), *dhātus* (minerals) and *kanda* (rhizomes and tubers). The *jaṅgamaviṣa* (poisonous animals) are of sixteen types.

Thus, ends the description of different types of poisons.

"मूलं तण्डुलवारिणा पिबति यः प्रत्यङ्गिरासम्भवम्।
निष्पिष्टं शुचिभद्रयोगदिवसे तस्याहिभीतिः कुतः ॥६०॥
दर्पादिव फणी यदा दशति तं मोहान्वितो मूलपम् ।
स्थाने तत्र तदैव[६६] याति नियतं वक्त्रं यमस्याचिरात् ॥६१॥

***Preventive Recipes***

The root of *pratyaṅgirā* (*kaṇṭaki śirīṣa*) should be made to a paste by triturating with *taṇḍulodaka* (rice-wash). If a person takes this paste on an auspicious day having sacred constellations, then he should not be afraid of snakes. If out of arrogance, a hooded snake bites such a person, the former (the snake) immediately succumbs to death.

मसूरं निम्बपत्राभ्यां खादेन्मेषगते रवौ ।
अब्दमेकं न भीतिः स्याद्विषात्तस्य न संशयः" ॥६२॥
(भैषज्यरत्नावली : विषाधिकार : ९)

When the sun is in *meṣarāśi* (Aries sign of the zodiac), one should take *masūra* along with neem leaves. He undoubtedly becomes immuned to snake-bite for one year.

"तण्डुलीयकमूलं[६७] तु पीतं तण्डुलवारिणा ।
तक्षकेणापि दष्टं[६८] च निर्विषं कुरुते नरम् ॥६३॥
(योगरत्नाकर : विषचिकित्सा : पृष्ठ ४६८)

The root of *taṇḍulīyaka* should be made to a paste by triturating with *tandulodaka* (rice-wash). Intake of this paste makes a person immuned to the poison of even *Takṣaka* type of snake.

लज्जावतीमूलविलिप्तं पाणिं बंध्वाथवा ।
तत्र तटीयमूलं गृह्णाति सर्पामतिघोररूपाम्[६९] ॥६४॥
हसन् सर्पणा प्रतिप्रभावः" ॥६५॥

The root of *lajjāvatī* should be made to a paste and applied over the hands. This makes a person immuned to the attacks of extremely venomous types of snakes. Tying the root of *lajjāvatī* in the hand or waste also produces this immunity. [The meaning of some words in this text is not very clear].

"दशंस्योपरि बध्नीयात्[७०] तत्क्षणाच्चतुरंगुले ।
क्षौमादिभिर्वेणिकया सिद्धैर्मंत्रैश्च मंत्रवित्[७१] ।
अंबुवत्सेतुबंधेन बंधेन स्तम्भते विषम्" ॥६६॥
न वहन्ति सिराश्चास्य मर्मसंधिगता अपि ।
न जायते विषाद्वेगो बीजनाशादिवांकुरः ॥६७॥

### *Tying Bandage*

A bandage should be tied on the proximal side (above) of the site of snake-bite leaving a space of four *angulas* (finger breadth). The bandage should be of silk, etc., or *veṇi* (breads of the hair). While tying the bandage, a person who has attained perfection in (reciting) the concerned *mantra* should recite it. By this, the spread of the poison gets arrested as the flow of water in a river gets arrested by the construction of a dam in it.

The blood in the vessels of the afflicted person do not flow even if these are located in the joints and vital organs. Therefore, the spread of the poison to the other parts of the body is arrested and it keeps the person free from poisoning effects like a sprout which does not grow if the seed itself is destroyed.

सत्वमालंब्य दंष्टव्यस्तत्क्षणादुरगो रिपुः ।
केवलं वा यद्यन्यच्च पेयमुष्णं घृतं गवाम् ॥६८॥

### *Biting the Snake*

The bitten person should muster courage and immediately bite the snake (by whom he is bitten) and drink warm cow's ghee alone or mixed with other anti-poison drugs. This makes him free from the poison.

वाच्यो वा नीलकण्ठोऽहं ध्येयं वा गारुडीतनुः ।
शून्यताध्यानमंत्रेण शून्यतां याति तद्विषम् ॥६९॥

### *Mantras, etc.*

He should recite the mantra *"Nīlakaṇṭho'haṃ"* and meditate over the body of *Garuḍa*. He should also recite *Śunyatā mantra* as a result of which he becomes free from poison.

"श्लेष्मणः कर्णगूथस्य वामानामिकया कृतः ।
लेपो हन्याद्विषं घोरं नृमूत्रं सेचनं तथा" ॥७०॥

(भैषज्यरत्नावली : विषाधिकार : १४)

### *Human-Urine*

With the help of the left ring finger saliva or ear-wax should be smeared over the site of the bite and over it human urine should be sprinkled which cures the poison.

“कूलिकामूलनस्येन कालदष्टोऽपि जीवति”[७२] ॥७१॥

(भैषज्यरत्नावली : विषाधिकार : १३)

*Root of Kūlikā*

Root of *Kūlikā* (*viṣatinduka* or *paṭola*) should be made to a paste. By the inhalation of this paste, the person, even if bitten by a deadly snake, survives.

पिण्डीतगरकमूल[७३] पुष्येणोत्पाट्य योजितं दंशे ।
मृतमपि दृष्टं पुरुषं चाल्यतीत्यत्रन्ते[७४] चित्रम् ॥७२॥

*Root of Piṇḍītagara*

Root of *piṇḍītagara* should be collected (uprooted) during *puṣya* constellation and made to a paste. If this is applied over the site of snake bite, even a dead person comes to life and moves. [There are mistakes in this verse.]

“शिरीषपुष्पस्वरसे सप्ताहं[७५] मरिचं सितम् ।
भावितं[७६] सर्पदष्टानां पाननस्याञ्जने[७७] हितम्” ॥७३॥

(भैषज्यरत्नावली : विषाधिकार : १५)

*Śveta Marica*

*Śveta marica* should be impregnated with the juice of *śirīṣa* flower for seven days. Use of this as *pāna* (drinking), *nasya* (inhalation) and *añjana* (collyrium) is useful for curing snake-bite cases.

“नक्तमालफलव्योषबिल्वमूलनिशाद्वयम्[७८-७९] ।
सौरसं पुष्पमाजं च[८०] मूत्रं बोधनमञ्जनम्” ॥७४॥

(भैषज्यरत्नावली : विषाधिकार : ३३)

*Recipe of Collyrium*

*Naktamāla* (fruit), *śuṇṭhī, pippalī, marica*, root of *bilva, haridrā, dāru haridrā* and flower of *surasā* should be made to a paste by triturating with goat's urine. Application of this paste as collyrium revives the consciousness of a patient of snake-bite.

"वन्ध्याकर्कोटकीमूलं[81] छागमूत्रेण भावितम् ।
नस्यं काञ्जिकसम्पिष्टं विषोपहतचेतसः"[82] ॥७५॥

(भैषज्यरत्नावली : विषाधिकार : १७)
(योगरत्नाकर : विषचिकित्सा : पृष्ठ ४६९)

*Vandhyā Karkoṭakī*

Root of *vandhyā karkoṭakī* should be impregnated with goat's urine and made to a paste by triturating with *kāñjī* (vinegar). Inhalation of this paste helps in the revival of the consciousness of a person bitten by the snake.

त्रिवृद्विशालो[83] मधुकं हरिद्रे ।
मंजिष्ठावर्गो लवणं च सर्वम् ॥७६॥
कटुत्रिकं चैव विचूर्णितानि ।
शृंगे निदध्यान्मधुसंयुतानि ॥७७॥
एषोऽगदो हन्त्युपयुज्यमानः ।
पानांजनाभ्यंजननस्ययोगैः ॥७८॥
अवार्यवीर्यो[84] विषवेगहन्ता ।
महागदो नाम महानुभावः ॥७९॥

***Mahāgada***

Powders of *trivṛt, viśālā, madhuka, haridrā, dāru haridrā*, drugs belonging to *Mañjiṣṭhādi varga*, five varieties of *lavaṇa, śuṇṭhī, pippalī* and *marica* should be mixed with honey and stored in a horn. Administration of this in *pāna* (as a drink), *añjana* (collyrium) and *abhyaṅga* (massage) cures acute form of poisoning. This recipe is called *Mahāgada*.

विषे त्वचि गते दंशे स्वेदश्वाससमाकुलम् ।
अर्कमूलमपामार्गफलिनीरक्तचन्दनम् ।
पाययेत् लेपयेन्मंत्री ततः स्वस्थो भवेदयम् ॥८०॥

*Affliction of Rasa Dhātu*

If the poison spreads from the site of the bite to *rasa dhātu*, then the patient gets perspiration and dyspnoea. This patient gets cured by the intake and external application of the paste of *arka* root, *apāmārga, phalinī* and *rakta candana.* Along with this recipe, *mantras* should be recited.

मस्तकवेदना तीव्रा साश्रु चक्षुर्द्वयं भवेत् ।
पक्वजंबूफलाकारा दंता रक्तगते विषे[८५] ॥८१॥
उशीरं चन्दनं रक्तं प्रियंगुं कुंकुमं नखम् ।
पानमालेपनं देयं ततः स लभते सुखम् ॥८२॥

*Affliction of Rakta Dhātu*

If, from the site of the bite, the poison spreads to *rakta dhātu*, then the patient gets acute form of headache; both his eyes become full of tears and his teeth become black like ripe fruits of jamun.

To this patient, *uśīra, rakta candana, priyaṅgu, kuṅkuma* and *nakha* should be given for internal use (drink) and external application. Thus, the patient gets cured.

"कटभ्यर्जुनशैरीयशेलुक्षीरिद्रुमत्वचः ।
कषायकल्कचूर्णाः स्युः कीटलूताविषापहाः"[८६] ॥८३॥

(भैषज्यरत्नावली : विषाधिकार : २८)

*Recipe for Spider-Poison*

The decoction, paste and powder of *kaṭabhi, arjuna, śairīya, śelu* and bark of *kṣīri druma* cure poisons of insects and spiders.

"आगारधूममञ्जिष्ठारजनीलवणोत्तमैः ।
लेपो जयंत्याखुविषं कर्णिकायाश्च पाचनम्"[८७] ॥८४॥

(भैषज्यरत्नावली : विषाधिकार : ३५)

*Recipe for Rat-Poison*

*Āgāradhūma* (house-shoot), *mañjiṣṭhā, haridrā* and *saindhava* should be made to a paste. Application of this cures rat-poison. It also causes suppuration of the *karṇikā* (a growth which takes place at the site of bite; Śivadāsa Sena has interpreted this term as "the sharp edge of the sting").

"यः कासमर्दकं मूलं वदने[८८] निक्षिप्य कर्णफूत्कारम्[८९]।
मनुजो ददाति शीघ्रं जयति विषं वृश्चिकानां सः" ॥८५॥
(भैषज्यरत्नावली : विषाधिकार : ३७)

*Recipes for Scorpion-Poison*

If a person keeps the root of *kāsamarda* in the mouth and blows air at the site of the scorpion-sting, then it insantaneously cures the patient.

पारावतशकृत्शुण्ठीमातुलुङ्गरसैः समैः ।
पथ्या कार्या ससंमिश्रैर्वृश्चिकस्य[९०] विषं जयेत् ॥८६॥

Stool of *pārāvata, śuṇṭhī* and pulp of *harītakī*, taken in equai quantities, should be made to a paste by triturating with the juice of *mātuluṅga*. Application of this paste cures scorpion-poison.

कुबेरकस्य[९१] बीजं तु क्षीरेणार्कस्य भावितम् ।
लेपमात्रे विषं याति वृश्चिकस्य न संशयः ॥८७॥

Seeds of *kuberaka* should be made to a paste by impregnating with the milky-latex of *arka*. Application of this paste cures scorpion poison.

"रजनीसैन्धवक्षौद्रसंयुक्तं घृतमुत्तमम् ।
पानं मूलविषार्त्तस्य दिग्धविद्धस्य[९२] चेष्यते" ॥८८॥
(भैषज्यरत्नावली : विषाधिकार : २१)

***Recipes***

If a person is injured by a weapon smeared with root-poison, then he should drink cow's ghee mixed with *haridrā, saindhava* and honey. He gets cured by this recipe.

'जैपाललेपो[१३] हन्त्याशु[१४] विषं वृश्चिकसंभवम् ॥८९॥

Application of the paste of *jayapāla* instantaneously cures scorpion poison.

नवसारहरितालं समभागान्वितं द्वयम्[१५] ।
ईषत्करञ्जं बीजं तु ताम्बूलैः सह भक्षयेत् ॥९०॥
शतवृश्चिकदष्टोऽपि तत्क्षणाज्जायते सुखम्' ।
चतुष्पद्भिर्द्विपद्भिर्वा नखदंतक्षतं तु यत् ।
सूयते पच्यते वापि स्रवति ज्वालयत्यपि ॥९१॥

*Navasāra* and *haritāla* should be taken in equal quantities and added with small quantity of the powder of *karañja* seed. It should be added to betel leaf and given to the patient to chew. It cures the patient instantaneously even if he is stung by hundreds of scorpions. It also cures injuries caused by the nails and teeth of quadruped and biped animals, even if there is swelling, suppuration, exudation and burning sensation.

"सोमवल्कोऽश्वकर्णश्च गोजिह्वा हंसपद्यपि ।
रजन्यौ गैरिकं लेपो नखदन्तविषापहः" ॥९२॥

(भैषज्यरत्नावली : विषाधिकार : ३६)

Poisoning caused by the nails and teeth of animals gets cured by the application of the paste of *somavalka, aśvakarṇa, gojihvā* and *haṃsapadı.*

"वचाहिङ्गुविडङ्गानि सैन्धवं गजपिप्पली ।
पाठा प्रतिविषाव्योषं काश्यपेन विनिर्मितम् ।
दशाङ्गमगदं पीत्वा सर्वकीटविषं जयेत्" ॥९३॥

(भैषज्यरत्नावली : विषाधिकार : ४६-४७)

***Daśāṅga Agada***

Intake of *vacā, hiṅgu, viḍaṅga, saindhava, gajapippalı, pāṭhā, prativiṣā, śuṇṭhī, pippalī* and *marica* cures all the insect poisons. This is called *Daśāṅga agada* and it was propounded by the sage Kāśyapa.

'दधिमधुनवनीत[१६] पिप्पलीशृंगवेरं
मरिचमपि च दद्यात्तत्सममं सैन्धवेन ।
यदि भवति सरोषतक्षकेनापि दष्टः
गदमह खलु पीत्वा निर्विषस्तत्क्षणेन ॥९४॥

*Recipes*

Curd, honey, butter, *pippalī, śṛṅgavera, marica* and *saindhava* should be taken in equal quantities and triturated. Intake of this potion instantaneously cures a person bitten even by an angry *takṣaka* (a type of celestial snake).

पारावतमलो वंशवल्कलं तालकं शिला ।
हिङ्गुकुक्कुटविष्ठा च कर्णिकारेण संयुता ।
मदनेनान्वितो लेपः सर्वलूताविषापहः ॥९५॥

Stool of *pārāvata*, bark of bamboo, *haratāla, manaḥsilā, hiṅgu*, stool of cock, *karṇikāra* and *madana* should be made to a paste. Application of this paste cures all types of spider-poison.

तण्डुलोदकपरिप्लुतं तथा
मूलमंबुदमवास्य घृताक्तं ।
पीयतानमखिलं च दारुणं
कृत्रिमगरलमाशु हन्ति तत्" ॥९६॥

Root of *mustā* should be impregnated with *taṇḍulodaka* (rice-wash) and mixed with ghee. Intake of this potion cures even serious type of *kṛtrima viṣa* (artificial poison).

"कीटदष्टक्रियाः सर्वाः समाना स्युर्जलौकसाम्" ॥९७॥
(भैषज्यरत्नावली : विषाधिकार : ३१)

Recipes prescribed for the treatment of insect poisoning should also be used for the treatment of poisoning by leeches.

छत्रीजर्जरपाणिश्च चरेद्रात्रौ तथा दिवा ।
तच्छायाशब्दवित्रस्ताः[९७] प्रणश्यन्ति भुजङ्गमाः ॥९८॥

*Use of Umbrella & Walking-Stick*

During day and night, one should walk along with umbrella and walking stick (*jarjara* = a stick which produces jingling sound). Because of their shadow and sound, snakes get scared and disappear.

विषं पित्ते गते पाणिपादौ[९८] पीते च लोचने[९९] ।
दष्टांगलक्षणं ज्ञात्वा नैव तं समुपेक्षयेत्[१००] ॥९९॥

*Pittagata Poison*

If *pitta* gets afflicted by the poison, then the hands and legs of the patient become yellow in colour and his eyes become yellow. In addition, other signs and symptoms of snake-bite will also appear. The patient having such signs should not be neglected.

पूतिगंधमुख[१०१] निद्रा श्वासकासौ निरन्तरम् ।
लालास्रावः स्खलज्जिह्वा विषे श्लेष्मगते भवेत् ॥१००॥
इन्द्रवारुणिका चित्रमार्द्रकत्रिफलान्वितम् ।
कटुकी[१०२]शतपत्रैश्च राजकोशातकीं पिबेत् ॥१०१॥

*Kaphagata Poison*

If *kapha* gets afflicted by the poison, then there will be foul smell in the mouth, excessive sleep, asthma, cough, salivation and stammering. Such a patient should be given the decoction of *indravāruṇī, citraka, ārdraka, harītakī, bibhītaka, āmalakī, kaṭukī, śatapatra* and *rāja kośātakī.*

श्वासो मूर्च्छा मुखं श्यामं गात्रसंकोचनं तथा ।
बुद्धेर्भ्रंशो भवेत्तस्य यस्य वायुगतं[१०३] विषम् ॥१०२॥

पारावताक्षिसंयुक्तं हरितालं मनःशिला ।
पानालेपे कृते दष्टः स्वस्थो भवति तत् क्षणात् ॥१०३॥

*Vāyugata Poison*

If *vāyu* gets afflicted by the poison, then the patient suffers from dyspnoea, fainting, brownish black coloration of the face, cramps in the body and delusion. If the paste prepared of the eyes of *pārāvata, haritala* and *manaḥśilā* is given both for *pāna* (internal use) and *lepa* (external application), the patient becomes normal instantaneously.

प्रणवादित्रिबीजेन नीलकंठेन मन्त्रवित् ।
मन्त्रणाददद्भुतं हन्ति विषं स्थावरजंगमम् ॥१०४॥
'ॐ प्रों त्री ढः[१०४] नीलकण्ठाय नमः स्वाहान्तः प्रणवादिरित्यर्थः' ॥१०५॥

*Mantras*

*Nīlakaṇṭha mantra* along with *praṇava* (*oṃ*) and three *bījas* (seed-letters) should be recited which makes a surprising cure of the patient afflicted by both the *sthāvara* (inanimate) and *jaṅgama* (animate) types of poison.

This *mantra* is "*Oṃ proṃ trī dhaḥ Nīlakaṇṭhāya namaḥ svāhā.*"

ॐ ह्रीं क्लीं हुं क्षूं ठः सर्पमुखबन्धनम् ॥१०६॥

"*Oṃ hrīṃ klīṃ, huṃ kṣūṃ ṭhaḥ.*" If this *mantra* is recited then the snake will not be able to open its mouth, i.e., it will not be able to bite a person.

ॐ हुं ठः ठः । गतिबंधः ॥१०७॥

"*Oṃ huṃ ṭhah ṭhaḥ.*" If this *mantra* is recited then it will arrest the movement of the snake. It will also arrest the spread of the poison from the site of bite.

'ॐ[१०५] ह्रीं क्षीं ठः । सर्पदृष्टिबंधः' ॥१०८॥

"*Oṃ hrīṃ kṣīṃ ṭhaḥ.*" If this *mantra* is recited then the snake will not be able to see through its eyes, i.e. it will become blind.

ॐ नमोऽनन्तहृदयाय धूतः[१०६] हुँ फट् स्वाहा ॥१०९॥
आत्ममुख'स्पर्शादृष्टावेशः[१०७] क्षपय[१०८] स्वाहा ॥११०॥
यत् किंचिदनेनाभिमंत्र्य गृहे क्षिपेत् ॥१११॥

"*Oṃ namo Anantahṛdayāya dhūtaḥ huṃ phaṭ svāhā. Ātmamukhasparśadṛṣṭāveśaḥ kṣapaya svāhā.*" Something like rice should be sanctified with this *mantra* and thrown in the house to prevent snakes coming into it.

ॐ नमो भगवते गरुडाय ठः सुपर्णमहामे'खलाय[१०९] स्वाहा ।
इंद नागस्य मुखबंधश्चक्षुर्बन्धः ॥११२॥
(नागमुखबंधः[११०])

"*Oṃ namo bhagavate Garuḍāya ṭhaḥ suparṇamahāmekhalāya svāhā.*" Recitation of this *mantra* makes a cobra snake incapable of opening its mouth and eyes. By implication, it will not be able to bite or see the prey.

आखुना भक्षितस्याथ नामोच्चार्य्य समुद्धरेत् ।
मार्गधूलिं क्षिपेद्दूरं ततस्तस्य सुखं भवेत् ॥११३॥

If a person is bitten by a poisonous rat, then while uttering the name of the patient, the dust from the road should be thrown at a long distance. This will make the patient free from the poisoning effect.

कटुत्रयं शिग्रुकरञ्जबीजं द्वयं निशायाः कपिकच्छुबीजम् ।
निहन्ति पानेन विलेपनेन विषं समस्तं[१११] गृहगोधिकायाः ॥११४॥

***Recipe for Poison of House-Lizard***

*Śuṇṭhī, pippalī, marica, śigru*, seeds of *karañja, haridrā, dāru haridrā* and seeds of *kapikacchu* should be taken internally [in the form of decoction] and used externally [in the form of paste] which cures poisoning by the bite of house lizard.

केशरं तगरं शुण्ठी मरिचं हि प्रलेपतः ।
मक्षिकाया विषं यद्वा घृतसैन्धवलेपतः ॥११५॥

*Bee-Poison*

Application of either the paste of *keśara, tagara, śunṭhī* and *marica* or ghee mixed with *saindhava* cures poisoning caused by the sting of bees.

वृकव्याघ्रशृगालार्क्षतरक्षुद्वीपिवाजिनाम्[११२] ।
रुधिरं स्रावयेद्दंशे दहेल्लोहशलाकया ॥११६॥

*Animal-Bite*

If a person is bitten by a wolf, tiger, jackal, bear, hyena, leopard or horse, the blood-letting therapy should be administered and *dāha* (cauterisation) should be performed over the site of the bite with the help of a hot iron rod.

धत्तूरस्य रसो दुग्धं पलं[११३] च गुडसर्पिषी ।
कुक्कुरस्य विषं हन्ति पानान्मत्तस्य दुःसहम् ॥११७॥

*Recipe for Mad Dog Bite*

If a person is bitten by a mad dog, then the patient should be given the juice of *dhattūra* (one *pala*) and milk (one *pala*) along with jaggery and ghee. This cures even serious type of such ailment.

कनकस्य फलैर्लेपः सबीजैस्तंडुलाम्भसा ।
'शुनकस्य[११४] विषं हन्ति पानान्मत्तस्य दुःसहम्' ॥११८॥

If a person is bitten by a mad dog, the site of bite should be smeared with the paste of *dhustūra* fruit. He should be given the seeds of *dhustūra* mixed with *taṇḍulāmbu* (rice-wash) to drink which cures even the serious type of such poisoning.

शुनकस्य विषं हन्ति गोजिह्वा मधुनाथ वा ॥११९॥

Intake of *gojihvā* along with honey cures poisoning by mad dog bite.

वटनिम्बशमीवल्ककषायो हन्ति लेपतः ।
निःशेषजीवजातीनां नखदन्तविषं द्रुतम् ॥१२०॥

*Recipes*

Application of the decoction of the barks of *vaṭa, nimba* and *śamī* instantaneously cures the poisoning by the nails and teeth of all animals.

एका वा हन्ति गोजिह्वा निःशेषप्राणिसम्भवम् ।
विंष मधुसमायुक्तं पिष्टं तन्दुलवारिणा ॥१२१॥

Use of *gojihvā* alone also cures poisoning by all types be animal-bite. It should be made to a paste by adding *taṇḍulodaka* (rice-wash) and should be taken along with honey.

'शर्क्कराचूर्णसंयुक्तं'[११५] चूर्णं ताप्यसुवर्णयोः ।
लेहः प्रशमयत्युग्रं सर्वोरगकृतं विषम् ॥१२२॥

***Recipes for Snake Bite***

*Bhasma* of *suvarṇa mākṣika* and *svarṇa* should be added with the powder of sugar and made to a paste. Intake of this cures serious type of poisoning caused by the bite of all types of snake.

नागरं गृहकपोतपुरीषं बीजपूरकरसो हरितालं सैन्धवं च।
विनिहन्ति निश्चितं एष लेप अलिज[११६]गरलं वा ॥१२३॥

Application of the paste of *śuṇṭhī*, stool of *gṛha kapota*, juice of *bījapūraka, haritāla* and *saindhava* undoubtedly cures poisoning by sanke-bite.

काकोदुम्बरिकामूलं धत्तूरकफलान्वितम् ।
पीतं तन्दुलतोयेन सारमेयविषापहम् ॥१२४॥

*Recipe for Mad Dog Bite*

Root of *kākodumbara* and fruit of *dhattūra* should be made to a paste by triturating with *taṇḍulodaka* (rice-wash). Intake of this potion cures poisoning by the bite of a mad dog.

शिरीषबीजैः कुलिशद्रसस्य[११७]
क्षीरेण पिष्टैः कृतलेपनानाम् ।
विषं व्रजत्यस्तमिह क्षणेन
मण्डूकदंशप्रभवं नराणाम् ॥१२५॥

*Recipe for Frog Bite*

Seeds of *śirīṣa* should be made to a paste by triturating with the milky latex of *snuhī*. Application of this paste cures the poisoning caused by the bite of poisonous frog.

कृष्णवेत्रस्य निःक्वाथः कल्को वा घृतमिश्रितम् ।
शृंगीमत्स्यविषं हन्ति बर्हिपत्रेण धूपितम् ॥१२६॥

*Recipe for Sting by Fish*

Poisoning caused by the sting of *śṛṅgī* type of fish is cured by the intake of the paste of decoction of *kṛṣṇa vetra* mixed with ghee. Fumigation with peacock feather also cures this type of poisoning.

अभ्यङ्गं दीपतैलेन दंशे खर्ज्जूरकस्य यः ।
करोति तत्क्षणेनैवविषं कर्षति निश्चितम् ॥१२७॥

If a person is stung by the *kharjūraka* type of scorpion, the affected site should be massaged with *dīpataila* (oil collected from a burning lamp; it is also the name of a recipe). It immediately draws out the poison and there should be no doubt about it.

मरिचं नागरोपेतं सिंधुसौवर्च्चलान्वितम् ।
फणिज्जकरसे हन्याल्लेपनाद्वरटीविषम् ॥१२८॥

*Recipe for Wasp Poison*

*Marica, śuṇṭhī, saindhava* and *sauvarcala* should be made to a paste by triturating with the juice of *phaṇijjhaka*. Application of this paste cures poisoning by sting of the wasp.

द्विवास्वप्नं व्ययामं च व्यवायं क्रोधमातपम् ।
सुरां तिलकपित्थांश्च वर्ज्जयेच्च विषातुरः' ॥१२९॥

*Prohibitions*

The patient suffering from poisoning should avoid sleep during day time, physical exercise, sexual intercourse, anger, exposure to sun ray, alcohol, sessame seeds and *kapittha*.

'विरुद्धाध्यशनक्रोधक्षुद्भयायासमैथुनम्[११] ।
वर्जयेद्विषमुक्तोऽपि दिवास्वप्नं विशेषतः ॥१३०॥

One should avoid *viruddhāśana* (intake of mutually contradictory food), anger, hunger (fasting), fear, strenuous work, sexual intercourse and day-sleep in special even after he is free from the effect of poisoning.

सोत्कम्पः पुलकावृतः प्रतिमुहुर्वक्रां समालोकते ।
दंतेनाधरपल्लवं दशति चेत्सीत्कारवत्कूजति ॥१३१॥
यस्तापं जडतां च याति नितरां दष्टः स उत्कण्ठते।
रन्तुं चास्थिसितामलांबरवन्ती रौद्री श्मशानस्थलीम्' ॥१३२॥

*Signs of Bad Prognosis*

If a poisoned person gets trembling and frequent horripilation, looks to the faces of persons with a fixed gaze, bites his lips with teeth, produces *sīt* or cooing sounds, becomes hot and stiff frequently and expresses anxiety, then he is destined to play with *raudris* having garlands of bones and white apparel in a crematorium, i.e. he succumbs to death.

अथ विषयुक्तान्नपानपरीक्षा लिख्यते राज्ञां तद्भूयादेव ॥१३३॥

### *Characteristics of Poisoned Food and Drinks*

Kings (rulers) should take appropriate precautionary measures against the administration of poisoned food and drinks; hence their examination methods are now being described.

"रिपवो विक्रमाक्रान्ता ये च स्वे[१२०] कृत्यतां गताः।
सिसृक्षवः क्रोधविषं विवरं प्राप्य तादृशम् ॥१३४॥
विषैर्निहन्युर्निपुणं नृपतिं दुष्टचेतसः।
स्त्रियो वा विविधान् योगान् कदाचित्सुभगेच्छया ॥१३५॥
विषकन्योपयोगाद्वा क्षणाज्जह्यादसून्नरः ।
तस्माद्वैद्येन सततं विषाद्रक्ष्यो नराधिपः[१२२] ॥१३६॥

When the enemy gets attacked by a powerful opponent, then the former out of anger search for loopholes to take revenge and mischievously adopt the method of secretly poisoning the powerful king to achieve his objectives. Similarly, ladies with a desire to get endowed with good fortune administer various things along with food to men-folk. Enemies also employ *viṣakanyā* (a beautiful young girl whose body is poisoned by the gradual administration of small doses of poisons; she herself remains free from the poisoning effect but the king who embraces her out of lust gets this effect) who causes instantaneous death of the opponent. Therefore, the physician should constantly protect the king from these various types of poisons.

यस्माच्च चेतोऽनित्यत्वमश्ववत् प्रथितं[१२३] नृणाम्[१२४]।
न विश्वसेत् तस्माद्राजा कदाचिदपि कस्यचित् ॥१३७॥

It is very difficult to control the human mind as it runs in different directions like a horse. Therefore, the king should never believe any body in any situation.

'अथ[१२५] योग्यवैद्य का विश्वास'

कुलीनं धार्मिकं स्निग्धं सुभृतं सततोत्थितम् ॥
अलुब्धमशठं भक्तं कृतज्ञं प्रियदर्शनम् ।
क्रोधपारुष्यमात्सर्यमायालस्यविवर्जितम् ॥१३८॥
'अध्यक्ष[१२६] कुर्यादिति शेषः' ॥१३९॥

*Characteristics of a Suitable Physician*

The king should put faith on a suitable physician having the following attributes :

(1) He should belong to a noble family;
(2) he should be religious minded, soft spoken, financially well-up and constantly attentive;
(3) he should not be greedy and treacherous;
(4) he should be loyal, greateful and pleasing in appearance;
(5) he should be free from anger; rustic behaviour, jealousy, deceptiveness and indolence.

Such a physician should be appointed as the Chief to protect the King.

जितेन्द्रियं क्षमावन्तं शुचिं[१२७]शीलदयान्वितम् ।
मेधाविनमसंभ्रान्तमनुरक्तं हितैषिणम् ॥१४०॥
पटुं प्रगल्भं निपुणं दक्षमालस्यवर्जितम्[१२८] ।
पूर्वोक्तैश्च गुणैर्युक्तं नित्यं सन्निहितागदम् ।
महानसे प्रयुञ्जीत[१२९] वैद्यं तद्विद्यपूजितम्[१३०] ॥१४१॥

*Chief Superviser of King's Kitchen*

The King should appoint a physician to supervise the kitchen and he should be endowed with the following attributes :

(1) He should have control over his senses;
(2) he should have the patience to forgive others;
(3) he should be clean, of good conduct and kind;
(4) he should be intelligent, he should not be confused and should be loyal;
(5) he should be the well-wisher of the king;

(6) he should be expert, efficient, experienced and proficient;
(7) he should be free from laziness and should be endowed with other attributes described in verse-138 above;
(8) he should be constantly keeping medicines with him; and
(9) he should be enjoying respect of other professional colleagues.

प्रशस्तदिग्देशकृतं[१३१] शुचिभाण्डं महच्छुचिः[१३२] ।
सजालकं गवाक्षाढ्यमात्मवर्गनिषेवितम्[१३३] ॥१४२॥
विकक्षसृष्टसंसृष्टं सवितानं कृतार्चनम् ।
परीक्षितस्त्रीपुरुषं भवेच्चापि महानसम् ।
तत्राध्यक्षं नियुञ्जीत प्रायो वैद्यं गुणान्वितम् ॥१४३॥

*Kitchen*

The kitchen should be located on an auspicious direction in an auspicious land. The vessels inside the kitchen should be clean. The kitchen should be specious and clean. It should have several windows fixed with wire-nets. It should have access to only family members of the king. It should have attached and adjecent rooms. It should have canopies. Prayers should be offered to fire-god in this kitchen regularly. Male and female employed in the kitchen should be properly scrutinised. The superviser of this kitchen should be a physician having appropriate qualities.

शुचयो दक्षिणा दक्षा विनीताः प्रियदर्शनाः[१३४] ।
संविभक्ताः[१३५] सुमनसो नीचकेशनखाः स्थिराः ॥१४४॥
स्नाताः दृढाः संयमिनः कृतोष्णीषाः सुसंयताः ।
तस्य चाज्ञा[१३६] विधेयाः स्युर्विविधाः परिकर्म्मिणः ॥१४५॥

*Kitchen Attendants*

Attendants in the kitchen should be clean, well disposed, experts, humble, pleasing in complexion, well categorised (experts in different types of work), of happy mind, having pruned hair and nails, regular, should be taking regular bath, strong, self-controlled, well turbaned and well disciplined. They should be obedient to the physician and should work according to his directions.

आहारस्थितयश्चापि भवन्ति प्राणिनो यतः ।
तस्मान्महानसे वैद्यः प्रमादरहितो भवेत् ॥१४६॥

*Need for Care*

The life of living beings is dependant upon the food. Therefore, the physician appointed to supervise the kitchen work should be very careful not to commit any mistake.

माहानसिकवोढारः सौपौदनिकपौपिकाः[१३७] ।
भवेयुर्वैद्यवशगा ये चाप्यन्येऽत्र[१३८] केचन" ॥१४७॥

(सुश्रुत : कल्पस्थान : १ : ४-१८)

*Subordination to Physician*

Cooks, kitchen assistants, persons engaged in cooking special items like rice, dals, cakes, and such other employees in the kitchen should be subordinate to and should obey the orders of the physician.

"केचिद्ब्रूयात् पार्थिवस्य त्वरिता वा तदाज्ञया ।
असतामपि सन्तोऽपि चेष्टां कुर्वन्ति मानवाः ॥
तस्मात् परीक्षणं कार्यं भृत्यानामादितो नृपैः ॥१४८॥

*Proper Scrutiny of Employees*

At times, even noble employees out of fear or in hurry to carry out the orders of the King exhibit irresponsibility. Therefore, at the time of appointment the King should get them examined very carefully.

अथ[१३९] विष अधिष्ठान-

अन्ने[१४०] पाने दन्तकाष्ठे तथाऽभ्यङ्गेऽवलेखने ।
उत्सादने कषाये च परिषेकेऽनुलेपने ॥१४९॥
स्रक्षु वस्त्रेषु शय्यासु कवचाभरणेषु च ।
पादुकापादपीठेषु पृष्ठेषु गजवाजिनाम् ॥१५०॥
विषजुष्टेषु[१४१] चान्येषु नस्यधूमाञ्जनादिषु ।
लक्षणानि प्रवक्ष्यामि चिकित्सामप्यनन्तरम् ॥१५१॥

### *Modes of Administering Poison*

Poisons can be administered to a person through his food, drinks, toothbrush (twig for brushing teeth), massage oil, combs, pastes of unction, decoctions, *pariṣeka* (water used for sprinkling over the body or bathing water), *anulepana* (pastes of aromatic items used for external application), garlands, apparel, beds, *kavaca* (mystic amulets or jackets used for potection), foot-wear, *pādapiṭha* (wooden pedestals), backs of elephants and horses, *nasya* (drugs used for inhalation), fumigation and collyriums and such other items. The enemy makes these items added with poisons. Characteristic features of such poisoned items will first be described. This will follow their treatment.

'अथ विषयुक्तभोजनपरीक्षा'

नृपभक्ताद्बलिं न्यस्तं सविषं भक्षयन्ति ये ।
तत्रैव[१४३] ते विनश्यन्ति मक्षिका वायसादयः ॥१५२॥
हुतभुक् तेन चान्नेन भृशं चटचटायते ।
'मयूरकण्ठप्रतिमो'[१४४] जायते चापि दुःसहः ।
'भिन्नार्चिस्तीक्ष्णधूमश्च'[१४५] न चिराच्चोपशाम्यति' ॥१५३॥
चकोरस्याक्षिवैराग्यं जायते क्षिप्रमेव तु ।
दृष्टाऽन्नं[१४६] विषसंसृष्टं म्रियन्ते जीवजीवकाः ॥१५४॥
कोकिलः[१४७] स्वरवैकृत्यं क्रौञ्चस्तु मदमृच्छति ।
हृष्येन्मयूरस्तूद्विग्नः[१४८] क्रोशतः शुकसारिके ॥१५५॥
हंसः[१४९] क्ष्वेडति चात्यर्थं भृङ्गराजस्तु कूजति ।
पृषतो विसृजत्यश्रुं विष्टां मुञ्चति मर्कटः ॥१५६॥
सन्निकृष्टांस्ततः कुर्याद्राज्ञस्तान् मृगपक्षिणः ।
वेश्मनोऽथ विभूषार्थं रक्षार्थं चात्मनः सदा ॥१५७॥

### *Examination of Poisoned Food*

Before the King takes his food, a portion of it is offered as *bali* (sacrifice). If the food is poisoned, then flies, crows, etc., who will eat this *bali* (sacrificed food) will die then and there. When this *bali* (sacrificial food) is offered to fire, there will be excessive crackling noise and its intolerably hot flame looks dark blue like the throat of a peacock. The flame will be scattared into different directions; the smoke coming out of the fire will be exceedingly pungent and it will take a long time to subside. If this food is given to a *cakora* bird, then just by seeing it, there will be instantaneous discoloration of its eyes. If a *jīvajīvaka* bird sees this poisoned food, then it succumbs to death. Seeing the poisoned food, the voice of the Koel bird becomes distorted, the *krauñca* bird gets intoxicated the peacock gets excited and irritated, parrots and myna birds produce quarelling noise, swan produces hoarse voice, *bhṛṁgarāja* bird produces kooing sound, *pṛṣata* produces tears and monkies void stool. Therefore, the king should keep these birds and animals near him. This helps in the decoration of the palace and protection of himself (King).

(अथ परोसे भोजन में विष परीक्षा)[१५०]
उष्णक्षिप्रस्य चान्नस्य वाष्पेणोर्ध्वं प्रसर्पता ।
हृत्पीडा भ्रान्तनेत्रत्वं[१५१] शिरोदुःखं च जायते ॥१५८॥

*Examination of Served Food*

If the poisoned food is already served to the King, then the steam that will come out of this hot food will cause cardiac pain, irritation in the eyes and headache.

तत्र नस्याञ्जने कुष्ठं लामज्ज[१५२] नलदं मधु ।
कुर्याच्छिरीषरजनीचन्दनैश्च प्रलेपनम् ॥१५९॥

*Management of the Poisoning*

The poisoning effects of the served food should be treated by the administration of the appropriate *nasya* (inhalation therapy) and *añjana* (application of medicated collyrium). For these therapies *kuṣṭha, lāmajjaka, nalada* and honey should be used. His body should be anointed with the paste of *śirīṣa, haridrā* and *candana*.

'हृदि[१५३] चन्दनैश्च प्रलेपनम्' ।
हृदि चन्दनलेपस्तु तथा सुखमवाप्नुयात् ॥१६०॥

### *Application of Sandal-Wood Paste*

Application of the sandal-wood paste in the cardiac region gives comfort to the patient suffering from food-poisoning.

पाणिप्राप्तं पाणिदाहं नखशातं[१५४] करोति च ।
अत्र[१५५] प्रलेपः श्यामेन्द्रगोपसोमोत्पलानि च ॥१६१॥

### *Touch of Poisoned Food*

If the person has already touched the poisoned food (as a prelude to eating), then there will be burning sensation in the hand and his nails get shrivelled. To treat such a patient, the paste of *śyāmā, indragopa, soma* and *utpala* should be applied.

(अथ[१५६] ग्रासविषपरीक्षा)

स चेत् प्रमादान्मोहाद्वा तदन्नमुपसेवते ।
अष्ठीलावत्ततो[१५७] जिह्वा भवत्यरसवेदिनी ॥१६२॥
तुद्यते दह्यते चापि श्लेष्मा चास्यात् प्रसिच्यते[१५८] ।
तत्र वाष्पेरितं[१५९] कर्म यच्च स्याद् दान्तकाष्ठिकम्[१६०] ॥१६३॥

### *Intake of Poisoned Food*

If by mistake or ignorance, he takes the poisoned food, then the tongue becomes hard like a stone and there will be no gustatory sensation. There will be pricking pain and burning sensation in the tongue and there will be excessive salivation. In such an event, therapies prescribed for inhaling poisoned steam and using poisoned *dantakāṣṭha* (twig used for brushing teeth) should be administered.

(आमाशयगतविषलक्षण[१६१])

मूर्छां छर्दिमतीसारमाध्मानं[१६२] दाहवेपथुः[१६३] ।
इन्द्रियाणां च वैकृत्यं कुर्यादामाशयं गतम् ॥१६४॥
तत्राशु[१६४] मदनालाबुबिम्बीकोशातकीफलैः ।
छर्दनं दध्युदश्विद्भ्यामथवा तण्डुलाम्बुना ॥१६५॥

### *Poisoned Food in Stomach*

If the poisoned food has already reached the stomach, then there will be fainting, vomiting, diarrhoea, flatulence, burning sensation, trembling and morbidity of sense organs. Such a patient should be immediately administered emetic therapy with the help of the fruits of *madana, alābu, bimbī* and *kośātakī* mixed with curd, buttermilk or *taṇḍulodaka* (rice-wash).

(पक्वाशयगतविषलक्षण[१६५])

दाहं मूर्च्छामतीसारं तृष्णामिन्द्रियवैकृतिम् ।
आटोपं पाण्डुतां कार्श्यं[१६६] कुर्यात् पक्वाशयं गतम् ॥१६६॥
'विरेचन[१६७] ससर्पिष्कं तत्रोक्तं नीलिनीफलम्' ।
दध्ना[१६८] दूषीविषारिश्च पेयो[१६९] मधुसमायुतः ॥१६७॥

### *Poisoned Food on Colon*

If the poisoned food has already reached the colon, then the patient suffers from burning sensation, fainting, diarrhoea, morbid thirst, morbidity of sense organs, abdominal distension, anemia and emaciation. To such a patient, purgation therapy with the help of *nīlinī* fruit mixed with ghee should be administered. Curd mixed with *Dūṣīviṣāri* (name of a recipe) and honey should be given to the patient.

(अथ पेयपदार्थविषपरीक्षा)

द्रवद्रव्येषु सर्वेषु क्षीरमद्योदकादिषु ।
भवन्ति विविधा राज्यः फेनबुद्बुदजन्म च" ॥१६८॥

(सुश्रुत : कल्पस्थान : १ : २३-४४)

### *Examination of Poisoned Drinks*

If poison is added to milk, alcohol and such other liquids used as drinks, then net-work of different colours, froth and bubbles will appear in such drinks.

नीला राजी रसे ताम्रा क्षीरे दधिनि दृश्यते।
श्यावा पीता सिता तक्रे घृते पानीयसन्निभा ॥१६९॥

मस्तुऽन्यपि कपोताभा राजी कृष्णा च सूदके[१७०]।
काली[१७१] मद्ये तथा क्षौद्रे हरित्तैलेऽरुणोपमा ॥१७०॥

If poison is added to fruit juice, then blue lines will appear over it; if added to milk or curd, then coppery coloured lines will appear; if added to butter-milk, then grayish, yellowish or blackish lines will appear; if added to ghee, then watery lines will appear; if added to *mastu* (thin butter-milk) then brownish (like dove) coloured lines will appear; if added to lentil-soup, then black coloured lines will appear; if added to alcoholic drinks, then balck lines will appear; if added to honey, then green coloured lines will appear; and if poison is added to oil, then reddish coloured lines will appear over its surface.

द्रव्याणामार्द्रशुष्काणां वैपरीत्यं च जायते ।
'मृदूनां कठिनानां च भवेत्स्पर्शविपर्ययः' ॥१७१॥

If poison is added to dry substance, then it will be wet and if it is added to a wet substance; then it will be dry. Similarly, if poison is added to a soft substance it will become hard to touch and if it is added to hard substance, then the latter will become hard to touch. Thus poison added substances will have opposite attributes.

"छायाश्चात्र न दृश्यन्ते यदि वा दृश्यन्ते पुनः ।
भवन्ति यमलाश्छिद्रास्तन्व्यो[१७२] वा विकृतास्तथा ॥१७२॥

If poison is added to a liquid (transparent) substance, then shadow will not be visible in it and even if it is visible, then there will be double shadow or there will be holes in the shadow or the shadow will either be thin or distorted.

शाकसूपान्नमांसानि क्लिन्नानि विरसानि च ।
'सद्यः[१७३] पर्युषितानीव विगन्धानि भवन्ति[१७४] च ॥१७३॥

*Poisoned Vegetables, etc.*

Poisoned vegetables, dals, boiled cereals and meat become sticky and tasteless. They will look stale even if freshly collected and foul smell comes out of these substances.

गन्धवर्णरसैर्हीनाः सर्वे भक्ष्याः फलानि च' ।
पक्वान्याशु विशीर्यन्ते पाकमामानि यान्ति च ॥१७४॥

*Poisoned Fruits*

When poisoned, all the edible fruits lose their smell, colour and taste. The ripe ones get immediately shrivelled and the green ones get ripened quickly.

(अथ[१७५] दातौनविषपरीक्षा)
विशीर्यते कूर्चकस्तु दन्तकाष्ठगते विषे।
'जिह्वादन्तौष्ठमांसानां[१७६] श्वयथुश्चोपजायते[१७७] ॥१७५॥
अथास्य धातकीपुष्पपथ्याजम्बूफलास्थिभिः' ।
सक्षौद्रैः प्रच्छिते[१७८] शोफे कर्त्तव्यं प्रतिसारणम् ॥१७६॥
अथवाऽङ्कोठमूलानि त्वचः सपृछदस्य वा ।
शिरीषसिन्दुवार[१७९] वा सक्षौद्रं प्रतिसारणम् ॥१७७॥

*Poisoned Dantakāṣṭha*

If the twig used for brushing teeth is poisoned, then the brush of the twig will get shrivelled. By brushing with the help of such a twig, there will be oedema in the tongue, teeth and lips. The swollen muscles of such a patient should be scratched and the powder of *dhātakī* flower, *harītakī*, seed pulp of *jambū*, etc., should be rubbed over it. Alternatively, the powder of the root of *aṅkoṭha* and bark of *saptacchada, śirīṣa* or *sinduvāra* mixed with honey should be rubbed over the oedematous tongue, etc.

जिह्वानिर्लेखकवलौ दन्तकाष्ठवदादिशेत् ॥१७८॥

*Poisoned Tongue-Scraper*

If a tongue-scraper or *kavala* (decoction of drugs used for gargling) is poisoned, then signs of poisoned tooth brush will appear and therapies described above should be administered.

(अथ[180] अभ्यङ्गगतविषलक्षण)

पिच्छिलो बहुलोऽभ्यङ्गो विवर्णश्च विषान्वितः ।
स्फोटजन्मरुजास्रावत्वक्पाकः स्वेद[181] एव च ॥१७९॥
दरणं चापि मांसानामभ्यङ्गे विषदूषिते[182] ।
तत्र शीताम्बुसिक्तस्य कर्त्तव्यमनुलेपनम् ॥१८०॥
चन्दनं तगरं कुष्ठमुशीरं वेणुपत्रिका ।
सोमवल्यमृता श्वेता पद्मं कालीयकं त्वचम्[183] ।
कपित्थरसमूत्राभ्यां[184] पानमेतच्च[185] युज्यते ॥१८१॥
उत्सादने परिषेके कषाये चानुलेपने[186] ।
शय्यावस्त्रतनुत्रेषु ज्ञेयमभ्यङ्गलक्षणैः[187] ॥१८२॥

*Poisoned Massage Oil*

If the massage oil is poisoned, it will be slimy, thick and discoloured. If massage is performed with such oil, then eruptions will appear over the skin, there will be pain, exudation and suppuration of the skin, and there will be profuse sweating and cracking of the muscle tissue. Such a patient should be sprinkled with cold water and his skin should be anointed with the paste of *candana, tagara, kuṣṭha, uśīra, veṇupatrika, somavallī, amṛtā, śvetā, padma, kālīyaka* and *tvak*. He should be given the juice of *kapittha* and cow's urine to drink.

*Poisoned Unction, etc.*

If *utsādana* (unction), *pariṣeka* (water used for sprinkling or bath), *kaṣāya* (drugs used for tanning nails & skin), *anulepana* (drugs used for external application), *śayyā* (bed), *vastra* (cloth) and *tanutra* (mystic amulet or protecting jacket) are poisoned, then the signs similar to those of poisoned massage oil will appear and similar treatment should be adopted.

केशशातः शिरोदुःखं खेभ्यश्च रुधिरागमः ।
ग्रन्थिजन्मोत्तमाङ्गेषु च विषजुष्टेऽवलेखने ॥१८३॥
तत्र प्रलेपो बहुशो भाविताः कृष्णमृत्तिकाः ।
ऋष्यपित्तघृतश्यामापालिन्दीतण्डुलीयकैः ॥१८४॥

गोमयस्य[१८८] रसो वाऽपि हितो वा मालतीरसः ।
रसो मूषिकपर्ण्या वा धूमो वाऽगारसंभवः ॥१८५॥

*Poisoned Comb*

Poisoned comb causes hairfall headache, bleeding from the orifices and appearance of nodules in the head. Black-mud frequently impregnated with *ṛṣyajihva*, ghee, *śyāmā*, *pālindī* and *taṇḍulīyaka* should be applied over the head. Application of the juice extracted from cow-dung or *mālatī* or *mūṣikaparṇī* is also useful in this condition. Application of the house-shoot is also useful in such cases.

शिरोभ्यङ्गः शिरस्त्राणं स्नानमुष्णीषमेव च ।
स्रजश्च विषसंसृष्टाः साधयेदवलेखनात् ॥१८६॥

*Poisoned Śirobhyaṅga, etc.*

If *śirobhyaṅga* (oil used for the massage of head), *śirastrāṇa* (umbrella), *snāna* (bath water), *uṣṇīṣa* (turban) and garland are poisoned, then signs similar to those of comb poisoning will appear, and the treatment prescribed above for comb-poisoning should be adopted.

मुखालेपे मुखं श्यावं युक्तमभ्यङ्गलक्षणैः[१८९] ।
पद्मिनीकण्टकप्रख्यैः कण्टकैश्चोपचीयते ॥१८७॥
तत्र क्षौद्रघृतपानं प्रलेपश्चन्दनं घृतम् ।
पयस्या मधुकं फञ्जी बन्धुजीवः पुनर्नवा ॥१८८॥

*Poisoned Mukhālepa*

If the unguent applied over the face is poisoned, the face becomes grayish black in colour and other signs similar to those of poisoned massage oil appear. The face becomes shrouded with pointed pimples of the nature of *padminīkaṇṭaka*. To such patients, honey and ghee should be administered and over his face the paste of sandal-wood, ghee, *payasyā*, *madhuka*, *phañjī*, *bandhujīva* and *punarnavā* should be applied.

अस्वास्थ्यं कुञ्जरादीनां लालास्रावोऽक्षिरक्तता ।
तत्राभ्यङ्गवदेवोक्ता यानवाहनयोः क्रिया ॥१८९॥

***Poisoning Elephants, etc.***

If the backs of elephants, etc., are poisoned, then that affects the health of the animal, more of saliva comes out of their mouth and their eyes become red. The person who rides on such poisoned animals suffers from pustular eruptions in the hips, anus, penis, scrotum and related joints. Therapies prescribed for poisoned massage oil should also be followed in this connection.

शोणितागमनं खेभ्यः शिरोरुक्कफसंस्रवः ।
'नस्यधूमगते'[१९०] लिङ्गमिन्द्रियाणां च वैकृतम् ॥१९०॥
तत्र दुग्धैर्गवादीनां सर्पिः सातिविषैः शृतम्' ।
पांने नस्ये च संस्वेदं हितं समदयन्तिकम्[१९१] ॥१९१॥

***Poisoned Nasya, etc.***

If the snuff and cigarettes are poisoned, then the person suffers from bleeding from orifices, headache, exudation of phlegm in excess and impairment of the functioning of sense organs. To such patients, ghee boiled with cow's milk and *ativiṣā* should be administered internally and used for inhalation therapy. Fomentation with *madayantikā* is useful in this condition.

गंधहानिर्विवर्णत्वं पुष्पाणां म्लानता भवेत् ।
जिघ्रतश्च शिरोदुःखं वारिपूर्णे च लोचने ।
तत्र वाष्पेरितं कर्म मुखालेपे च यत् स्मृतम्॥१९२॥

***Poisoned Flower***

If the flower is poisoned, then it loses its aroma, becomes discolored and feds away quickly. Smell of such a poisoned flower causes headache and lachrymation. Such patients should be treated on the lines suggested for poisoned gases and poisoned *mukhālepa* (paste of drugs anointed over the face).

(अथ[१९२] कर्णतैलविष)

कर्णतैलगते श्रोत्रवैगुण्यं शोफवेदने ।
कर्णस्रावश्च तत्राशु कर्त्तव्यं प्रतिपूरणम् ॥१९३॥

स्वरसो बहुपुत्रायाः सघृतः क्षौद्रसंयुतः ।
सोमवल्करसो 'वाऽपि सुशीतो'[१९३] हित इष्यते ॥१९४॥

*Poisoned Ear-Drop*

Use of poisoned *karṇa taila* (medicated oil used as ear drop) causes impairment in hearing, swelling and pain in the ears and exudation of pus from the ear. To such a patient, medicated oils should be given as ear drop. The juice of *bahuputrā* along with ghee and honey is useful. Cooled juice of *somavalka* is also useful for such patients.

अश्रूपदेहो दाहश्च 'वेदना'[१९४] दृष्टिविभ्रमः ।
अञ्जने विषसंसृष्टे भ'वेदान्ध्यमथापि च ॥१९५॥
तत्र सद्यो घृतं पेयं तर्पणं च समागधम् ।
अञ्जनं मेषशृङ्गस्य'[१९५] निर्यासो वरुणस्य च ॥१९६॥
मुष्ककस्याजकर्णस्य फेनो गोपित्तसंयुतः ।
कपित्थमेषशृङ्गचोश्च पुष्पं भल्लातकस्य च ।
एकैकं कारयेत् पुष्पं बन्धूकाङ्कोठयोरपि ॥१९७॥

*Poisoned Collyrium*

If the collyrium is poisoned, then the person using such collyrium may become blind. Such a person should be given freshly prepared ghee along with *pippalī* to drink. The juices of *meṣaśṛṅga, varuṇa, muṣkaka* and *arjaka* should be mixed with *samudra phena* and *gorocanā* and used as collyrium. Similarly, collyrium should be prepared of the flowers of either *kapittha, meṣaśṛṅgī, bhallātaka, bandhūka* or *aṅkoṭha* and applied over the eyes.

शोथः स्रावस्तथा स्वापः पादयोः स्फोटजन्म च ।
भवन्ति विषजुष्टाभ्यां पादुकाभ्यामसंशयम् ॥१९८॥
'उपानत्पादपीठानि'[१९६] पादुकावत् प्रसाधयेत्' ॥१९९॥

*Poisoned Foot-Wear*

By wearing poisoned foot-wear, a person undoubtedly suffers from oedema, exudation, numbness and pustular eruptions in the feet. Similar signs appear if the shoes and wooden pedestal are poisoned.

भूषणानि हतार्चींषि न विभान्ति यथा पुरा।
स्वानि स्थानानि हन्युश्च दाहपाकावदारणैः ॥२००॥

*Poisoned Ornaments*

If poisoned, ornaments lose their glaze and they do not appear as before. The person wearing such poisoned ornaments gets burning sensation, suppuration and cracks in the sites where these are used.

पादुकाभूषणेपूक्तमभ्यङ्गविधिमाचरेत् ॥२०१॥

To get rid of the poisoning effects of foot-wears and ornaments, one should use medicated oil for massage.

विषोपसर्गो वाष्पादिर्भूषणान्तो य ईरितः ।
उपद्रवांस्तत्र[१९१] वीक्ष्य विदधीत चिकित्सितम्" ॥२०२॥
(सुश्रुत : कल्पस्थान : १ : ४५-७६)

*Treatment of Complications*

Complications which arise because of the poisoned ingredients beginning with poisoned steam (vide verse no. 158) and ending with poisoned ornaments (vide verse no. 201) should be carefully ascertained and their treatment should be performed.

"मूषिकाऽजरुहा वाऽपि हस्ते बद्धा तु भूपतेः ।
करोति निर्विषं सर्वमन्नं विषसमायुतम्" ॥२०३॥
(सुश्रुत : कल्पस्थान : १ : ७८-७९)

*Antidote for Poisoned Food*

If the King uses the amulet of *mūṣikā* (name of a plant) and *ajaruhā* in his hand, then this makes the poisoned food nontoxic.

"विषघ्नानि च सेवेत भक्ष्यभोज्यानि बुद्धिमान् ।
पिप्पलीमधुकक्षौद्रशर्करेक्षुरसाम्बुभिः ।
छर्दयेद्रुप्रहृदयः[१९८] प्राश्नीयाद् यदि वै विषम्" ॥२०४॥

(सुश्रुत : कल्पस्थान : १ : ८४-८५)

The wise person should take eatable food by adding antidotes to keep him free from any such possible poisoning effects. If it comes to his knowledge that he has already consumed poisoned food, then he should take such measures as to protect his heart, and thereafter, take emetic therapy consisting of *pippalı, madhuka*, honey, sugar, sugarcane juice and water.

युक्तसेनस्य नृपते परानभिजिगीषतः[१९९] ।
भिषजा रक्षणं कार्यं यदा तदुपदेक्ष्यते ॥२०५॥

*Protection of King*

When the King along with his soldiers invades an enemy, then the physician should protect him by the prescribed measures.

विजिगीषुः सहामात्यैर्यात्रा युक्तः प्रयत्नतः ।
रक्षितव्यो विशेषेण विषादेव नराधिपः ॥२०६॥

When the King, along with his Ministers, proceedes on a war for victory, the physician should be very careful to specially protect the King from poisons.

पंथानमुदकं छायां भक्तं यवसमिंधनम्[२००] ।
दूषयंत्यरयस्तस्माज्जानीयाच्छोधयेद्भिषक् ॥२०७॥

The physician should be well aware of the fact that in the path of his war journey, enemies specially arrange to poison the road, water by the side of the journey path, shades of trees where the King and his retinue are likely to take rest, food, animals and fuel. The physician should take measures to purify all these poisons by antidotes.

एकोत्तरं मृत्युशतमथर्व्वाणि प्रचक्षते ।
तत्रैकः काल संयुक्तः[201] शेषास्त्वागंतवः स्मृताः ॥२०८॥

*Types of Death*

According to the *Atharvānas* (followers of the *Atharva veda*), there are one hundred and one modes of death. One of these varieties of death is *kālamṛtyu* (timely death) and the remaining one hundred varieties are untimely death which are caused by extraneous factors (*āgantavaḥ*).

दोषागंतुनिमित्तेभ्योः[202] रसमन्त्रविशारदौ ।
रक्षेतां नृपतिं नित्यमन्नैर्वैद्यपुरोहितौ[203] ॥२०९॥

The King should always be protected from both these types of death, viz., *doṣaja* (caused by the vitiated *doṣas*) and *āgantuja* (caused by the extraneous factors). For this purpose, the physician who is proficient in the knowledge of different types of drugs (*rasa*) and food ingredients (*anna*) and the priest who is proficient in the practice of *mantras* should be held responsible.

ब्रह्मा वेदांगमष्टांगमायुर्वेदमभाषत ।
तस्मात्पुरोहितमते वर्त्तेत भिषगात्मवान् ॥२१०॥

*Priest and Physician*

Ayurveda having eight specialized branches, is one of the *aṅgas* (limbs) of the Vedas, and it was propounded by the Lord Brahmā. Therefore, the practitioner of Ayurveda, i.e. the physician should be self-controlled and act according to the instructions of the priest (who is proficient in the practice of the Vedic *mantras*).

सङ्करः सर्ववर्णानां प्रणाशोऽधर्मकर्मणाम् ।
प्रजानामपि चोच्छित्तिः नृपव्यसनहेतुतः ॥२११॥

*King's Luxury*

It is because of the King's indulgence in the luxury of life and paying scant attention to the welfare of his subjects then *saṅkaras* (mixed-breed offsprings) take birth from the consumation of men and women belonging to different castes. This irreligious act which is sinful leads to the anihilation of the society and destruction of the people (subjects) in the kingdom.

पुरुषाणां नृपाणां च केवलं तुल्यमूर्त्तिता ।
राज्ञां त्यागः क्षमा धैर्यं विक्रमश्चाप्यमानुषः ॥२१२॥

*King and Ordinary Man*

Both the King and the ordinary man in his state are physically similar. The only difference between them is that the King has a special designation, he can sacrifice, he exercises forbearance and he demonstrates courage as well as valour which are of superhuman nature.

तस्मादेवमिवाभीक्ष्णं वाङ्मनःकर्मभिः शुभैः ।
चिन्तयेन्नृपतिं वैद्यः श्रेयांसीच्छन् विचक्षणः ॥२१३॥

Therefore, the physician desirous of his own welfare and the welfare of the society, should be a constant wellwisher of the King in his (physician's) speech, thought and action.

स्कन्धावारे च महति राजगेहादनन्तरम् ।
भवेत्संनिहितो वैद्यः सर्वोपकरणान्वितः ॥२१४॥
तत्रस्थमेनं ध्वजवत् यशःख्यातिसमुच्छ्रितम् ।
उपसर्पन्त्यमोहेन विषशल्यामयार्दिताः ॥२१५॥

*Residence of Physician*

The physician well equipped with all the instruments and drugs should be made to constantly reside in a spacious house in front of the royal palace in the capital of the country. The physician located there works like a flag of exalted fame and celebrity, and to his house there should be unrestricted access for all those patients who are suffering from poisons, injury by weapons and other diseases.

॥ तथा[२०४] च ॥

राज्ञोऽरिदेशे[२०५] रिपवस्तृणाम्बुमार्गांश्च[२०६] भक्तानि च दूषयन्ति ।

तानि[२०७] प्रदुष्टानि भिषग्विपश्चिद्विशोधयेदागमितार्थसूत्रः ॥२१६॥

*Additional Information*

When, during wars, the King is moving in the country of the enemy, then the local people (enemies) put poisons in the grass, water, road and food. A wise physician should ascertain this and purify such poisoned items by antidotes.

दुष्टं जलं पिच्छिलमुग्रगन्धि फेनावृतं[२०८] राजिभिरावृतं च।

मण्डूकमत्स्याश्च[२०९] तथा म्रियंते मत्ताश्च सानुपचरा भ्रमन्ति ॥२१७॥

मज्जन्ति[२१०] ये चात्र नराश्वनागास्ते छर्दिमोहज्वरदाहशोफान् ।

क्षिप्रं लभन्ते त्वपरांश्च[२११] रोगान्[२१२] दुष्टं जलं शोधयितुं यतेत ॥२१८॥

*Poisoned Water*

If the water is poisoned then it becomes slimy, foul smelling and frothy. and net-work of different colours appears over its surface. Frogs and fish inside the pond (water reservoir) die and float on the surface of the water. Animals inhabiting the banks of the reservoir become mad and move here and there. If human beings, horses and elephants take bath in this water, then they immediately suffer from vomiting, unconsciousness, fever, burning sensation, oedema and such other diseases. The physician should make efforts to purify the water of such reservoirs.

धवाश्वकर्णासनपारिभद्र-

सपाटलाशिग्रुकमुष्ककं[२१३] च ।

दग्ध्वा सराजद्रुमसोमवल्कं[२१४]

तद्भस्म शीतं विकिरेत्[२१५] सुखाय ।

भस्माञ्जलिश्चापि घटे निधाय

विशोधयेदीप्सितमेवमम्भः ॥२१९॥

*Purifying Poisoned Water-Reservoir*

The ash collected by burning trees like *dhava, aśvakarṇa, asana, pāribhadra, pāṭalā, śigru, muṣkaka, rājadruma* and *somavalka* should be made cool and sprinkled over this poisoned water reservoir for purification. If a small quantity of water is required to be purified, then the required quantity should be kept in a jar and the ash, mentioned about should be added into it which purifies the water.

क्षितिप्रदेशं विषदूषितं वा
तीर्थं[२१६] शिलां वाप्यरिभिः स्थलीं[२१७] वा ॥२२०॥
स्पृशन्ति गात्रेण च[२१८] येन गाव-
उष्ट्राश्च नागाः पुरुषा स्त्रियो वा ।
तदाशु[२१९] सूयते विदह्यते[२२०] च
विशीर्यते रोमनखं तदैव[२२१] ॥२२१॥
तत्राप्यनन्तां सहसर्वगन्धैः
स्वच्छाभिरद्भिः[२२२] सह योज्य मार्गान् ।
सिञ्चिदथाद्भिस्त्वमृतान्विताभि[२२३]
विडङ्गपाठाकटभीजलैर्वा
मार्गोऽस्ति चान्यो यदि तेन गच्छेत् ॥२२२॥

**Poisoned Land, etc.**

If the land, *tirtha* (steps leading to a water reservoir), slab of stone and *sthali* (open space of sitting together) are poisoned by the enemy and if the bodies of cows, camels, elephants, men and women come into contact with this poisoned land, etc. then there will be immediate swelling, burning sensation and shrivelling of the hair and nails. On this road (land), etc., clean water boiled with *ananta* and drugs belonging to *Sarvagavdha* group should be sprinkled. Similarly the water boiled with *amṛtā, viḍaṅga, pāṭhā* and *kaṭabhi* should be sprinkled over this road, etc., to make them free from poisons. If however, another safe-road is available, the king should procede through that.

तृणेषु भक्तेषु च दूषितेषु
मूर्च्छन्ति सीदन्ति वमन्ति चान्ये

विडभेदमायांत्यथ[२२४] वा म्रियन्ते ॥२२३॥
तेषां चिकित्सां प्रयतेत कर्त्तुं
विषापहैश्चाप्यगदैः[२२५] प्रलिप्य ।
वाद्यानि सर्वान्यनुवादयेत ।

(सुश्रुत : कल्पस्थान : ३ : ६-१४)

वाद्यस्य शब्देन हि तानि[२२६] नाशं
विषाणि घोराण्यपि यानि तत्र[२२७] ॥२२४॥

*Poisoned Grass, etc.*

If the grass and food on the way are poisoned, then the animals eating such grass, etc., get fainting, depression, vomiting and diarrhoea. Ultimately such animals may succumb to death. The physician should attempt to correct their maladies with appropriate therapies. Drums, etc., smeared with anti-poison drugs (antidotes) should be beaten to counteract these poisons. By the sound of such drums, even serious types of poisons lose their effects.

धूमेऽनिले वा विषसंप्रयुक्ते
मृगाः[२२८] श्रमार्ताः प्रपतन्ति भूमौ ॥२२५॥
कासप्रतिश्यायशिरोरुजश्च
भवन्ति तीव्रा नयनामयाश्च ।
लाक्षाहरिद्रातिविषाभयाब्दहरेणुकैलादलवक्रकुष्ठम् ।
प्रियङ्गवश्चाप्यनिले[२२९] निधाय
धूमानिलौ तेन[२३०] विशोधयेत ॥२२६॥

(सुश्रुत : कल्पस्थान : ३ : १५-१७)

*Poisoned Smoke*

If the smoke or air is poisoned, then deers feel exhausted and fall on the ground. It also causes cough, cold, headache and serious types of eye diseases. To counteract this, fumigation should be performed with the help of *lākṣa, haridrā, ativiṣā, abhayā, mustā, hareṇu, elā, patra, tagara, kuṣṭha* and *priyangu* by which the smoke and the air get purified (become free from poisons).

इति श्रीमहाराजाधिराजश्रीटोडरमल्लविरचिते टोडरानन्दे आयुर्वेदसौख्ये विषनिदानचिकित्साकथनं नाम षट्सप्ततितमो हर्षः ।

Thus, end the 76th chapter dealing with the diagnosis and treatment of poisons in the *Āyurveda saukhya* of *Ṭoḍarānanda* composed by the great King Ṭoḍaramalla.

## NOTES AND REFERENCES

१. (क) This is the beginning of 80th chapter of *Āyurveda saukhya* in *Ṭoḍarānanda* and the invocation reads as follows :
"निहत्य कंसं सुरिपुं नराणां मुदं ददौ यां पितरौ विमुच्य ।
कृष्णस्तयोः सामरयोर्नरेन्द्रे तां टोडरे विप्रमुदि प्रदद्यात् ॥
(ख) 'निहत्य ...... प्रदद्यात्' पाठोऽयं चतुर्थषष्ठपुस्तकयोः नोपलभ्यते ।
२. दाहपाकं इति आकरे पंचमपुस्तके च पाठः ।
३. 'स्थावरं ...... विषम्' पाठोऽयं षष्ठपुस्तके नोपलभ्यते ।
४. ततश्चान्योन्यमिक्ष्यते इति पंचमपुस्तके पाठः ।
५. मोहः इति पञ्चमपुस्तके पाठः ।
६. फलविषैः प्रलापो मोह एव च इति प्रथमपुस्तके पाठः ।
७. तु इति आकरे पाठः ।
८. गुरुगात्रता इति माधवनिदाने पाठः ।
९. मित्रैर्व्रणैर्यस्य इति पंचमपुस्तके पाठः ।
१०. सपीतं इति आकरे पाठः ।
११. 'योऽतिसार्यते ...... रूपिणः' पाठोऽयं चतुर्थपुस्तके नोपलभ्यते ।
१२. समाख्यातं इति प्रथमपुस्तके पाठः ।
१३. विकारतत् इति पंचमपुस्तके पाठः ।
१४. (क) मंडलितः इति चतुर्थपुस्तके पाठः ।
(ख) मंडलजः इति षष्ठपुस्तके पाठः ।
१५. विकारकृत् इति चतुर्थपुस्तके पाठः ।
१६. स्निग्धो. इति आकरे पाठः ।

१७. दष्टाः इति आकरे पाठः ।

१८ नरामर्म. इति प्रथमपुस्तके पाठः ।

१९ पित्तातपपीडितेषु इति आकरे पाठः ।

२०. (क) कुष्ठयुक्ते इति आकरे पाठः ।

(ख) कुष्ठयुष्टे रूक्षोऽबले इति प्रथमपुस्तके पाठः ।

(ग) कुष्ठपृष्ठे कुक्षगलेऽबले इति षष्ठपुस्तके पाठः ।

२१. रक्तमेति राज्यो इति आकरे पाठः ।

२२. 'राज्यो.........रोमहर्षो' पाठोऽयं पंचमपुस्तके नोपलभ्यते ।

२३. वतिद्यता यस्य निरैतिवक्त्रादूक्तं स्रवेदूर्धमधश्च इति षष्ठपुस्तके पाठः ।

२४. (क) दंष्ट्राभिपाता. इति प्रथमपुस्तके पाठः ।

(ख) दंष्ट्राभिधाता. इति चतुर्थपुस्तके पाठः ।

२५. कफावृतं इति आकरे पाठः ।

२६. .वैरस्य मुखः इति आकरे पाठः ।

२७. मूर्च्छन् वमन् गद्गदवाग्विषण्णो भवेच्च दुष्योदरलिङ्गजुष्टः इति आकरे पाठः ।

२८. तत्र इति आकरे पाठः ।

२९. मण्डलकोठमोहान् इति आकरे पाठः ।

३०. धातुक्षयं इति आकरे पाठः ।

३१. वैवर्ण्यमूर्च्छाविषमज्वरान् वा कुर्यात् प्रवृद्धां प्रबलां तृषां वा इति सुश्रुते पाठः ।

३२. कुर्यात् प्रवृद्धिं इति माधवनिदाने पाठः ।

३३. संवत्सरोत्थितम् इति आकरे पाठः ।

३४. .ग्निर्गरश्चास्यो. इति आकरे पाठः ।

३५. मर्मप्रध्वंसमाध्मानं इति प्रथमपुस्तके पाठः ।

३६. यस्माल्लूतं इति षष्ठपुस्तके पाठः ।

३७. दंशमध्ये इति आकरे पाठः ।

३८. (क) जालकावृतम् इति प्रथमपुस्तके पाठः ।

(ख) जालककृतम् इति षष्ठपुस्तके पाठः ।

३९. उर्ध्वाकृति इति आकरे पाठः ।

४०. (क) क्लेदशोषेकरोधिकाम् इति षष्ठपुस्तके पाठः ।

(ख) .ज्वरान्वितम् इति आकरे पाठः ।

४१. स्तद्दष्टमिति निर्दिशेत् इति आकरे पाठः ।

४२. सर्पणामेव विण्मूत्रकीटाः स्युः जस्नुताः । दूषीविषाः घाणहराद्रत संक्षोम तोयना । इति चतुर्थपुस्तके अधिकः पाठः ।

४३. प्राणान्तिकाश्च जायन्ते श्वासहिक्काशिरोग्रहः इति आकरे पाठः ।

४४. शिरोज्वरः इति षष्ठपुस्तके पाठः ।

४५. दाहश्च पाण्डुदूषी विषार्दितै इति षष्ठपुस्तके पाठः ।

४६. (क) .मंदशुतिज्वरः इति प्रथमपुस्तके पाठः ।
(ख) शब्दश्रुति इति आकरे पाठः ।

४७. .मूषिकैः इति आकरे पाठः ।

४८. काग्नां इति षष्ठपुस्तके पाठः ।

४९. (क) श्यावत्वमथवा इति आकरे पाठः ।
(ख) शोथत्वगादीनां इति चतुर्थपुस्तके पाठः ।

५०. वा इति आकरे पाठः ।

५१. भेदः दध्रे स्यात्कृकलासकैः इति प्रथमपुस्तके पाठः ।

५२. तु भिदंती इति प्रथमपुस्तके पाठः ।

५३. पश्चात्तु इति आकरे पाठः ।

५४. दृष्टो साध्यस्त हृध्वण. इति षष्ठपुस्तके पाठः ।

५५. पर्वाद्भिरत्यर्थं इति प्रथमपुस्तके पाठः ।

५६. वा इति पंचमपुस्तके पाठः ।

५७. करभैर्दष्टे दंशश्चैवावशीर्यति इति षष्ठपुस्तके पाठः ।

५८. पीतकस्तृषा इति प्रथमपुस्तके पाठः ।

५९. (क) सविषाश्च इति प्रथमपुस्तके पाठः ।
(ख) ह्यरुचि इति षष्ठपुस्तके पाठः ।

६०. रुजां इति प्रथमपुस्तके पाठः ।

६१. विकाऽशुद्दुत् इति पंचमपुस्तके पाठः ।

६२. श्रूयते इति प्रथमपुस्तके पाठः ।

६३. प्रशान्तदोषं इति आकरे पाठः ।

६४. मन्नाभिकांक्षं इति पंचमपुस्तके पाठः ।

६५. "स्थावरं ...... स्मृतः" पाठोऽयं प्रथमपुस्तके नोपलभ्यते ।

६६. स एव इति आकरे पाठः ।

६७. "तण्डुलीयकमूलं ..... प्रभावः" पाठोऽयं प्रथमपंचमपुस्तकयोः नोपलभ्यते ।

६८. सर्पानियापार रूपान् इति षष्ठपुस्तके पाठः ।

७०. दंशोपरि निबध्नीयात् इति आकरे पाठः ।

७१. मन्त्रयेत् इति आकरे पाठः ।

७२. जावपि इति षष्ठपुस्तके पाठः ।

७३. पिंडतगरकमूलं पुष्येनोत्पाट्य प्रयोजितं दंशे इति षष्ठपुस्तके पाठः ।

७४. बोलयतित्पत्रन्तो इति षष्ठपुस्तके पाठः ।

७५. भावितं मरिचं सितम् इति आकरे पाठः ।

७६. सप्ताहं इति आकरे पाठः ।

७७. नस्याञ्जने इति आकरे पाठः ।

७८. नक्तमालफलं व्योषं विल्वमूलं इति आकरे पाठः ।

७९. निशाह्वयम् इति पंचमपुस्तके पाठः

८०. वा इति आकरे पाठः ।

८१. "मांसीहरेणु त्रिफला मुरुंगी रक्तांल्पता य.ष्टिपत्रकानि विडङ्गकासीस" पाठोऽयं चतुर्थषष्ठपुस्तकयोः अधिकमुपलभ्यते ।

८२. विषोपहतचेतसाम् इति चतुर्थषष्ठपुस्तकयोः पाठः ।

८३. सोमराजीफलं मुख्यं कदली सिंधुवारकः । चोरकी करणाः (चोरको चरणः) कुष्ठं सर्पगन्धा ससप्तला । पुनर्नवा शिरीषश्च पुष्पमारग्वधार्कजं। श्यामांवष्टे विडङ्गानि तथा चाश्मंतकानि च । भूमीकदम्बकश्चैव गण एष रसः स्मृतः । एकशो द्वित्रिशो वापि प्रयोक्तव्यो विषापहः ।' पाठोऽयं चतुर्थषष्ठपुस्तकयोः अधिकमुपलभ्यते ।

८४. अवाच्च योगा विषवेगहन्ता इति चतुर्थषष्ठपुस्तकयोः पाठः ।

८५. विषम् इति षष्ठपुस्तके पाठः ।

८६. कीटलूताव्रजापहाः इति षष्ठपुस्तके पाठः ।

८७. (क) पातनम् इति आकरे पाठः ।
(ख) पाततः इति षष्ठपुस्तके पाठः ।

८८. वदने निफूत्कारं इति षष्ठपुस्तके पाठः ।

८९. कर्णेफूत्कारम् इति आकरे पाठः ।

९०. संसयुक्तैवृश्चिकस्य इति षष्ठपुस्तके पाठः ।

९१. कुठेरकस्य इति षष्ठपुस्तके पाठः ।

९२. दग्धविद्धस्य इति प्रथमपुस्तके पाठः ।

९३. 'जेपाललेपो ...... सुखम्' पाठोऽयं प्रथमपंचमपुस्तकयोः नोपलभ्यते ।

९४. जललेपो निंहत्याशु इति षष्ठपुस्तके पाठः ।

९५. दशम इति आदर्शपुस्तकेषु पाठः ।

९६. 'दधि ..... तत्' पाठोऽयं प्रथमपंचमपुस्तकयोः नोपलभ्यते ।

९७. तच्छायाशब्दर्वत्रस्ताः इति प्रथमपुस्तके पाठः ।

९८. विषपिते गते पाणि इति षष्ठपुस्तके पाठः ।

९९. चक्षुषी इति षष्ठपुस्तके पाठः ।
१०० समुपलक्षयेत् इति षष्ठपुस्तके पाठः ।
१०१. पूतिगंधं मुखे इति चतुर्थपुस्तके पाठः ।
१०२. कटुकां इति षष्ठपुस्तके पाठः ।
१०३. चायुगतं इति षष्ठपुस्तके पाठः ।
१०४. 'ॐ ....... रित्यर्थः' पाठोऽयं प्रथमपुस्तके नोपलभ्यते ।
१०५. 'ॐ ....... बंधः' पाठोऽयं षष्ठपुस्तके नोपलभ्यते ।
१०६. (क) धुतः इति प्रथमपुस्तके पाठः ।
(ख) नमोनंतश्च ह्रं फट् स्वाहा इति षष्ठपुस्तके पाठः ।
१०७. 'स्पर्शा ....... महामे' पाठोऽयं चतुर्थपुस्तके नोपलभ्यते ।
१०८. क्षयमस्राहा इति षष्ठपुस्तके पाठः ।
१०९. सुवर्णमहामेखलाय इति षष्ठपुस्तके पाठः ।
११०. पाठोऽयं षष्ठपुस्तके नोपलभ्यते ।
१११. समुत्थं इति चतुर्थषष्ठपुस्तकयोः पाठः ।
११२. (क) शृगालऋक्षतरक्षुद्वीपि इति पंचमपुस्तके पाठः ।
(ख) शृगालानां तरक्षुद्वीपि इति चतुर्थषष्ठपुस्तकयोः पाठः ।
११३. फलं षष्ठपुस्तके पाठः ।
११४. 'शुनकस्य ....... दुःसहम्' पाठोऽयं पंचमपुस्तके अधिकमुपलभ्यते ।
११५. (क) 'शर्क्करा. ..... विषात्तुरः' पाठोऽयं प्रथमपंचमपुस्तकयोः नोपलभ्यते ।
(ख) सटीचूर्णसंयुक्तं इति षष्ठपुस्तके पाठः ।
११६. अलिभं इति षष्ठपुस्तके पाठः ।
११७. कुत्राद्वशस्य इति षष्ठपुस्तके पाठः ।
११८. चूर्णितम् इति षष्ठपुस्तके पाठः ।
११९. 'विरुद्धा ....... स्थलीम्' पाठोऽयं चतुर्थषष्ठपुस्तकयोः नोपलभ्यते ।
१२०. स्वौ कृत्यता गत्याः इति षष्ठपुस्तके पाठः ।
१२१. विषकल्पोपयोगाच्च इति आदर्शपुस्तकेषु पाठः ।
१२२. महीपतिः इति चतुर्थपुस्तके पाठः ।
१२३. पटितं इति षष्ठपुस्तके पाठः ।
१२४. नृषु इति प्रथमपुस्तके पाठः ।
१२५. पाठोऽयं पंचमपुस्तके अधिकमुपलभ्यते ।
१२६. पाठोऽयं पंचमपुस्तके नोपलभ्यते ।
१२७. (क) शीलशौचदयान्वितम् इति प्रथमपुस्तके पाठः ।
(ख) स शीतं च दयान्वितम् इति षष्ठपुस्तके पाठः ।

१२८. (क) दक्षं चालस्य इति प्रथमपुस्तके पाठः ।
(ख) दक्षं पैशून्यवर्जितम् इति चतुर्थपुस्तके पाठः ।
(ग) दक्षं मायाविवर्जितम् इति पंचमपुस्तके पाठः ।

१२९. नियुञ्जीत इति प्रथमपुस्तके पाठः ।

१३०. तद्विधं पूजितम् इति षष्ठपुस्तके पाठः ।

१३१. (क) प्रसन्नदिग्देशकृतं इति प्रथमपुस्तके पाठः ।
(ख) प्रशस्तदिग्दोषकृतं इति षष्ठपुस्तके पाठः ।

१३२. महत्शुचं इति षष्ठपुस्तके पाठः ।

१३३. गवाक्षाद्यमात्मवर्ग. इति प्रथमपुस्तके पाठः ।

१३४. शुभदर्शनाः इति प्रथमपुस्तके पाठः ।

१३५. संधियुक्ताः इति चतुर्थषष्ठपुस्तकयोः पाठः ।

१३६. (क) चाज्ञाभिधेयास्युर्विविधाः इति प्रथमपुस्तके पाठः ।
(ख) राज्ञा विधेयास्युः वित्रिधा परिकर्म्मिणाः इति षष्ठपुस्तके पाठः ।

१३७. (क) महनसिकवोढारः इति प्रथमपुस्तके पाठः ।
(ख) महानासिकवाढारस्तथौदनिक इति षष्ठपुस्तके पाठः ।

१३८. चाप्यन्ये तु इति पंचमपुस्तके पाठः ।

१३९. पाठोऽयं पंचमपुस्तके अधिकमुपलभ्यते ।

१४०. दंतकाष्ठान्नपाने च तथाभ्यंगे च भक्षणे इति प्रथमपुस्तके पाठः ।

१४१. (क) विषदिग्धेषु इति प्रथमपुस्तके पाठः ।
(ख) विषयुक्तेषु इति चतुर्थषष्ठपुस्तकयोः पाठः ।

१४२. पाठोऽयं पंचमपुस्तके अधिकमुपलभ्यते ।

१४३. (क) तत्रैतेपि विनश्यन्ति इति प्रथमपुस्तके पाठः ।
(ख) तैव ते विनस्यन्ति इति पंचमपुस्तके पाठः ।

१४४. 'मयूरकण्ठप्रतिमो ...... तु' पाठोऽयं प्रथमपुस्तके पाठः ।

१४५. 'भिन्नार्चि. ...... .शाम्यति' पाठोऽयं चतुर्थपुस्तके अधिकमुपलभ्यते ।

१४६. दुष्टान्नं इति पंचमपुस्तके पाठः ।

१४७. उद्वेगमाति मर्ज्जारः क्रौंचस्तु इति चतुर्थषष्ठपुस्तकयोः पाठः ।

१४८. (क) हृष्येन्मयूर उद्विध्नः इति आकरे पाठः ।
(ख) हृष्यन्मयूरस्तूद्विग्ने इति प्रथमपुस्तके पाठः ।
(ग) हृष्यं मयूरश्चोद्विग्नः इति चतुर्थषष्ठपुस्तकयोः पाठः ।

१४९. हंसस्खलति इति चतुर्थषष्ठपुस्तकयोः पाठः ।

१५०. पाठोऽयं पंचमपुस्तके अधिकमुपलभ्यते ।

१५१. श्रान्तनेत्रत्वं इति पंचमपुस्तके पाठः ।

१५२. रामठं इति पंचमपुस्तके पाठः ।

१५३. पाठोऽयं पंचमपस्तके नोपलभ्यते ।

१५४. नखश्यावं कर इति षष्ठपुस्तके पाठः ।

१५५. तत्र प्रलेपः इति प्रथमपुस्तके पाठः ।

१५६. पाठोऽयं पंचमपुस्तके अधिकमुपलभ्यते ।

१५७. ततोस्याषीलिवाद्जिह्वाभवत्यरसवेदिनी इति प्रथमपुस्तके पाठः ।

१५८. प्रवर्त्तते इति प्रथमपुस्तके पाठः ।

१५९. (क) वक्येरितं इति प्रथमपुस्तके पाठः ।
(ख) बाह्येरितं इति षष्ठपुस्तके पाठः ।

१६०. (क) स्यादान्तकाधिकम् इति प्रथमपुस्तके पाठः ।
(ख) स्याघृतकाष्टिकम् इति षष्ठपुस्तके पाठः ।

१६१. पाठोऽयं पंचमपुस्तके अधिकमुपलभ्यते ।

१६२. छर्दिसमोहाद्वाहृदाहासहमेव च इति चतुर्थषष्ठपुस्तकयोः पाठः ।

१६३. दाहमेव च इति प्रथमपुस्तके पाठः ।

१६४. तत्रापि इति प्रथमपुस्तके पाठः ।

१६५. पाठोऽयं पंचमपुस्तके अधिकमुपलभ्यते ।

१६६. काष्ण्यं इति प्रथमपुस्तके पाठः ।

१६७. (क) 'विरेचनं ..... फलं' पाठोऽयं प्रथमचतुर्थषष्ठपुस्तकेषु नोपलभ्यते ।
(ख) तत्र नीलीफलं श्रेष्ठं सर्पिष्कं विरेचनं इति प्रथमपुस्तके पाठः ।

१६८. दद्याददुषि. इति षष्ठपुस्तके पाठः ।

१६९. लेपो इति चतुर्थषष्ठपुस्तकयोः पाठः ।

१७०. मोदके इति चतुर्थषष्ठपुस्तकयोः पाठः ।

१७१. कालामद्याम्भसोः क्षौद्रे हरि तैलेरुणोपमा इति चतुर्थषष्ठपुस्तकयोः पाठः ।

१७२. अन्या वा विकृतास्तथा इति प्रथमपुस्तके पाठः ।

१७३. 'सद्यः ....... फलानि च' पाठोऽयं प्रथमपुस्तके नोपलभ्यते ।

१७४. विरसानि च इति पंचमपुस्तके पाठः ।

१७५. पाठोऽयं पंचमपुस्तके अधिकमुपलभ्यते ।

१७६. 'जिह्वादन्तौष्ठमांसनां ......... जम्बूफलास्थिभिः' पाठोऽयं प्रथमपुस्तके नोपलभ्यते ।

१७७. ॐ दन्तौ विषवान् सान्द्रोयात्यविश्राव्यतामिव । चिरेण पच्यते पक्वां भवेत् पर्युषितोपमः । हीयते गन्धवर्णाद्यैः क्रियते चन्द्रिकां चितः । व्यञ्जनान्याशु शुष्यन्ति ध्मानक्वाथानि तत्र च । हीनातिरिक्ता विकृता

छाया दृश्यते नैव वा । फेनोर्द्धरात्री सीमन्तं ततं बुद्वुद्सम्भवः । विछिन्न विरसा रागाः षाडवाः शाक सामिषम् । अथास्य धातकी पुष्पपथ्याजम्बूफलं निशा' । पाठोऽयं चतुर्थषष्ठपुस्तकयोः अधिकमुपलभ्यते ।

१७८. क्वथिते शोथे इति प्रथमपुस्तके पाठः ।

१७९. (क) शिरीषमाषका वाऽपि सक्षौद्राः इति पंचमपुस्तके आकरे च पाठः ।
(ख) सिरीषसिन्धुना क्षौद्रं इति षष्ठपुस्तके पाठः ।

१८०. पाठोऽयं पंचमपुस्तके अधिकमुपलभ्यते ।

१८१. स्वेदनं ज्वरः इति आकरे पाठः ।

१८२. विषसंयुते इति आकरे पाठः ।

१८३. विषम् इति षष्ठपुस्तके पाठः ।

१८४. कपित्थरसमूत्राश्च इति चतुर्थषष्ठपुस्तकयोः पाठः ।

१८५. पानमेतत्प्रशस्यते इति प्रथमपुस्तके पाठः ।

१८६. सानुलेपने इति प्रथमपुस्तके पाठः ।

१८७. ज्ञेयमभ्यङ्गलक्षणं इति प्रथमपुस्तके पाठः ।

१८८. गोमयस्वरसो इति आकरे पाठः ।

१८९. ज्ञेयमभ्यङ्गलक्षणैः इति षष्ठपुस्तके पाठः ।

१९०. 'नस्यधूमगते ...... शृतम्' पाठोऽयं चतुर्थषष्ठपुस्तकयोः नोपलभ्यते ।

१९१. समधुयष्टिकम् इति प्रथमपुस्तके पाठः ।

१९२. पाठोऽयं पंचमपुस्तके अधिकमुपलभ्यते ।

१९३. (क) 'वाऽपि सुशोतो' पाठोऽयं चतुर्थपुस्तके नोपलभ्यते ।
(ख) सशीतो प्रथमपुस्तके पाठः ।

१९४. 'वेदना ....... संसृष्टेभ.' पाठोऽयं चतुर्थपुस्तके नोपलभ्यते ।

१९५. मेखशृग्याश्च इति प्रथमपुस्तके पाठः ।

१९६. 'उपानत् ...... प्रसाधयेत्' पाठोऽयं प्रथमपुस्तके नोपलभ्यते ।

१९७. समीक्ष्योपद्रवांस्तस्य इति पंचमपुस्तके आकरे च पाठः ।

१९८. भक्षितं इति आकरे पाठः ।

१९९. परानधिजिगीषतः इति प्रथमपुस्तके पाठः ।

२००. जवसमिंधनम् इति पंचमपुस्तके पाठः ।

२०१. संज्ञस्तु इति पंचमपुस्तके पाठः ।

२०२. दोषागंतुजमृत्युभ्योः रसमन्त्रविशारदौ इति पंचमपुस्तके पाठः ।

२०३. यत्नाद्वैद्यपुरोहितौ इति पंचमपुस्तके पाठः ।

२०४. भवन्ति चात्र इति आकरे पाठः ।

२०५. राज्ञोनिदेशेश्पिवोजलानि इति आदर्शपुस्तकेषु पाठः ।

२०६. मार्गान्निधूमश्वसनान् विषेण इति आकरे पाठः ।

२०७. संदूषयन्त्येभिरतिप्रदुष्टान् विज्ञाय लिङ्गैरभिशोधयेत्तान् इति आकरे पाठः ।

२०८. फेनान्वितं इति आकरे पाठः ।

२०९. मण्डूकमत्स्यं म्रियते विहङ्गा मत्ताश्च सानूपचरा भ्रमन्ति इति आकरे पाठः ।

२१०. मूर्च्छति इति प्रथमपुस्तके पाठः ।

२११. ऋच्छन्ति तेषामपहृदय इति आकरे पाठः ।

२१२ दोषान् इति आकरे पाठः ।

२१३. .परिभद्रान् सपाटलान् सिद्धकमोक्षकौ च इति आकरे पाठः ।

२१४. .सोमवल्कां स्तद्भस्म इति आकरे पाठः ।

२१५. वितरेतु सरःसु इति आकरे पाठः ।

२१६. शिलातलं तीर्थमथेरिणं वा इति आकरे पाठः ।

२१७. स्थलावा इति चतुर्थपुस्तके पाठः ।

२१८. तु येन येन गोवाजिनागोष्ट्रखरानरा वा इति आकरे पाठः ।

२१९. तच्छूनतां यात्यथ दह्यते इति आकरे पाठः ।

२२०. 'नृपते ...... विदह्यते' पाठोऽयं षष्ठपुस्तके नोपलभ्यते ।

२२१. तथैव इति आकरे पाठः ।

२२२. पिष्ट्वा सुराभिर्विनियोज्य मार्गम् इति आकरे पाठः ।

२२३. सिञ्चेत् पयोभिः सुमृदन्वितैस्तं विडङ्गपाठाकटभीजलैर्वा इति आकरे पाठः ।

२२४. विड्भेदमृच्छन्त्यथवा म्रियन्ते तेषां चिकित्सां प्रणयेद्यथोक्ताम् इति आकरे पाठः ।

२२५. विषापहैर्वाऽप्यगदैर्विलिप्य वाद्यानि चित्राण्यपि वादयेत इति आकरे पाठः ।

२२६. यान्ति इति आकरे पाठः ।

२२७. सन्ति इति आकरे पाठः ।

२२८. खगाः इति षष्ठपुस्तके आकरे च पाठः ।

२२९. प्रियङ्गुकां चाप्यनले इति आकरे पाठः ।

२३०. चापि इति आकरे पाठः ।

# CHAPTER IX

## ॥ अथ रसायनाधिकारः ॥

*(Rejuvenation Therapy)*

"दीर्घमायुः[१] स्मृतिं मेधामारोग्यं तरुणं वयः ।
प्रभावर्णस्वरौदार्यं देहेन्द्रियबलोदयम्[२]" ॥
(भैषज्यरत्नावली : रसायनाधिकार : ३)
नरः सम्यगवाप्नोति सेव्यमानो रसायनम् ॥१॥

*Utility of* ***Rasāyana*** ***Therapy***

A person who takes *rasāyana* (rejuvenation) therapy gets endowed with longevity, memory, intellect, positive health, youthfulness, complexion, good colour of the skin, voice, magnanimity and strength of the body as well as sense organs in an appropriate manner.

'यज्जराव्याधिविध्वंसि[३] भेषजं तद्रसायनम्[४] ॥२॥

***Definition***

The therapy (medicine) which anihilates old age (aging process) and which makes the body free from diseases is called *rasāyana* (rejuvenation therapy).

"पूर्वे वयसि मध्ये वा शुद्धकायः[४] समाचरेत्" ॥३॥

(योगरत्नाकर : रसायनाधिकरण : पृष्ठ ४९८)

*Time of Administration*

Rejuvenation therapy should be administered to a person during his youth or to a middle-aged person. Before administering this therapy his body should be purified (cleansed of morbidities).

"अविशुद्धशरीरस्य[५] युक्तो रासायनो विधिः ।
न[६] भाति वाससि क्लिष्टे रङ्गयोग इवाऽर्पिताः[७] ॥४॥

(योगरत्नाकर : रसायनाधिकरण : पृष्ठ ४९८)
(भैषज्यरत्नावली : रसायनाधिकार : १-२)

*Need for Body-Purification*

If the rejuvenation therapy is administered to a person whose body is impure (not free from morbid factors), then it becomes incapable of exhibiting its excellence as a dirty cloth, when painted, does not look beautiful.

"सिन्धूत्थशर्कराशुण्ठीकणामधुगुडैः क्रमात् ।
वर्षादिष्वभयाभ्यस्ता[८] रसायनगुणैषिणा" ॥५॥

(योगरत्नाकर : रसायनाधिकरण : पृष्ठ ४९९)
(भैषज्यरत्नावली : रसायनाधिकार : २६)

*Use of Harītakī*

A person desirous of rejuvenating effect should habitually take *harītakī* along with different vehicles in various seasons as follows :

| Season | Vehicle to be used along with *harītakī* |
|---|---|
| (1) Rainy season | *saindhava* |
| (2) Autumn | sugar |
| (3) Early winter | ginger |
| (4) Late winter | *pippalī* |

(5) Spring honey
(6) Summer jaggery

"त्रैफलेनायसं[9] पात्रं कल्केनालेपयेन्नवम्[10] ।
तमहो[11]रात्रिकं लेपं पिबेक्षौद्रोदकाप्लुतम् ॥६॥
प्रभूतस्नेहमशनं जीर्णे तस्मिन्प्रयोजयेत् ।
अजरोऽरुक्समाऽभ्यासाज्जीवेच्चापि समाः शतम्" ॥७॥

(चरक : चिकित्सा : १(३) : ४३-४४)

*Use of Triphala*

A new iron vessel should be smeared with the paste (*kalka*) of *triphalā* (fruit pulp of *harītakī, bibhītaka* and *āmalakī*) and kept for the day and night (24 hours). The paste should then be taken with honey and water. After the digestion of this potion, the person should take a lot of fat. By using this recipe continuously for one year, one can live for one hundred years free from old age and diseases.

"मण्डूकपर्ण्याः स्वरसः प्रयोज्यः
क्षीरेण यष्टीमधुकस्य चूर्णम् ।
रसो गुडूच्यास्तु समूलपुष्प्याः
कल्कः प्रयोज्यः खलु शंखपुष्प्याः ॥८॥
आयुः प्रदान्यामयनाशनानि
बलाग्निवर्णस्वरवर्द्धनानि ।
मेध्यानि चैतानि रसायनानि
मेध्या विशेषेण तु शङ्खपुष्पी ॥९॥

(चरक : चिकित्सा : १(३) : ३०-३१)
(भैषज्यरत्नावली : रसायनाधिकार : ८-९)

*Rejuvenating Recipes*

Four rejuvenating recipes are given below :

(1) Juice of *maṇḍūkaparṇī*;
(2) powder of *yaṣṭimadhu* mixed with honey;

(3) juice of *guḍūcī* along with its root and flowers; and
(4) paste of *śaṅkhapuṣpī*.

These recipes promote longevity, cure diseases and enhance strength, *agni* (power of digestion and metabolism), *varṇa* (complexion) and *svara* (voice). These rejuvenating recipes are *medhya* (wholesome for intellect). Among them, *śaṅkhapuṣpī* is the drug *par excellence* for the promotion of intellect.

"ये मासमेकं[१२] स्वरसं पिबन्ति
दिने दिने भृङ्गराजः समुत्थम् ।
क्षीराशिनस्ते बलवर्णयुक्ताः
समाः शतं जीवितमाप्नुवन्ति" ॥१०॥

॥ भृङ्गराजकल्पः[१३] ॥

(भैषज्यरत्नावली : रसायनाधिकार : ७)

(योगरत्नाकर : रसायनाधिकरण : पृष्ठ : ४९९)

*Bhṛṅgarāja Kalpa (First Recipe)*

If a person takes the juice of *bhṛṅgarāja* every day for one month, and while using this recipe, lives on milk diet, then he lives for one hundred years endowed with strength and complexion.

असिततिलविमिश्रान्पल्लवान्[१४] भक्षयेद्यः
सततमथ पयाशी भृङ्गराजस्य मासम् ।
भवति सचिरजीवी व्याधिभिर्मुक्तदेहो
भ्रमरसदृशकेशः कामचारी मनुष्यः ॥११॥

॥ भृङ्गराजकल्पः[१५] ॥

*Bhṛṅgarāja Kalpa (Second Recipe)*

If a person takes the leaves of *bhṛṅgarāja* mixed with the black sessame for one month, and while using this recipe, lives on wholesome food, then he lives a long life with his body free from any disease. His hair becomes black like a *bhramara* (black-bee) and he becomes capable of moving wherever he likes.

"पीताश्वगन्धा पयसार्द्धमासं
घृतेन तैलेन सुखाम्बुना वा ।
कृशस्य पुष्टिं वपुषो बिभर्त्ति[16]
बालस्य शस्यस्य यथाम्बुवृष्टिः ॥१२॥
॥ अश्वगन्धाकल्पः[17] ॥

*Aśvagandhā Kalpa*

Intake of *aśvagandhā* with either milk, ghee, oil or lukewarm water for fifteen days causes plumpness of the body of an emaciated person as a tender plant gets envigorated by rain-water.

धात्रीतिलान्[18] भृङ्गराजोविमिश्रान्
ये भक्षयेयुर्मनुजाः क्रमेण ।
ते कृष्णकेशा विमलेन्द्रियाश्च
निर्व्याधियोप्यामरणा[19] भवेयुः" ॥१३॥
॥ धात्रीकल्पः[20] ॥
(भैषज्यरत्नावली : रसायनाधिकार : १०-११)

*Dhātrī Kalpa*

If a person takes *āmalakī* mixed with *tila* and *bhṛṅgarāja* in a gradually increased dose, then his hair become black, his senses become sharp (clear), he becomes free from diseases and he lives for a long time (for one hundred years).

मासं[21] वचामप्युपसेवमानाः
क्षीरेण तैलेन घृतेन वापि ।
भवन्ति रक्षोभिरधृष्यरूपा
मेधाविनो निर्मलमिष्टवाचः ॥१४॥
॥ वचाकल्पः[22] ॥

*Vacā Kalpa*

If a person takes *vacā* along with milk, oil or ghee for one month, then his complexion becomes excellent, he becomes intelligent and his voice becomes clear and sweet to hear.

"वृद्धदारकमूलानि[२३] श्लक्ष्णचूर्णानि कारयेत् ।
शतावर्या रसेनैव सप्तवारांश्च भावयेत् ॥१५॥
अक्षमात्रं तु[२४] तच्चूर्णं सर्पिषा सह योजयेत् ।
मासमात्रोपयोगेन मतिमान् जायते नरः ।
मेधावी स्मृतिमांश्चैव वलीपलितवर्जितः ॥१६॥
॥ वृद्धदारककल्पः[२५] ॥

*Vṛddhadāra Kalpa*

Roots of *vṛddhadāru* should be made to a fine powder, and it should be impregnated with the juice of *śatāvarī* for seven times. This powder in the dose of one *akṣa* should be taken along with ghee. By the use of this recipe only for one month, the person becomes endowed with strong will-power, intellect and memory. His body becomes free from wrinkles and gray hair.

हस्तिकर्णरजः खादेत् प्रातरुत्थाय सर्पिषा ।
यथेष्टाहारचारोपि[२६] सहस्रायुर्भवेन्नरः ॥१७॥
मेधावी बलवान् कामी स्त्रीशतानि व्रजत्यसौ ।
मधुना त्वश्ववेगः[२७] स्याद् बलिष्ठः स्त्रीसहस्रगः ।
अयं मन्त्रः[२८] प्रयोक्तव्यो भिषजा चाभिमन्त्रणे ॥१८॥
ॐ नमो महाविनायकाय अमृतं रक्ष रक्ष मम ।
फलसिद्धिं देहि रुद्रवचनेन स्वाहा" ॥१९॥
॥ हस्तिकर्णकल्पः[२९] ॥
(भैषज्यरत्नावली : रसायनाधिकार : १२-१५)

*Hastikarṇa Kalpa*

One should take the powder of *hastikarṇa* (*palāśa*) along with ghee early in the morning after getting up from the bed. He may resort to food and regimens as he likes. By doing so he lives long (lit. for one thousand years). He becomes endowed with intellect, strength and sex-passion inasmuch as he becomes capable of having sexual intercourse with many (lit. one hundred) women. If he takes this potion with honey, then he becomes capable of running like a horse and strong, and he could have sexual intercourse with many (lit. one thousand) women. This recipe should be impregnated by the physician with the following *mantra*: "*Oṃ namo mahāvināyakāya amṛtaṃ rakṣa rakṣa mama phalasiddhiṃ dehi rudravacanena svāhā.*"

"पुनर्नवस्यार्द्धपलं नवस्य
पिष्टं पिबेद्यः पयसाऽर्द्धमासम् ।
'मासद्वयं तद्द्विगुण[३०] समां वा
जीर्णोऽपि भूयः स[३१] पुनर्नवः स्यात्' ॥२०॥
॥ पुनर्नवाकल्पः[३२] ॥
(योगरत्नाकर : रसायनाधिकरण : पृष्ठ ४९९)

### *Punarnavā Kalpa*

Half *pala* of the freshly collected (roots of) *punranavā* should be made to a paste by triturating with milk. Intake of this for fifteen days, or two months or four months or one year makes even an old person very young.

"धात्रीचूर्णस्य कंसं स्वरसपरिगतं क्षौद्रसर्पिःसमांशं
कृष्णेमानी सिताष्टप्रसृतियुतमिदं[३३] स्थापितं भस्मराशौ ॥२१॥
वर्षान्ते तत्समश्नन् भवति विपलितो रूपवर्णप्रभावै-
र्निर्व्याधिर्बुद्धिमेधास्मृतिवचनबलस्थैर्यसत्त्वैरुपेतः ॥२२॥
॥ बृहद्धात्रीकल्पः[३४] ॥

### *Bṛhat Dhātrī Kalpa*

One *kaṃsa* of the powder of *āmalakī* shou-d be impregnated with *āmalakī*-juice. To this, one *kaṃsa* of each of honey ghee and *pippalī* powder, and eight *prasṛtis* of sugar should be added. It should be kept inside a heap of ash for one year. Thereafter, it should be taken out of the heap of ash and taken. Intake of this makes a person free from gray hair, and endows him with excellent complexion and colour. He becomes free from diseases and he possesses wisdom, intellect, memory, power of speech, strength, courage and strong will-power.

गुडूच्यपामार्गविडङ्गशङ्खिनी-
वचाभयाकुष्ठशतावरी समा ।
घृतेन लीढा प्रकरोति मानवं
त्रिभिर्दिनैः ग्रन्थसहस्रधारिणम्" ॥२३॥

॥ प्रज्ञाकर[३५] चूर्णम् ॥

(भैषज्यरत्नावली : रसायनाधिकार : २२-२३)

*Prajñākara Cūrṇa*

*Guḍūcī, apāmārga, viḍaṅga, śaṅkhinī, vacā, abhayā, kuṣṭha* and *śatāvarī*—all these drugs taken in equal quantities should be added with ghee. Intake of this linctus for three days enables a person to memorise many (lit. thousands of) texts.

"ब्राह्मीवचाभयावासापिप्पल्यो मधुसैन्धवम् ।
अस्य प्रयोगेन[३६] सप्ताहात्किन्नरैः सह गीयते ॥२४॥

Intake of *brāhmī, vacā, abhayā, vāsā* and *pippalī* along with honey and rock-salt for one week makes the voice of a person like that of a *kinnara* (celestial musicians).

हन्त्यम्लपित्तवमनारुचिदाहमोह[३७]-
खालित्यमेहतिमिरव्रणशुक्रदोषान्[३८] ।
भुक्त्वा नरः सततमामलकीरसेन
वृद्धोऽपि तेन च भवेत्तरुणीरिरंसुः" ॥२५॥

(योगरत्नाकर : रसायनाधिकार : पृष्ठ ५०१)

Intake of food regularly with the juice of *āmalakī* cures *amlapitta* (hyperacidity), vomiting, anorexia, burning sensation, unconsciousness, wrinkling of the skin, *meha* (obstinate urinary disorders including diabetes), *timira* (cataract) and *savraṇa śukla* (corneal ulcer). By the intake of this potion, even an old man becomes capable of having sexual intercourse with a young woman.

तीव्रेण कुष्ठेन परीतमूर्त्तिः
यः सोमराजीं नियमेन खादेत् ।
संवत्सरं कृष्णतिलद्वितीयां
स सोमराजीवपुषाधिशेते ॥२६॥
॥ सोमराजीकल्पः[३९] ॥

*Somarājī Kalpa*

If a person is suffering from serious type of *kuṣṭha* (obstinate skin diseases including leprosy), he should take *somarājī* or (alternatively) black variety of *tila* for one year. By doing so, his body becomes beautiful like a moon.

"पञ्च[४०] भल्लातकांश्छित्त्वा साधयेद्विधिवज्जले[४१] ।
कषायं त[४२] पिबेच्छीतं घृतेनाक्तोष्ठतालुकम् ॥२७॥
पञ्चवृद्ध्या पिबेद्यावत्सप्ततिं ह्रासयेत्ततः ।
जीर्णेऽद्यादोदनं शीतं घृतक्षीरोपसंहितम् ॥२८॥
एतद्रसायनं मेध्यं वलीपलितनाशनम् ।
कुष्ठार्शःकृमिदोषघ्नं दुष्टशुक्रविशोधनम्"[४३] ॥२९॥
(योगरत्नाकर : रसायनाधिकार : पृष्ठ ५००)

*Use of Bhallātaka*

Five fruits (seeds) of *bhallātaka* should be rubbed out of their outer skin and boiled in water according to the prescribed procedure. This decoction should be made cool. The person should smear his lips and palate with ghee and take this decoction. The quantity of *bhallātaka* should be increased by five fruits (seeds) every day till it reaches the number of seventy. Thereafter, the number of *bhallātaka* should be reduced (by five fruits every day). After the decoction is digested, the person should be given cooled rice mixed with ghee and milk to take. This rejuvenating recipe promotes intellect and cures wrinkles and graying of hair. It also cures *kuṣṭha* (obstinate skin diseases including leprosy), piles, parasitic infestation and vitiation of semen.

तैलं भल्लातकानां यः पिबेन्मांसं यथाबलम्।
सर्वोपतापान्निर्मुक्तो जीवेद् वर्षशतं दृढम् ॥३०॥
॥ इति भल्लातककल्पः[४४] ॥

*Bhallātaka Kalpa*

If a person takes oil extracted from *bhallātaka* in appropriate dose in accordance with his strength for one month, then he becomes free from all diseases, becomes strong and lives for one hundred years.

कासश्वासातिसारज्वरपिटककटी-[४५]
कुष्ठकोष्ठप्रदोषान्[४६] ।
मूत्राघातोदरार्शःश्वयथुगलशिरः-
कर्णशंखाक्षिरोगाः[४७] ॥३१॥
ये चान्ये वातपित्तक्षतजकफकृता
व्याधयः सन्ति जन्तोः ।
तांस्तानभ्यासयोगादपहरति पयः
पीतमन्ते निशायाः ॥३२॥
॥ दुग्धपानगुणाः[४८] ॥

*Milk*

Intake of milk habitually at bed time in the night cures cough, asthma, diarrhoea, fever, pimples, pain in the lumber region, *kuṣṭha* (obstinate skin diseases including leprosy), disorders of the colon, anuria, *udara* (obstinate abdominal disorders including ascites), piles, oedema, diseases of throat, head, ears, temples and eyes and such other diseases caused by *vāyu, pitta, kapha* and consumption.

॥ अन्यच्च[४९] ॥

विगतघननिशीथे प्रातरुत्थाय नित्यं
पिबति खलु नरो यो नासारंध्रेण[५०] वारि ।
स भवति मतिपूर्णः चक्षुषा तार्क्ष्यतुल्यो
वलिपलितविहीनः सर्वरोगैर्विमुक्तः ॥३३॥

*Nāsā-jala-pāna*
*(Taking Water Through Nose)*

When the nights are free from cloud, a person should get up from the bed and take water through the nostrils [of the nose] regularly. This makes the person strong-willed, his eye sight becomes sharp like the mythical bird *garuḍa* and he becomes free from wrinkles, graying of hair and all the diseases.

अम्भसः प्रसृतीनष्टौ रवावनुदिते पिबेत् ।
वातपित्तगदान्[५१] हन्ति जीवेद्वर्षशतं नरः ॥३४॥

***Uṣaḥ Pāna (Taking Water During Dawn)***

If a person takes eight *prasṛtis* of water every day before sun-rise, then he becomes free from diseases caused by *vāyu* and *pitta*, and he lives for one hundred years.

"व्यङ्गवलीपलितघ्नं पीनसवैस्वर्यकासशोथहरम् ।
रजनीक्षयेऽम्बुनस्यं रसायनं दृष्टिजननं च" ॥३५॥

(भैषज्यरत्नावली : रसायनाधिकार : २४)

***Water Inhalation at Dawn***

Inhalation of water at the end of the night (during dawn) is rejuvenating and promoter of eyesight. It cures *vyaṅga* (black pigmented patches in the face), wrinkles, graying of hair, chronic cold, hoarseness of voice, cough and oedema.

तत् त्रिफलाम्बु निशीथं पलितहरं दृष्टिदं श्रेष्ठम् ।
प्रसृतित्रयं तु पातव्यं नासया नाधिकं मतम् ॥३६॥

*Intake of Triphalā Water*

*Triphalā* powder should be soaked in water, kept over night, strained and taken through the nostrils early in the morning. It cures graying of hair and promotes eye sight. One should not drink more than three *prasṛtis* of this water.

"न केवलं दीर्घमिहायुरश्नुते
रसायनं यो विधिवन्निषेवते ।
गतिं स देवर्षिनिषेवितां शुभां
प्रपद्यते ब्रह्म तथैव चाक्षयम्"[५२] ॥३७॥

(चरक : चिकित्सा : १(१) : ७६)
(योगरत्नाकर : रसायनाधिकार : पृष्ठ ५०२)

*Significance of Rejuvenation Therapy*

A person who makes use of this rejuvenation therapy, according to the prescribed procedure, not merely enjoys long life in this world, but also after death he enjoys the auspicious life of the *devas* and *ṛṣis* and gets submerged in the immutable Brahman.

क्षाराम्लमद्यकटुतैलतुषोदकाम्ल-
नीवारकोद्रवकिलाटदधिप्रमेदान्[५३] ।
स्त्रीसंगजागरविचिन्तनदुष्टशाक[५४]-
गव्यांस्त्यजेदपि रसायनकृत्सदैव[५५] ॥३८॥

॥ रसायनाधिकारः[५६] ॥

*Prohibitions*

A person taking rejuvenation therapy should always avoid the following food & regimens :

(1) Intake of alkalies, sour things, alcohol, pungent substance and oil;

(2) intake of sour *tuṣodaka* (a sour drink), *nīvāra, kodrava, kilāṭa* (cheese), curd and excessively fatty substance;
(3) sexual intercourse, remaining awake at night and excessive worry; and
(4) intake of polluted vegetables and such other substances.

'इति'[१७] श्रीमहाराजाधिराजश्रीटोडरमल्लविरचिते
टोडरानन्दे आयुर्वेदसौख्ये रसायनकथनो
नाम सप्तसप्ततमो हर्षः' ॥

Thus, ends the 77th chapter dealing with the description of Rejuvenation therapy in the *Āyurveda saukhya* of *Ṭoḍarānanda* composed by the great King Ṭoḍaramalla.

NOTES AND REFERENCES

१. (क) This is the beginning of eighty first chapter of *Āyurveda saukhya* in *Ṭoḍarānanda* and the invocation reads as follows :
'निहत्य कंसं सुरिपुं सुराणां मुदं ददौ यो पितरौ विमुच्य ।
कृष्णस्तयोः सामरयोर्न्नरेन्द्रे तां टोडरे विप्रमुदिं प्रदद्यात् ॥
(ख) द्रष्टव्यम् ..... चरक : चिकित्सा : १(१) : ७ ।
२. .बलप्रदम् इति षष्ठपुस्तके पाठः ।
३. 'यज्जराव्याधि. ...... तद्रसायनम्' पाठोऽयं प्रथमपुस्तके नोपलभ्यते ।
४. मनुष्यस्य रसायनम् इति आकरे पाठः ।
५. नाविशुद्धशरीरस्य इति आकरे पाठः ।
६. आभाति इति आकरे पाठः ।
७. (क) इवाऽऽहितः इति आकरे पाठः ।
(ख) द्रवापर्तिः इति चतुर्थषष्ठपुस्तकयोः पाठः ।
८. .भया सेव्या इति चतुर्थषष्ठपुस्तकयोः आकरे च पाठः ।
९. वैफलेनायसं पात्रं कल्केनालिंपये भवाम् इति षष्ठपुस्तकेपाठः।
१०. (क) त्रयम् इति चतुर्थपुस्तके पाठः ।
(ख) तयाम् इति पंचमपुस्तके पाठः ।
११. तेमहो रात्रकं लेपं सिता क्षौद्रोदकाह्युतम् इति षष्ठपुस्तके पाठः ।

१२. "पाठामूलं मुखे क्षिप्तं खड्गे सैन्यं न चारयेत् ।
तदेव सर्पिषा पीतं विषं सर्पस्य नाशयेत् ।
विखलानं (विदुभ्यातं) तथा षंड्भकखद्वं शिखास्थितम् ।
दिव्यस्तंभं प्रियत्वं च सर्वेषा कुरुते तथा ।
विचर्चिकां प्रलेपेन छागमूत्रेण संयुताः ।
कर्ण चक्षुःशिरा(शिरो)रोगान्हन्ति छागलसर्पिषा ।
ॐ नमो माहेश्वरी वंध हूँ फट स्वाहा ।

॥ पाठाकल्पः ॥

पाठोऽयं चतुर्थषष्ठपुस्तकयोः अधिकमुपलभ्यते ।

१३. पाठोऽयं प्रथमपंचमपुस्तकयोः नोपलभ्यते ।

१४. अशिततिल. इति प्रथमपुस्तके पाठः ।

१५: पाठोऽयं प्रथमपंचमपुस्तकयोः नोपलभ्यते ।

१६. विधत्ते इति आकरे पाठः ।

१७. अश्वगन्धारसायनम् इति आकरे पाठः ।

१८. एतदनन्तरं षष्ठपुस्तके विषचिकित्सात्मकं पाठं विद्यते । प्रमादपूर्णोऽयं नोद्धृतम् ।

१९. निर्व्याधयो वर्षशतं भवेयुः इति आकरे पाठः ।

२०. पाठोऽयं षष्ठपुस्तके अधिकमुपलभ्यते ।

२१. धात्रीकल्पः शंखचूर्णं पुटे दग्धं घृष्टंमी संयुतम् ।
एतल्लिप्ताः वचाः कृष्णाजायं तेषेवदोपमाः केशरम् । पाठोऽयं चतुर्थषष्ठपुस्कयोः अधिकमुपलभ्यते ।

२२. पाठोऽयं चतुर्थपुस्तके अधिकमुपलभ्यते ।

२३. 'रुदन्ती नाम विख्याता जराव्याधिविनाशिनी ।
चणकसदृशपत्रैः युक्ता (माविंदुरूपिणी)
चतुर्विधा तु सा ज्ञेया रक्तापीता सितासिता ।
रोदिनीवजनान् दृष्ट्वा जरया जर्जरीकृतान् ।
तामौषधिं समादाय शुक्लपक्षे शुभे दिने ।
पत्रमूलान्वितां प्राज्ञः छायाशुष्कां तु कारयेत् ।
विरेकं वमनं कृत्वा विडालपदमात्रया भक्षयेन्मधुसर्पिभ्यां मासमेकं सहौषधीम् ।
जीर्णायां भोजनं कुर्यात् क्षीरान्नैनैव संयमी ।
दृढकायोति तेजस्वी परमायुर्भवेन्नरः ।

॥ रुदतीकल्पः ॥

पत्रैः खर्जूरपत्राभैर्मुशली नाम कीर्तितम् ।
मूलं तस्याः समुद्धृत्य छायाशुष्कं सुचूर्णितम् ।
मधुसर्पिर्युतं भुक्तं देहशुद्धौ शुभे दिने ।
जीर्णे क्षीरेण भोक्तव्यं वातलान्नं विवर्ज्जयेत् ।
पलितैर्वलिभिर्मुक्तो मासयोगेन जायते ।
घृतेन मधुना युक्ताः सर्वकुष्ठविनाशिनी ।
तत्र गोमूत्रसंयुक्ता शूलं हर्षाश्च नाशयेत् ।

॥ मुशलीकल्पः ॥'

पाठोऽयं चतुर्थषष्ठपुस्तकयोः अधिकमुपलभ्यते ।

२४. माषद्वयन्तु इति आकरे पाठः ।

२५. वृद्धदारकरसायनम् इति आकरे पाठः ।

२६. यथेष्टाहारचेष्टोऽपि इति आकरे पाठः ।

२७. (क) त्वस्यवेगः इति प्रथमपुस्तके पाठः ।
(ख) स्वस्यवेगः इति चतुर्थपुस्तके पाठः ।

२८. मन्त्रश्चासौ इति आकरे पाठः ।

२९. योगनामोऽयं आकरे नोपलभ्यते ।

३०. तत्त्रिगुणं इति आकरे पाठः ।

३१. 'मासद्वयं ...... स्यात्' पाठोऽयं पंचमपुस्तके नोपलभ्यते ।

३२. (क) पाठोऽयं प्रथमपंचमपुस्तकयोः नोपलभ्यते ।
(ख) पुनर्नवायोग इति आकरे पाठः ।

३३. मधुयुतं इति चतुर्थषष्ठपुस्तकयोः पाठः ।

३४. (क) पाठोऽयं प्रथमपंचमपुस्तकयोः नोपलभ्यते ।
(ख) आमलकी रसायनम् इति आकरे पाठः ।

३५. पाठोऽयं प्रथमपंचमपुस्तकयोः नोपलभ्यते ।

३६. प्रयोगात्सप्ताहात्किन्नरैः इति आकरे पाठः ।

३७. ब्राह्मीमुण्डीवचाशुण्ठीपिप्पलीमधुसंयुतम् (ता) । सप्तरात्रमिदं सेव्यं किन्नरै सह गीयते ॥ पाठोऽयं चतुर्थषष्ठपुस्तकयोः अधिकमुपलभ्यते ।

३८. तिमिरार्मसशुक्रदोषान् इति आकरे पाठः । ।

३९. पाठोऽयं चतुर्थषष्ठपुस्तकयोः अधिकमुपलभ्यते ।

४०. यः कुष्ठचूर्णं रजनीविरामे
मध्वाज्यमवह्यसंमिश्रितमत्ति नित्यम् ।
समं च मातंगबलः सुगंधिः

वाङ्भीच्चिरायुश्च भवेन्मनुष्यः ॥

॥ कोष्ठकल्पः ॥ पाठोऽयं चतुर्थषष्ठपुस्तकयोः अधिकमुपलभ्यते ।

४१. शोधयेद्विधिवज्जले इति आकरे पाठः ।

४२. च इति आकरे पाठः ।

४३ दृष्टं शुक्रविवर्द्धनम् इति षष्ठपुस्तके पाठः ।

४४. पाठोऽयं प्रथमपुस्तके नोपलभ्यते ।

४५. .विटपकटी. इति षष्ठपुस्तके पाठः ।

४६. .पृष्ठकोष्ठ. इति षष्ठपुस्तके पाठः ।

४७. कर्णनासाक्षिरोगान् इति चतुर्थषष्ठपुस्तकयोः पाठः ।

४८. पाठोऽयं प्रथमपुस्तके नोपलभ्यते ।

४९. पाठोऽयं षष्ठपुस्तके नोपलभ्यते ।

५०. (क) घ्राणरंध्रेण वारि इति चतुर्थपुस्तके पाठः ।
(ख) घ्राणरंध्रे तु नीरम् इति षष्ठपुस्तके पाठः ।

५१. वातपित्तकफा इति चतुर्थषष्ठपुस्तकयोः पाठः ।

५२. तथेति चाक्षरम् इति आकरे पाठः ।

५३. .दध्निप्रसेदान् इति पंचमपुस्तके पाठः ।

५४. विष्टिम्भदुष्टशाक इति पंचमपुस्तके पाठः ।

५५. 'भल्लातकानां च वनोदधृतां वृतं च्युतानां च पदाढकं स्यात् । तच्चेष्टकाचूर्णकणैर्विघृष्य प्रक्षालयित्वा विसृजेत् प्रवाते शुष्कं पुनस्त द्विदलीकृतं च विपाचयेदप्सु चतुर्गुणासु । पादावशेषं परिपूतशीतं क्षीरेण तुल्यं नी वचा (न विषा) च येतत् । पादावशेषे पुनरेव (रैव) शीतं घृतेन तुल्येन पुनः पचेच्च । तदर्द्धया शर्क्करया सयेतं ततः स्वजेनोत्क्वथितं विधाय । त्रिजातक त्र्यूष्णजीरवांशीः (वोशीः) । सितार्द्धतोतस्त्रिण (स्तृण) राजशीर्षं । तृवच्च मांसीत्रिफलासमेतं कर्पूरयुक्तं खदिरामृतं च । सु (स) चन्दना कल्लकचीनवाससदेवपुष्पंमुशली द्वयं च । कंक्कोलमोचाह्वयदीप्ययुग्मं नतं समातंगकणाविदारी । मेदाद्वयं लोहरसेन्द्रवंगमन्नं (द्व) त तथा कुंकुमकं च कर्षं । जातिफलं मस्तकि जातिपत्री तत्सप्तरात्रादुपजातवीर्य्यं । सुधारसादप्यधिकत्वयेति । प्रातर्विशुष्द्धः कृतदेव कार्यो मात्रां लिहेदात्मशरीरयोग्यां । न चान्निपाने परिहार्य्यमस्ति न चातपेनाध्वनि मैथुने वा । यथेष्टचेष्टोऽभिहि तोय (भि) योगा दवेन्नरः । कांचनराशिगौरः तुल्यमेधाः नरसिंहवञ्चीदामाः सुखं (क्षुरधं) गच्छति सत्वयुक्तः । दंताश्च शीर्णाः पुनरुम्द (द्ध) वंति

केशाश्च शुक्लाः पुनरेव कृष्णाः । नीलांजनालिप्रतिमा भवन्ति त्वचो विवर्णा पुनरेव दिव्याः (ध्याः) । विशीर्णं कर्णागुंलिनासिकोऽपि कृम्यर्छितो भिन्नगलोपिकुष्टी । सोऽपि क्रमादंकुरिता दशाखस्तरुर्यथा भाति अथाम्बु सिक्तः । पुष्टान्म (पुष्टांत्म) परान् (परां) जयति स्वेरण बलेन नागं तुरगं जवेन । रसायनस्यस्य नरः प्रयोगाद्व(ध) ह्स्यते (ह्स्थने) रण्यधिकः स्वबुध्या । ग्रन्थं विशालं पुनरुक्तदोषं गृह्णाति शीघ्रं (शिप्रं) खलुजश्म (खलुतथ्य) मेतत् । कुर्वीतेमं (सं) कल्पमवल्य (कल्पनल्प) बुद्धिर्ज्जी (नि) वेन्नरो वर्णशतानि पञ्जराजानमुग्रं च रसायनां । च नाचाकास्योर (कारयो) गभ्दग (गाद्धय) वानगल्पः (त्यः) ।

॥ इति भेडादमृतभल्लातककल्पः ॥

॥ इति रसायनाधिकारः ॥

पाठोऽयं चतुर्थषष्ठपुस्तकयोः अधिकमुपलभ्यते ।

५६. पाठोऽयं षष्ठपुस्तके नोपलभ्यते ।

५७ 'इति ..... ड्र्षः' पाठोऽयं पंचमपुस्तके अधिकमुपलभ्यते ।

# CHAPTER X

## ।। अथ वाजीकरणाधिकारः ।।

*(Aphrodisiac Therapy)*

"तैस्तैर्भावैरहृद्यैस्तु[१] रिरंसोर्मनसि क्षते ।
ध्वजः पतत्यतो नृणां क्लैव्यं समुपजायते" ।।१ ।।

(योगरत्नाकर : क्लैव्यनिदान : पृष्ठ ४७९)

*Etiology (Psychic Factors)*

If a person desires to have sexual intercourse but his mind is hurt by several *ahṛdya* (not congenial for the heart or the mind) factors, then this leads to the non-erection of the male genital organ which gives rise to impotency.

अन्नैरम्लोष्णलवणैरतिमात्रोपसेवितैः[२] ।
सौम्यधातुक्षयो[३] दृष्टः 'क्लैव्य'[४] तदपरं स्मृतम् ।।२ ।।

*Etiology (Physical Factors)*

Excessive intake of sour, hot and saline food leads to the diminution of semen which is another factor responsible for impotency.

"अतिव्यवायशीलो वा' न च वाजीक्रियारतः ।
ध्वजभङ्गमवाप्नोति तच्छुक्रक्षयहेतुकम्" ॥३॥
(योगरत्नाकर : क्लैव्यनिदान : पृष्ठ ४७९)

If a person excessively indulges in sex without using aphrodisiacs, then this causes excessive loss of semen which results in *dhvajabhanga* (non-erection of penis).

असाध्यं सहज' क्लैव्यं मर्मच्छेदाच्च यद्भवेत् ।
साध्यानामवशिष्टानां कार्यो वाजीकरो विधिः ॥४॥

*Prognosis*

Congenital impotency and the impotency caused by the injury (lit. cut) to *marma* (vital part) are incurable. Other types of impotency are curable and such cases should be treated by the administration of aphrodisiac therapy.

"पिप्पलीलवणोपेतौ बस्ताण्डौ क्षीरसर्पिषा ।
साधितौ भक्षयेद्यस्तु स गच्छेत् प्रमदाशतम्" ॥५॥
(भैषज्यरत्नावली : वाजीकरणाधिकार : १८)

*Goat's Testicles*

Testicles of a goat should be mixed with *pippalī* and salt, and then cooked by adding milk and ghee. A person which takes this recipe becomes capable of having sexual intercourse with many (lit. one hundred) women.

शाल्मलीपुष्पचूर्णं तु क्षौद्रं कर्षं लिहेदनु ।
दुर्बलो बलमाप्नोति मासैकेन यथा शशी ॥६॥

*Śālmalī Flower*

By the intake of the powder of *śālmalī*-flower (one *karṣa*) along with honey for one month, a weak person becomes strong (and beautiful) like a full-moon.

कुष्ठमांसीहरिद्राभिर्मुराशैलेयपंचकैः
'वचाकर्चूरमुस्तैश्च'[6] सर्वौषधिगणः स्मृतः ॥७॥

*Sarvauṣadha Group of Drugs*

*Kuṣṭha, jaṭāmāṃsī, haridrā, murāmāṃsī* and *śaileya* —these five drugs added with *vacā, karcūra* and *mustā* constitute *Sarvauṣadhi gaṇa* (group).

सर्वौषधिकसंमिश्रा संशुष्कामलकत्वचः[7] ।
सुगन्धामलकानीति निर्दिश्यन्ते विचक्षणैः' ॥८॥
स्नानं कृत्वा नरेन्द्रार्हं सौमनस्यं प्रजायते ।
सर्वदोषग्रहघ्नं च वाजीकरणमुत्तमम्[8] ।
'सौमनस्य[9] भवेत्तेन प्रमदानां प्रियो भवेत् ॥९॥

*Sugandhāmalaka*

The pulp of dried *āmalaka* mixed with drugs belonging to *Sarvauṣadhi* group is called *Sugandhāmalaka*. Bath with the decoction of these drugs is suitable for Kings. It causes happiness of the mind. It removes afflictions by all the evil planets including evil spirits. It is an excellent aphrodisiac therapy. The bath with this decoction gives pleasure and makes a person lovable by ladies.

"बस्ताण्डसिद्धे[10] पयसि भावितान्[11] सकृत्तिलान् ।
यः खादेत्स पुमान्[12] गच्छेत् स्त्रीणां शतमपूर्ववत् ॥१०॥

*Sessame Seeds*

Sessame seeds should be frequently impregnated with the milk boiled by adding goat's testicles. Intake of this, makes a person capable of indulging sexual intercourse with many (lit. hundred) women.

चूर्णं विदार्याः सुकृतं स्वरसेनैव भावितम् ।
'सर्पिः[13] क्षौद्रयुतं लीढ्वा[14] शतं गच्छेन्नरोऽङ्गनाः ॥११॥

***Vidārikanda***

The powder of *vidārikanda* should be impregnated with its juice (of *vidārikanda*). Intake of this powder mixed with gheee and honey enables a person to indulge in sex with many (lit. hundred) women.

एवमामलकं चूर्णं स्वरसेनैव भावितम् ।
शर्करामधुसर्पिर्भिर्युक्तं लीढ्वा पयः पिबेत् ।
एतेनाशीतिवर्षोऽपि युवेव परिहृष्यति ॥१२॥

***Āmalakī***

The powder of *āmalakī* should be impregnated with its juice. This should be taken along with sugar, honey and ghee. Thereafter, one should take milk. By doing so, even an eighty year old person gets sexually excited like a young person.

विदारिकन्दकल्कं[१५] तु घृतेन[१६] पयसा नरः ।
उदुम्बरसमं खादेत् वृद्धोऽपि तरुणायते ॥१३॥

***Vidārikanda (Second Recipe)***

The paste of *vidārikanda* should be mixed with ghee and milk. Intake of this along with the powder of *udumbara* makes even an old person young.

स्वयंगुप्तेक्षुरकयोर्बीजचूर्णं सशर्करम् ।
धारोष्णेन नरः पीत्वा पयसा न क्षयं व्रजेत् ॥१४॥

***Ātmagupta***

If a person takes the powder of the seeds of *ātmagupta* and *ikṣuraka* along with sugar, and thereafter, if he drinks warm milk freshly collected (*dhāroṣṇa*), his semen never gets ejaculated by sexual intercourse, i.e. he becomes capable of indulging in sex for a long time.

उच्चटाचूर्णमप्येवं क्षीरेणोत्तममुच्यते ॥१५॥

***Uccaṭā***

The powder of *uccaṭā* should similarly be taken along with milk which promotes virility.

शतावर्युच्चटाचूर्णं पेयमेवं सुखाम्बुना[१७] ॥१६॥

*Śatāvarī*

The powder of *śatāvarī* and *uccaṭā*, if taken along with luke-warm water, promotes virility.

कर्ष[१८] मधुकचूर्णस्य घृतक्षौद्रसमन्वितम् ।
पयोऽनुपान[१९] यो लिह्यान्नित्यवेगः स ना भवेत् ॥१७॥

*Madhuka*

One *karṣa* of the powder of *madhuka* should be mixed with ghee and honey, and taken along with milk. The person using this recipe gets sexual urge every day.

गोक्षुरकः क्षुरकः शतमूली वानरि नागबलातिबला च।
चूर्णमिदं पयसा निशि पेयं यस्य गृहे प्रमदाशतमस्ति" ॥१८॥

(भैषज्यरत्नावली : वाजीकरणाधिकार : १९-२६)

*Gokṣuraka, etc.*

The powder of *gokṣuraka, kṣuraka, śatamulī, vānari, nāgabalā* and *atibalā* should be taken with milk at night by a person (King) who has many (lit. hundred) women at home.

मुशलीकन्दचूर्णं च गुडूचीसत्त्वसंयुतम् ।
वानरीगोक्षुराभ्यां च शाल्मलीशर्करामलैः[२०] ।
आलोड्य घृतदुग्धाभ्यां पाययेत्कामवृद्धये ॥१९॥

*Muśalīkanda, etc.*

The powder of *muśalīkanda* should be added with *guḍūcī sattva, vānarī, gokṣura* and *śālmalī* (powders) and boiled with ghee and milk. Intake of this potion promotes sexual strength.

कपिकच्छुकमूलं तु अजाक्षीरेण तं पिबेत् ।
तेनैव जायते शुक्रं कामयेत् स्त्रीसहस्रशः ॥२०॥

### *Ātmaguptā (Second Recipe)*

Goat's milk boiled with the root of *ātmaguptā* should be taken for the promotion of semen and it makes a person capable of indulging in sex with many (lit. hundred) women.

वाराहीकन्दशृंगाटं पलयुगल[21] चूर्णितम् किंचिदाज्ये भृष्टम् ।
कल्के दलत्वक्सुरकुसुमकणाकेसराणां च[22] श्वेताम् ॥२१॥
सर्वैः समानां पयसि दशगुणे साधु पक्त्वा महिष्याः।
कामोद्बोधा तदनु[23] चटकाः कामुकैः[24] शुक्रवृद्धयै[25] ॥२२॥
एतान्सदा सेव्यमानो वृद्धोऽपि तरुणायते ।
तरुणीनां शतं याति तरुणानां च का कथा ॥२३॥

### *Vārāhīkanda, etc.*

Two *palas* of each of *vārāhīkanda* and *śṛṅgāṭa* should be made to a powder and fried with ghee. To this, equal quantities of each of *dala, tvak, lavaṅga, pippalī, kesara* and sugar should be added and boiled by adding ten times of buffalo-milk. After taking this milk, one should take the eggs of sparrow. This promotes semen. Intake of this recipe regularly endows youthfulness even in an old person, what to speak of young people. He becomes capable of indulging in sex with many (lit. hundred) of young women.

लघुशाल्मलिमूलेन तालमूलीं च चूर्णिताम् ।
सर्पिषा पयसा पीत्वा रतौ चटकवद्भवेत् ॥२४॥

### *Śālmalī Root*

Powders of the root of an young *śālmalī* tree and *tālamūlī* should be mixed with ghee and milk. Intake of this recipe makes a person sexy like a sparrow.

वृद्धशाल्मलिमूलस्य रसं शर्करया पिबेत् ।
एतत्प्रयोगेन सप्ताहाज्जायते रेतसोंऽबुधिः[26] ॥२५॥

The juice of the root of an old *śālmalī* tree should be taken by adding sugar. By the intake of this recipe for seven days, the semen of a person increases considerably (lit. like a sea).

सितावानरिकंदकृतं पयसा यः प्रपिबेन्ननु चूर्णवरम् ।
स भवेद्वनिताशतसौख्यकरः सुरते सततं तरुणीषु रतः ॥२६॥

*Recipes*

If a person takes sugar and the powder of the root of *ātmagupta* along with milk, he becomes capable of providing sex-satisfaction to many (lit. hundred) young women.

भीरुक्षीरविदारिका कुडवकः श्वेतार्द्धकार्द्धार्धिकम्[२७] ।
प्रस्थं शाल्मलिमूलजातरसतो नीत्वा तथाऽग्नौ पचेत् ॥२७॥
चातुर्जातपलान्वितो मधुयुतः कार्यः परं शुक्रलम् ।
लेहोऽयं पलितान्तको बलकरः ख्यातो वलीनाशनः ॥२८॥
॥ शतावर्यवलेहः[२८] ॥

*Śatāvaryavaleha*

One *kuḍava* of each of *śatāvarī* and *kṣīravidārī*, one and half *kuḍava* of sugar and one *prastha* of the juice of *śālmalī*-root should be cooked together over fire. To this, one *pala* of each of *tvak, elā, patra, kesara* and honey should be added. Intake of this promotes semen. It cures graying of hair, promotes strength and removes wrinkles.

कंकोलकं पूगफलं लवंगकुसुमानि च ।
जातिफलानि कर्पूरमेतत् पंचसुगन्धिकम् ॥२९॥
भक्षयेत्तु नरेन्द्राणां सौमनस्यं प्रजायते ।
आस्यं विशदतामेति प्रमदानां वशं करम् ।
ताम्बूलैश्च युतं ह्येतत् भक्ष्येत्सुखदं नृणाम् ॥३०॥

*Betel-Nut and Betel-Leaf*

*Kaṅkolaka, pūga* fruit, *lavaṅga* flower, *jātiphala* and *karpūra,* these five drugs taken together are called *Pañca sugandhika* (five aromatics). Use of these by King give pleasure and make him capable of indulging in sex with women. These drugs, taken along with betel-leaf endows happiness to people.

माषदालि[२९] घृतैर्युक्तं पायसं तत्तु कारयेत् ।
घृतशर्करया युक्तं रतिमिच्छन्तु भक्षयेत् ।
अक्षयं जायते शुक्रं कामयेत्स्त्रीशतान्यपि ॥३१॥

*Māṣa*

Grains (dals) of *māṣa* should be fried with ghee and made to a *pāyasa* by boiling with milk. Intake of this, by adding ghee and sugar promotes sexual strength. His semen does not get reduced and he becomes capable of indulging in sex with many (lit. hundred) women.

शतावरीगोक्षुरकेण दर्भशृंगाटको नागबलात्मगुप्ता[३०] ।
सिता समानं निशि चूर्णमेषां दुग्धेन पीतं प्रकरोति पुंस्त्वम् ॥३२॥

*Recipes*

*Śatāvarī, gokṣuraka, darbha, śṛṅgāṭaka, nāgabalā, ātmaguptā* and sugar should be taken in equal quantities and made to a powder. Intake of this powder with milk promotes virility.

शतावरीरजः[३१] प्रस्थं प्रस्थं गोक्षुरकस्य च ।
वाराह्याः विंशतिपलं गुडूच्याः पंचविंशतिः ॥३३॥
भल्लातकानां द्वात्रिंशत् चित्रकस्य दशैव तु।
तिलानां लुंचितानां च प्रस्थं दद्याच्च[३२] चूर्णितम् ॥३४॥
त्र्यूषणस्य पलान्यष्टौ शर्करायाश्च सप्ततिः ।
माक्षिकं शर्करार्द्धेन मधुनोर्द्धेन[३३] वै घृतम् ॥३५॥
शतावरीसमं देयं विदारीकन्दचूर्णकम् ।
एतानि सूक्ष्मचूर्णानि स्निग्धे भाण्डे निधापयेत् ॥३६॥

पलार्द्धमुपयुंजीत[३४] यथेष्टं चात्र[३५] भोजनम् ।
एषा[३६] मासोपयोगेन रुजं हन्ति जरामपि ॥३७॥
वलीपलितखालित्यप्लीहषा[३७]ढ्यांध्यपीनसान् ।
भगन्दरान्मूत्रकृच्छ्रानश्मरींश्च भिनत्यपि ॥३८॥
अष्टादशानि[३८] कुष्ठानि तथाष्टावुदराणि च ।
प्रमेहांश्च महाव्याधीन् पंचकासान् सुदुस्तरान् ॥३९॥
अशीतिर्वातजान् व्याधीन् चत्वारिंशच्च पैत्तिकान् ।
विंशतिं श्लैष्मिकांश्चैव संसृष्टान्[३९] सान्निपातिकान् ।
एताः सर्वा रुजो[४०] हन्ति वृक्षमिंद्राशनिर्यथा ॥४०॥
स कांचनाभो मृगराजविक्रमः तुरङ्गमादप्यति[४१]याति वेगतः ।
स्त्रीणां शतं गच्छति सोऽतिरम्यः[४२] सुहृष्टपुष्टश्चटको यथा तथा
॥४१॥
पुत्राञ्जनयते[४३] वीरान् नरसिंहपराक्रमान् ।
नारसिंहेति विख्यातः[४४] चूर्णो रोगगणापहः ॥४२॥
॥ नारसिंहचूर्णम् ॥

(भारतभैषज्यरत्नाकर : तृतीय भाग : पृष्ठ १६८)
(भैषज्यरत्नावली : वाजीकरणाधिकार : ३०-३९)

*Nārasiṃha Cūrṇa*

Powders of *śatāvarī* (one *prastha*), *gokṣuraka* (one *prastha*), *vārāhīkanda* (20 *palas*), *guḍūcī* (25 *palas*), *bhallātaka* (32 seeds), *citraka* (10 *palas*), dehusked *tila* (one *prastha*), *śuṇṭhī* (8 *palas*), *pippalī* (8 *palas*), *marica* (8 *palas*), sugar (70 *palas*), honey (35 *palas*), ghee ($17^1/_2$ *palas*) and powder of *vidārīkanda* (one *prastha*) should be stored in a jar smeared with ghee. This recipe should be taken in a dose of half *pala*. The person using this recipe can take any type of food he desires. Intake of this recipe for one month prevents aging process, wrinkles, graying of hair and baldness and cures splenic disorders, blindness, impotency, chronic cold, fistula-in-ano, dysuria, stone in kidneys, eighteen types of *kuṣṭha* (obstinate skin diseases including leprosy), eight *udaras* (obstinate abdominal diseases including ascites), *prameha* (obstinate urinary disorders including diabetes), five varieties of cough, eighty varieties of *vātika* diseases, forty varieties of *paittika* diseases, twenty varieties of *kaphaja* diseases and other such diseases caused by the simultaneous vitiation of two or three *doṣas*. These serious diseases are cured by the recipe as a tree gets destroyed by the thunderbolt of Indra. The person using this recipe looks like gold and he gets the strength of a lion. He becomes capable of running faster than a horse. He appears lovable, strong and stout and like a sparrow, he indulges in sex with many (lit. hundred) women. He produces sons who are brave and strong like Lord Narasiṃha. This recipe which cures several diseases is called *Nārasiṃha cūrṇa*.

"पलं[४५] गोक्षुरबीजस्य[४६] द्विपलं कपिकच्छुरा ।
पलं नागबलामूलं[४७] पलमेकं शतावरी ॥४३॥
विदारीकन्दचूर्णं तु पलमेकं तथैव च ।
पलार्द्धं[४८] त्रपुषीबीजं वाजिगन्धा पलत्रयम् ॥४४॥
त्रिसुगन्धं[४९] कणा धात्री लवङ्गं नागकेसरम् ।
वासकं[५०] तालमज्जा च गुडूची रक्तचन्दनम् ॥४५॥
एतानि कर्षमात्राणि सूक्ष्मचूर्णानि कारयेत् ।
बलाशाल्मलिकाद्रावैर्भावयेदेकविंशतिः[५१] ॥४६॥
कुशकाशं[५२] तथा सप्तशर्करा समयोजिता ।
नष्टशुक्रा[५३]स्तु ये पुंसा मूत्रकृच्छ्रांस्तथैव च ॥४७॥
वृद्धमूत्रं जयेत् दुष्टं धन्वन्तरिकृतालयम् ।
शतं गच्छेत्तु नारीणां कामतुल्यं सवीर्यवान् ।
क्षीरानुपानभोजी च वर्जयेत्कटुकादिकम् ॥४८॥
॥ इति कामदेवचूर्णम्[५४]" ॥

(भारतभैषज्यरत्नाकर प्रथमभाग पृष्ठ २१४)

**Kāmadeva Cūrṇa**

*Gokṣura*-seed (one *pala*), *kapikacchu* (two *palas*), root of *nāgabalā* (one *pala*), *śatāvarī* (one *pala*), *vidārīkanda* (one *pala*), seeds of *trapuṣa*

(1/2 *pala*), *aśvagandhā* (3 *palas*), and one *karṣa* of each of *tvak*, *elā*, *patra*, *pippalī*, *āmalakī*, *lavaṅga*, *nāgakesara*, *vāsaka*, *tālamajjā*, *guḍūcī* and *raktacandana* should be made to a fine powder. This should be impregnated for 21 times in the decoction (or juice) of each of *balā* and *śālmalī*. It should then be added with the powders of *kuśa*, *kāśa* and sugar (seven *palas*). It cures seminal pollution, dysuria and anuria like the blessings of Lord Dhanvantari. The person taking this recipe becomes beautiful like *Kāmadeva* (the god of sex) and strong. It makes him capable of indulging in sex with many (lit. hundred) women. The person taking this recipe should take milk as food and he should avoid pungent spices, etc.

"[५५]हरार्कायोवङ्गाभ्रकबलिकलैकद्विजलधि
द्विपादास्त्रिशद्भिर्मिलितमनलेंऽशैर्मृदि पुनः ॥४९॥
द्व्यहं पक्वं कूप्यां भवति सिकतायन्त्रजुषित-
स्तलस्थः षण्ढत्वप्रलयकृदयं षण्मुखरसः ॥५०॥
॥ षण्मुखरसः" ॥

(भारतभैषज्यरत्नाकर : पञ्चमभाग : पृष्ठ १८८)

***Ṣaṇmukha Rasa***

*Pārada* (16 parts), *tāmra bhasma* (one part), *lauha bhasma* (two parts), *vaṅga bhasma* (four parts), *abhraka bhasma* (1/2 part) and *gandhaka* (30 parts) should be mixed together, kept in a glass bottle and cooked in *Vālukā yantra* for two days. The medicine, settled at the bottom of the bottle should be collected and used. It effectively cures impotency and it is called *Ṣaṇmukha rasa*.

"पृथग्द्वौ हाटकं चन्द्रं त्रयो वङ्गाहिकान्तजम् ।
चत्वारः सूतमभ्रं च प्रवालं मौक्तिकं तथा ॥५१॥
भावना दुग्धि गव्येक्षुवासाश्रीद्विजलैर्निशा[५६] ।
मोचकन्दरसैः सप्तक्रमाद्भाव्यं पृथक्पृथक् ॥५२॥
शतपत्ररसेनैव मालतीकुसुमैस्तथा[५७] ।
पश्चान्मृगमदैर्भाव्यः सुसिद्धो[५८] रसराड् भवेत् ॥५३॥

कुसुमाकरविख्यातो वसन्तपदपूर्वकः ।
वल्लद्वयमितः सेव्यः सिताज्यमधुसंयुतः ॥५४॥
वलिपलितहृन्मेध्यः कामदः सुखदः सदा ।
मेहघ्नः पुष्टिदः श्रेष्ठः परं वृष्यो रसायनम् ॥५५॥
आयुर्वृद्धिकरं पुंसां प्रजाजननमुत्तमम् ।
क्षयकासतृषोन्मादश्वासरक्तविषार्तिजित् ॥५६॥
सिताचन्दनसंयुक्तमम्लपित्तादिरोगजित् ।
शुक्लपाण्ड्वामयान् शूलान्मूत्राघाताश्मरीं हरेत् ॥५७॥
योगवाही त्विदं सेव्यं कान्तिश्रीबलवर्धनम् ।
सुसात्म्यमिष्टभोजी च रमयेत्प्रमदाशतम् ॥ ॥५८॥

॥ वसन्तकुसुमाकर रसः" ॥

(भारतभैषज्यरत्नाकर : चतुर्थभाग : पृष्ठ ७३२)

***Vasnta Kusumākara***

*Svarṇa bhasma* (2 parts), *raupya bhasma* (2 parts), *vaṅga bhasma* (3 parts), *nāga bhasma* (3 parts), *kānta lauha bhasma* (3 parts), *rasa sindūra* (4 parts), *abhraka bhasma* (4 parts), *pravāla bhasma* (4 parts) and *muktā bhasma* (4 parts) should be mixed together, triturated and impregnated with (1) cow's milk, (2) sugar-cane juice, (3) juice of *vāsā*, decoctions of (4) *śveta candana*, (5) *hrībera*, (6) *uśīra* and (7) *haridrā*, (8) juices of the underground stem of *moca*, (9) *kamala* and (10) flower of *mālatī* and (11) *kastūrī*, for seven days in each. This excellent preparation is called *Vasanta kusumākara*. It should be used in the dose of two *vallas* along with sugar, ghee and honey. It cures wrinkles and graying of hair. It promotes intellect, sex-passion and happiness. It cures *meha* (obstinate urinary disorders including diabetes). It provides nourishment. It is an excellent recipe for promoting virility and rejuvenation. It promotes longevity and helps one to get progeny. It cures tuberculosis, cough, morbid thirst, insanity, asthma, diseases of blood and poisoning. If taken with sugar and sandalwood paste, then it cures diseases like *amlapitta* (hyperacidity), anemia, colic pain, dysuria and stone in the urinary tract. It is *yogavāhī* (which promotes the effects of other added medicines). It promotes complexion, auspiciousness and strength. The person using this recipe should take wholesome and sweet food. It enables the person to have sexual intercourse with many (lit. hundred) women.

भ्रमक्लमो रुग्दौर्बल्यं बलधात्विंद्रियक्षयः ।
अकालमरणं च स्यात् विशेषेणातिमैथुनात् ॥५९॥

*Ill-Effects of Excess Sex*

If a person indulges in sex in excess, then he suffers from giddiness, fatigue, weakness in the thighs and reduction in strength, tissue elements and the power of sense organs. It leads to untimely death of a person.

आयुष्मंतो मंदजरा वपुर्वर्णबलाधिकाः ।
स्थिरोपचितमांसाश्च भवन्ति स्त्रीषु संयताः ॥६०॥

*Good Effects of Celebacy*

Persons who control themselves and abstain from sex indulgence with women live long; their aging process becomes slow, their bodies become full of complexion and strength; and their musculature becomes stable and plumpy.

त्र्यहाद्वसंते शरदि पक्षाद्वृष्टिनिदाघयोः ।
सेवेत कामतः कामं नरो वाजीकृतो हिमे ॥६१॥

*Frequency of Sex in Different Seasons*

One should indulge in sex intercourse once in three days during spring and autumn and once in fifteen days in the rainy season and summer. In winter season one may indulge in sex as frequently as he likes provided he has taken aphrodisiac drugs.

"कूष्माण्डकात् पलशतं सुस्विन्नं निष्कुलीकृतम् ।
प्रस्थञ्च घृततैलस्य तस्मिंस्तप्ते निधापयेत् ॥६२॥
त्वक्पत्रधान्यकव्योषजीरकैलाद्वयानलम् ।
ग्रन्थिकं चव्यमातङ्गपिप्पलीविश्वभेषजम् ॥६३॥

शृङ्गाटकं कशेरुञ्च प्रवाल[६०] तालमस्तकम् ।
चूर्णीकृतं पलांशञ्च गुडस्य तुलया पचेत् ॥६४॥
शीते भूते पलान्यष्टौ मधुनः सम्प्रदापयेत् ।
कफपित्तानिलहरं मन्दाग्नीनाञ्च शस्यते ॥६५॥
कृशानां बृंहणं श्रेष्ठं वाजीकरणमुत्तमम् ।
'प्रमदासु[६१] प्रसक्तानां ये च स्युः क्षीणरेतसः ॥६६॥
क्षयेण तु गृहीतानां परमेतद् भिषग्जितम्' ।
कासं श्वासं ज्वरं हिक्कां हन्तिच्छर्दिमरोचकम् ॥६७॥
गुडकूष्माण्डकं[६२] ख्यातमश्विभ्यां समुदाहृतम्'' ।
खण्डकूष्माण्डवत् पात्रं स्विन्नकूष्माण्डकद्रवः ॥६८॥
॥ गुडकुष्माण्डकावलेहः[६३] ॥

(भैषज्यरत्नावली : वाजीकरणाधिकार : ८१-८६)

***Guḍa Kuṣmāṇḍāvaleha***

One hundred *palas* of *kūṣmāṇḍa*, free from its skin and seeds, should be steam-boiled and its juice should be squeezed out. The pulp should then be fried by adding one *prastha* each of ghee and oil. Thereafter, the juice should be added and boiled with the powder of *tvak, patra, dhānyaka, śuṇṭhī, pippalī, marica, jīraka, elā, kṣudrailā, citraka, granthika, cavya, gajapippalī, ārdraka, śṛṅgāṭaka, kaśeru, pravāla* and *tālamastaka*, one *pala* each, and one hundred *palas* of jaggery should be added and cooked. When the preparation becomes cool after cooking, 8 *palas* of honey should be added. The recipe alleviates *kapha* and *pitta*. It is useful for persons having suppressed power of digestion. It nourishes emaciated persons and it is an excellent aphrodisiac recipe. Persons who are attached to women and indulge in excess of sex suffer from diminution of semen and tuberculosis. It is an excellent recipe for such persons. It also cures cough, asthma, fever, hiccup, vomiting and anorexia. It is called *Guḍa kūṣmāṇḍaka* and in the days of yore, it was propounded by the Aśvins.

यत्किञ्चिन्मधुरं स्निग्धं बृंहणं जीवनं गुरु ।
हर्षणं मनसश्चैव सर्वं तद्वृष्यमुच्यते ॥६९॥

*Attributes of Aphrodisiacs*

All such substances which are sweet, unctuous, nourishing, promoter of longevity and heavy and which cause exhileration of the mind are called *vṛṣya* (aphrodisiac).

शुभेह्नि देशे सम्भूतं पलं शतं सम्यगश्वगन्धायाः ।
पुष्येऽहूनि संक्षुन्नं विपचेद्द्रोणेम्भसि च विद्वान् ॥७०॥
ज्ञात्वाष्टभागशेषं गृहूणीयात्तद्रसं सुपरिपूतम् ।
द्वे चैवात्र पलशते दद्याच्छागस्य शुद्धमांसस्य ॥७१॥
सर्पिः प्रस्थमथैकं गव्यं पयश्चतुर्थकं दद्यात् ।
कल्कानक्षसमांसानूर्ध्वमतः सम्प्रवक्ष्यामि ॥७२॥
काकोलीद्वयमृद्धिद्वे मेदे जीवकं च द्वयम् ।
संयुक्तं ऋषभकमेलामधुकं मृद्वीकाम् ॥७३॥
संजीवनी मधुकुल्यां बलां विदारी शतावरी च ।
दत्त्वा सम्यग्विपचेत् सर्पिरथोद्धृत्य पीत्वा च ॥७४॥
मधुशर्करयोः कुडवं दत्त्वा भाण्डस्थितमुद्धृतम् ।
लीढ्वा तत्पाणितलं यथेच्छ्वाहारमश्नीयात् ॥७५॥
क्षीणक्षतशिशुवृद्धाः क्षीणेन्द्रिया हीनमांसाश्च प्राश्य प्राप्नुयुः।
सद्यः बलारोग्यतेजांसि उपयुज्य सर्पिरेतत् सप्तति वर्षोयुरेवम् ॥७६॥
भूत्वा बहुश स्त्रियोधिगच्छति न चापि शुक्रक्षयं लभते।
पुत्रार्थिनी च नारी लभते पुत्रान् वयस्यतीतेऽपि वंध्यापि ॥७७॥
लभते पुत्रं प्राश्यैतदश्वगंधाद्यं उपयुक्तेयं यत्वर्षः ।
त्रिमासं सार्द्धसामं वा नारीशतं संगच्छेन्नैव भजेत योषितस्तृप्तिम्
॥७८॥
खालित्यवलीपलितैर्न चास्य देहेभिभूयते क्षिप्रम् ।
वातव्याधिभिरात्तस्तथैव हृद्वस्तिरोगार्त्ताः ।
भुञ्जीतमिदं नराः न रोगार्त्ताः भवन्ति ॥७९॥

एवं जगद्धितार्थं सर्पिरिदं वाजिगन्धायाः ।
श्रेष्ठं वाजीकरणं निर्दिष्टं पूर्वमश्विभ्याम् ॥८०॥

॥ अश्वगन्धाघृतम् ॥

*Aśvagandha Ghṛta*

Roots of *aśvagandha* growing in a sacred place should be collected on an auspicious day during the *Puṣya* constellation. These roots should be coarsely pounded and boiled by adding one *droṇa* of water till one eighth of water remains. The decoction should then be filtered out. To this, two hundred *palas* of goat-meat (free from bones), one *prastha* of ghee and four *prasthas* of cow's milk should be added. In addition, the paste of one *akṣa* each of *kākolī, kṣīrakākolī, ṛddhi, vṛddhi, medā, mahāmedā,* two varieties of *jīvaka, ṛṣabhaka, elā, madhuka, mṛdvīkā, sañjīvanī* (drugs belonging to *Jīvanīya* group), *madhukulyā, balā, vidārī* and *śatāvarī* should be added to this recipe and cooked. After it is properly cooked, the ghee should be strained, and to this, one *kuḍava* of each of honey and sugar should be added. The recipe should then be stored in a jar. This medicated ghee should be administered in the dose of one *paṇitala*. While taking this recipe, the patient can take any type of food he desires. By using this, persons suffering from consumption, children, old persons and persons having weakness of their sense organs and wasting of muscles instantaneously acquire strength, health and complexion. Even a person of seventy years of age, by taking this medicated ghee, becomes capable of having sexual intercourse with many women and does not get his semen reduced. Even an aged woman or a sterile woman gets the desired son by the intake of this recipe. This is called *Aśvagandhādya* [*ghṛta*] and it should be used for one year, for three months or for one and half months. By taking this recipe a person gets satisfied only by having sexual intercourse with many (lit. hundred) women and he becomes free from baldness, wrinkles and gray hair. It cures *vātika* diseases and diseases of the heart and urinary bladder. This medicated ghee prepared of *aśvagandha* is an excellent aphrodisiac recipe and it was propounded in the age of yore by the Aśvins for the benefit of mankind. [There are many mistakes in the text].

'शतावरी[६४] विदारीमुशलीहयगन्धाबलारसैः ।
शाल्मलीकन्दगुडूची भृङ्गिकारेतैः क्वथितैः ॥८१॥

पाचयेत्प्रस्थं विशुद्धं गव्यसर्पिषो ततः ।
पंचगुणे सिद्धे दुग्धे माहिषे विजयारसे ॥८२॥
तुल्ये समार्द्रकरसे जीवन्तीनां रसे ततः ।
द्विगुणे क्वथिते तत्र क्षिपेन्मृद्वग्निसाधितम् ॥८३॥
क्षुद्रमीनाजवाह्पललातरसं त्रिधा ।
तुल्यांश्च बस्ताण्डकयोः चटकाण्डांश्च निक्षिपेत् ॥८४॥
वानरीबीजविजयाबलाबीजगोक्षुरम् ।
प्रस्थं पादमितां स्तत्र कल्कातं मृद्रा पाचयेत् ॥८५॥
चातुर्जातकपंचकोलमरीचान् द्वे जीरके चित्रकम् ।
कुंकुमचन्दनाकरकराजातीफलं नागरम् ॥८६॥
कङ्कोलं कमलं लवङ्गद्यकुलान् कंशांशिकान् भावयेत् ।
कल्कान् वसनेन पूतमथवाद्भ्राद्यविचित्रं घृतम् ॥८७॥
तुल्यांशास्तु शिवामृगमदं कर्पूरकाश्मीरजैः ।
मृद्वीकां नवनारिकेलवचसीखर्जूरकान्प्रक्षिपेत् ॥८८॥
सिद्धं सर्पि गदं मनोरमं जरं सीमन्तनी मोहजम् ।
त्रैलोक्यप्रथितं घृतो तमगुणं कन्दर्पबाणाभिधम् ॥८९॥
स्थविरास्तरुणायंते हीनवीर्याबलोद्धताः ।
पलैकं भक्षणादस्य क्लीवो चापि पुरुषायते ॥९०॥
॥ शतावर्याद्यं घृतम्' ॥

(There are errors in these verses; hence left untranslated).

"चन्दनं कुङ्कुमोशीरं प्रियङ्गुत्रुटिरोचनाः ।
तुरुष्कागरुकस्तूर्यः कर्पूरं जातिपत्रिका ॥९१॥
जातिकङ्कोलपूगानां लवङ्गस्य फलानि च ।
नलिका नलदं कुष्ठं हरेणुस्तगरः प्लवम् ॥९२॥

नखं व्याघ्रनखं स्पृक्वा बोलो दमनको मुरा ।
स्थोणेयकं चोरकं शैलेयं सैलवालुकम् ॥९३॥
सरलः सप्तपर्णश्च लाक्षा तामलकी तथा ।
लामज्जकं पद्मकं च धातक्याः कुसुमानि च ॥९४॥
प्रपौण्डरीकं कर्चूरः समांशैः शाणमात्रकैः ।
महासुगन्धमित्येतत्प्रस्थं तैलस्य साधयेत् ॥९५॥
प्रस्वेदमलदौर्गन्ध्यकण्डूकुष्ठहरं परम् ।
अनेनाभ्यक्तगात्रः स्याद् वृद्धः सप्ततिकोऽपि वा ॥९६॥
'युवा[६५] भवति शुक्राढ्यः स्त्रीणां चात्यन्तवल्लभः ।
सुभगो दर्शनीयश्च गच्छेच्च प्रमदाशतम् ॥९७॥
वन्ध्यापि लभते गर्भं षण्ढोऽपि पुरुषायते ।
अपुत्रः पुत्रमाप्नोति जीवेच्च शरदां शतम्' ॥९८॥
॥ महासुगंधितैलम्' ॥

(भारतभैषज्यरत्नाकर : चतुर्थभाग : पृष्ठ ११२)

***Mahāsugandhi Taila***

One *prastha* of oil should be cooked by adding one *śāṇa* of each of *candana, kuṅkuma, uśīra, priyaṅgu, truṭi (elā), gorocanā, turuṣka, aguru, kastūrī, karpūra, jātipatrī, jātiphala, pūga, lavaṅga, nalikā, nalada, kuṣṭha, hareṇu, tagara, plava, nakha, vyāghranakha, spṛkkā, bola, damanaka, murā, sthauṇeyaka, coraka, śaileya, elavāluka, sarala, saptaparṇa, lākṣā, tāmalakī, lāmajjaka, padmaka,* flowers of *dhātakī, prapauṇḍarīka* and *karcūra.* This is called *Mahāsugandha taila.* It cures excessive perspiration, dirt in the skin, foul smell of the body, itching and *kuṣṭha* (obstinate skin diseases including leprosy). By the massage of this medicated oil even a seventy years old person becomes young. He gets excess of semen and becomes lovable by ladies. He becomes auspicious and beautiful. It enables a person to have sexual intercourse with many (lit. hundred) women. Even a sterile woman conceive and an impotent man becomes virile by the use of this recipe. It helps in getting a male progeny and the person lives for one hundred years by the use of this recipe.

मल्लिका वार्षिका जाती वासन्ती ग्रीष्मचम्पकौ ।
तरण्यौ यूथिका कुंदः सामिलानोतिमुक्तकः ॥९९॥
बकुलः[६६] किंकिरातश्च तिलकाशोककिंशुकाः ।
पुष्पाण्येतानि संगृह्य वृष्यसौगंध्यमिच्छता ॥१००॥
॥ इति वृष्यसुगन्धिपुष्पाणि[६७] ॥

*Aromatic Flowers having Aphrodisiac Effect*

Flowers of *mallikā, vārṣikā, jātī, vāsantī, grīṣma, campaka,* two varieties of *taraṇī, yūthikā, kunda, āmilā, atimuktaka, bakula, kiṅkirāta, tilaka, aśoka* and *kiṃśuka* are to be used for their aphrodisiac properties.

सनालानि तु पद्मानि क्षीरेणाजेन पेषयेत् ।
गुटिकां छायया शुष्कां नारीयोनौ प्रवेशयेत् ।
दशवारप्रसूता च कन्यावज्जायते पुनः ॥१०१॥

*Recipes for Strengthening Vaginal Muscles*

Lotus flower along with its stalk should be made to a paste by triturating with goat's milk. Pills made out of this paste should be dried in the shade. By keeping this pill inside the vagina, the vaginal opening of a lady who had even delivered ten children, becomes like that of virgin girl.

खञ्जरीटस्य मांसं तु मधुना सह पेषयेत् ।
अनेन योनिलेपेन पतिर्दासो भवत्यलम् ॥१०२॥

The meat of *khañjarīṭa* should be made to a paste by triturating with honey. Application of this paste in the vagina makes her husband a slave.

सुरूपा[६८] यौवनस्था या लक्षणैर्या विभूषिता ।
या च वश्या शिक्षिता च सा स्त्री वृष्यतमा मता ॥१०३॥

*Aphrodisiac Woman*

A woman who is beautiful, young and endowed with auspicious

signs, who is submissive and who is well versed in different sexual performances is aphrodisiac *par excellence.*

नर्त्ते वै[61] षोडशाद्वर्षात्सप्तत्याः परतो न च ।
आयुःकामो नरस्त्रीभिः संयोगं कर्त्तुमर्हति ॥१०४॥

*Age of Woman*

A person desirous of longevity should not indulge in sexual intercourse with a woman who is below the age of sixteen or who is above seventy years of age.

पुष्पार्कसंकोचं परिकापिण्डकूर्मजलूका शशिकीटा विड ।
संकोच समभागचूर्ण वटी कृत्वा ध्वजलेपं कारयेत् ।
पश्चास्त्रिप्यते सा स्त्री वंधकी भवति ॥१०५॥

*Contraceptive Recipes*

[There are many mistakes in this verse; hence left untranslated.]

खसफलशुण्ठीक्वाथः षोडशशेषे गुडेन निशि पीतः ।
कुरुते रते न पुंसो रेतःपतनं विनाम्लेन ॥१०६॥

Pods of *khasa* and *śuṇṭhi* should be boiled by adding water and reducing to $^1/_{16}$th part. Intake of this decoction at night along with jaggery makes a person not to ejaculate semen during sexual intercourse unless he takes sour food.

आर्द्रे वरटीछत्रे न व्ये कंदे सुदर्शनाख्यस्य[70] ।
साधितमतसीतैलं विंदुरयं नाभिलेपतो धत्ते ॥१०७॥

Oil of *atasi* cooked with the fresh and wet *chatra* (parasol-shaped hive) of a wasp and the root of *sudarśana* should be applied over the umbilicus of the male partner. By doing so during sexual intercourse, the man does not ejaculate semen.

'मुनिवररससंयुक्तं'[71] टङ्कणलेपाद्वसीकुरुते ॥१०८॥

*Ṭaṅkaṇa* (borax) should be triturated by adding the juice of *agasti* and made to a paste. Application of this paste in the umbilicus prevents ejaculation of semen during sexual intercourse.

भुजेषु चणागयतु सकणयणि हे भुंजि गुडयुतम् ।
जैजाव इणिमेलासि चिरसमये रमसि तरुणीनाम्' ॥१०९॥

[The meaning of this verse is not clear; hence left untranslated].

'शशिसूतकटंकणमागधिकं'[72] मुनिपुष्परसेन ।
हिरण्यरसं मधुसूरणसंयुतलेपमिदं ।
प्रमदामदमर्दनं वश्यंकरम्' ॥११०॥

*Karpūra, pārada, taṅkaṇa* and *pippalī* should be made to a paste by triturating with the juice of *agasti*. Application of this paste [on the umbilicus] during sexual intercourse prolongs the period before seminal ejaculation. Similarly, the paste of the juice of *dhustūra*, honey and *sūraṇa* should be applied for prolonging the sex-act.

जातीफलार्ककरहाटलवंगशुण्ठीकङ्कोलम् ।
कुङ्कुमकणाहरिचन्दनानि एतैः समानमहिफेनम् ।
तुल्यां श्वेतां निधाय मधुना वटकं विदध्यात् ॥१११॥
माषद्वयोन्मितमिमं निशि भक्षयित्वा ।
मृष्टं पयः तदनु माहिषं चाशु पीत्वा ॥११२॥
कुर्वन्ति कामुकजनाः न तु विन्दुपातम् ।
चेतांसि चापि चकितानि कलावतीनाम् ॥११३॥

One part of each of *jātiphala, arka, karahāṭa, lavaṅga, śuṇṭhī, kaṅkola, kuṅkuma, pippalī* and *haricandana*, nine parts of *ahiphena* and nine parts of sugar should be triturated by adding honey. From out of this paste, pills of two *māṣas* each should be prepared. Taking one such pill at night and taking buffalo-milk immediately after that causes retention of semen during sexual intercourse and gives surprising sex-satisfaction even to a sexy-woman.

चटकाण्डं तु संगृह्य नवनीतेन पेषयेत् ।
तेन लेपयेत् पादौ शुक्रस्तम्भः प्रजायते ।
यावन्तः स्पृहते[73] भूमिं तावत्स्यान्नात्र संशयः ॥११४॥

Sparrow-eggs should be made to a paste by triturating with butter. Application of this paste in the soles of feet during sexual intercourse causes seminal retention. The retention power continues till the man touches the ground with his feet and there should be no doubt about it.

'॥ नामा[74] ॥ वृतमध्यस्थितं नामतद्बात्येद्वत् चतुष्टयं ।
तद्बहिः क्ष्मायुरद्वन्द्वं लिखिता शिलपाखिलं ।
शुभनक्षत्र सद्वारे स्थापितं मधुनि ध्रुवं ।
स्त्रियमाकर्षयेत्क्षिप्रं यन्त्रमेतत्त्वसंशयः' ॥११५॥

***Yantra for Seminal Retention***

[Meaning of this verse is not clear; hence left untranslated].

खसतिलफलमेकं शुण्ठीकर्षः सितापलद्वन्द्वम् ।
एतच्चूर्णं पयसा पीतं रेतोरयं ध्रुवं धत्ते ॥११६॥

***Recipes***

One fruit of *khasatila*, one *karṣa* of *śuṇṭhī* and two *karṣas* of sugar should be made to a fine powder. Intake of this powder along with milk certainly prevents ejaculation of semen during sexual intercourse.

कांचनस्य फलदन्तानां पूगचूर्णसहितेन रसेन ।
लिङ्गलेपमसकृत्प्रहरार्द्धं बिन्दुवेगधारणाय कुरु त्वम् ॥११७॥

Juice of the seeds of *dhustūra* and the powder of *pūga* should be triturated together and made to a paste. Frequent application of this paste over the male genital organ and keeping it for half *prahara* (one and half hours) prevents the urge for seminal ejaculation during sexual intercourse.

अहिफेनं दुग्धशुद्धं रक्तिकात्रितयोन्मितम् ।
बिन्दुवेगं ध्रुवं धत्ते सितया निशि भक्षितम् ॥११८॥

*Ahiphena* should be purified by adding milk. Intake of this in the dose of three *rattis* along with sugar at night certainly retains the urge for seminal ejaculation during sexual intercourse.

श्वेतार्कतूलवद्वर्त्या वराहवसया सह ।
तद्वर्त्या दीपकं दद्यात् ध्वजस्तंभो भवेदिति ॥११९॥

A wick should be prepared of the root of the white variety of *arka* by adding the fat of pig. A lamp should be lighted with the wick in the bed room as a result of which the male genital organ remains erected.

मेदसा क्षौद्रमिश्रेण वराहस्य प्रलेपितम् ।
सम्यक् लिङ्गं रतांतेऽपि स्तम्भतां न विमुंचति ॥१२०॥

Application of the paste of pig-fat and honey keeps the male genital organ erect even after the sexual intercourse.

क्षौद्रेण सह संपिष्टं पुण्डरीकस्य केशरात् ।
तस्य इच्छास्तु यावन्तं मेढ्रस्तावत्स्थिरीभवेत् ॥१२१॥

Stamen of lotus should be made to a paste by triturating with honey. Application of this paste keeps the male genital organ erect as long as the person desires.

'नागवल्ली''दलद्रवैः सप्ताहं शुद्धसूतकम् ।
मर्द्दयेत्क्षालयेच्चाम्लैश्चतुर्निष्कप्रमाणतः ॥१२२॥

विषकन्दगतं सूतं विषेणैव निरोधयेत् ।
ततः शूकरमांसस्य गर्भे कृत्वा तु शोधयेत् ॥१२३॥
संध्याकाले बलिं दद्यात्कुक्कुटं मद्यसंयुतम् ।
ततश्चुल्यां लोहपात्रि तैले धतूरसम्भवे ॥१२४॥
क्षिप्त्वा वंशानले पाच्यं यावन्मांसस्य पिण्डकम् ।
संध्यामारभ्य मंदाग्नौ यावत्सूर्योदयो भवेत् ॥१२५॥
हठाज्जागरणं कुर्यात् अन्यथा नैव सिध्यति ।
प्रातरुत्थाय गुटिकां क्षीरभाण्डे विनिःक्षिपेत् ॥१२६॥
तत्क्षीरं पीयते क्षिप्रं जायते प्रत्ययं महत् ।
रतिकाले मुखे धार्या गुटिका वीर्यरोधिनी ॥१२७॥
क्षीरं पीत्वा रमेद्रामाकुलैः कामी कलान्वितः ।
मुखस्था गुटिका यावत् तावद्वीर्यं न मुंचति ॥१२८॥
॥ निरसगुटिका ॥

*Nirasa Guṭikā*

Purified mercury should be impregnated with the juice of betel-leaf for one week. Then it should be triturated and washed with sour vinegar. In a dose of four *niṣka*, mercury should be kept inside the root of aconite (*viṣakanda*) and it should be covered with another piece of it. This should be packed inside a bolus of pork and again purified. In the evening, *bali* (sacred sacrifice) of chicken and alcohol should be offered. Then it should be cooked in an iron pan containing *dhustūra* oil and kept over an oven. Bamboo should be used as fuel for this cooking and it (cooking) should be continued till the bolus of pork has become hard.

The cooking should be continued from the evening till the next sun-rise by applying mild fire. Then the bolus should be very hot and suddenly it should be immersed in a pot of milk. Any delay will not make the recipe effective. Intake of this milk promotes the strength of a person suddenly. If the pill of mercury is kept inside the mouth during sexual intercourse it stops ejaculation of semen. One can enjoy sexual intercourse with woman after taking this milk.

धत्तूरकस्य पुष्पाणि कर्पूरेण समन्वितम् ।
एतेन लेपयेत् लिङ्गं प्रमदानां वशंकरम् ॥१२९॥

Flowers of *dhustūra* should be added with camphor and made to a paste. Application of this paste over the male genital organ gives sexual satisfaction to women.

मधुसैन्धवसंयुक्तं पारावतमलान्वितम् ।
एतल्लिप्तेन्द्रियो रामा दासीव कुरुते रतिम् ॥१३०॥

Stool of *pārāvata* should be added with honey and rock-salt. By the application of this paste in the male genital organ, the woman behaves like a slave during sexual intercourse.

मूषकविष्ठायाः लिङ्गे लेपः कृतो रत्यवसरे ।
द्रावयति वारवनितां अपि वारं वारं नियतम् ॥१३१॥

Application of the stool of rat in the form of a paste over the penis enables a person to have frequent sexual intercourse which exhausts even a prostitute.

चूर्णितैर्मधुसंयुक्तैर्महाराष्ट्रीफलच्छदैः ।
लिङ्गलेपेन सुरते द्रवो भवति योषिताम् ॥१३२॥

Skin of the fruit of *mahārāṣṭrī* (*kaṇṭakārī*) should be made to a powder and mixed with honey. Application of this paste over the penis exhausts a woman during sexual intercourse.

'कण्टकारी'[76] रसालेपं सकर्पूरं यदा नरः ।
कुरुते शीघ्रमेवासौ द्रावयेद्वनिताशतम् ॥१३३॥

The juice of *kaṇṭakārī* should be added with camphor and applied over the penis which enables a man to make many (lit. hundred) female partners exhausted during sexual intercourse.

भृङ्गं कर्पूरसंयुक्तं मधुना सह मिश्रितम् ।
द्रावयेद्वनितालक्षं तदेकाग्रमनां सदा ॥१३४॥

*Bhṛṁgarāja* should be added with camphor and honey. Application of this paste over the penis makes many (lit. one lakh) women exhausted during sexual intercourse.

टङ्कणं च सकर्पूरं महाराष्ट्री समाक्षिकम् ।
लिङ्गलेपेन वै कुर्याद्वश्याः पातालयोषितः' ॥१३५॥

*Ṭaṅkaṇa, karpūra, mahārāṣṭrī* (*kaṇṭakārī*) and honey should be made to a paste by triturating together. Application of the paste over the penis makes even the females of *pātāla loka* satisfied during sexual intercourse.

घनसारभागमेकं टंकणभागद्वयेन संचूर्ण्य ।
लिङ्गलेपान्मधुना द्रवंति वनिता रते नियतम् ॥१३६॥

One part of *karpūra* and two parts of *ṭaṅkaṇa* should be made to a powder. Application of this powder mixed with honey over the penis certainly makes women exhausted during sexual intercourse.

एक एव महाद्रावी मालतीसंभवो रसः ।
किं पुनस्त्रयसंयुक्तो मधुकर्पूरपारदैः ॥१३७॥

Application of the juice of *mālatī*-flower over the penis is excellent to exhaust the women in sexual intercourse. Its effect is considerably enhanced if added with honey, camphor and mercury.

मालतीपुष्परसः निम्बूफले गुग्गुलुधूपितं तु ।
रसन्यसेद्वृश्चिककण्टकं वा इदं ततो मुद्रितमाशु दद्यात् ।
आद्यघ्राणतः स्त्री द्रवति भक्षणेन कौतुकाय ॥१३८॥

Juice of *mālatī*-flower or lemon should be fumigated with the smoke of *guggulu.* A scorpion-sting should be inserted into the juice inside the lemon and fumigated with the smoke of *guggulu.* By the inhalation of the smell of this fruit and by the intake of this juice, women get exhausted during sexual intercourse. [There are errors in this verse.]

कीटकाः काकजङ्घाया बुद्धया दत्त्वा अधोमुखाः।
सद्रवां कुरुते कामं वारवामामपि ध्रुवम् ॥१३९॥

[The meaning of this verse is not clear; hence left untranslated.]

कर्चूरभल्लातकशङ्खचूर्ण[77] क्षारं यवानां समनःशिलालम्[78]।
तैलं विपक्वं हरितालरजोविमिश्रं निर्मूलरोमानि[79] करोति सद्यः ॥१४०॥

### Recipe for Depilation

Oil cooked with *karcūra, bhallātaka, śaṅkha bhasma, yava kṣāra, mahaḥśilā* and *haritāla* and mixed with the powder of *haritāla*, if applied, causes instant depilation of all hair.

'सूर्यांशुतप्तं[80] घृतमंगनायाः योन्यां गतं हन्ति वरांगगन्धम्' ॥१४१॥

### Recipe for Removing Foul Smell

Ghee heated in the rays of sun, if applied in the vagina, makes the genital tract free from foul smell.

ब्रह्मदण्डी मुरामांसी दध्ना च सह संयुतः।
अनेनोद्वर्त्तिता नारी सा मृतेप्यनुगच्छति ॥१४२॥

*Brahmadaṇḍī, murāmāṃsī* and curd should be used for unction by a lady to remove foul smell of her body. [The text appears to be incorrect.]

हरितालचूर्णकलिकालेपात्तप्तेन वारिणा सद्यः।
निपतंति केशाद्यः कौतुकमिदमद्भुतं कुरुते ॥१४३॥

Application of the powder of *haritāla* along with hot water surprisingly removes hair instantaneously.

'संयोजित[८१]पल्लवपंचकेन जातिप्रसूनं मधुकान्वितम्' ॥१४४॥

[The text is incomplete; hence not translated.]

कुङ्कुमनारंगत्वक्केसरराजीवकेसरैर्विहितः ।
लेपोयं मलपिण्डका दौर्गन्ध्यस्वेदनाशनः ॥१४५॥
॥ प्रथितः ॥

*Kuṅkuma*, skin of *nāraṅga, nāga kesara* and *padma kesara* should be made to a paste and applied. It cures dirt, pimples, foul smell and excessive perspiration.

शाल्मलीकंटकारिष्टपत्रलोध्रकुलत्थकैः ।
उद्वर्त्तनमिदं नित्यं स्वेददौर्गन्ध्यनाशनम् ॥१४६॥

Unction prepared of *śālmalī kaṇṭaka*, leaf of *nimba, lodhra* and *kulattha* should be used regularly. It cures excessive perspiration and foul smell of the body.

अलक्तकेन विहितो मृतवंगलेपो ।
व्यङ्गं पिनष्टिवदने[२-८३] कुरुते च वर्णम् ॥१४७॥

Application of the paste of *vaṅga bhasma* and *alaktaka* (lac) cures *vyaṅga* (black pigmented patches in the face) and promotes facial complexion.

यूका व्रजन्ति खलु पारदनागवल्ली-
दलरसैः शिरसिजाश्च शरीरजाश्च ॥१४८॥

Application of mercury triturated with betel-leaf-juice cures lice of the head and body.

'केतकीपुष्पसम्भूतं[४] रजस्तैलेन पाचितम् ।
तेन लिप्ताऽबलायोनिर्गाढा स्यादतिविस्तृता ॥१४९॥

Pollens of *ketakī* flower should be boiled with oil. Application of this medicated oil causes contraction of the dilated vaginal canal in a woman.

चूर्णं तलपलाशस्य भूतिलोमिकदंबकम् ।
शरच्चन्द्रेन्दुभागेन मेलि हन्ति च लेपतः ॥१५०॥

[The meaning of this text is not clear; hence not translated.]

लोमसंघसमुत्पाटच्च तत्प्रदेशे विलेपयेत् ।
कुसम्भबीजतैलं च न कदाचित्तदुद्भवः' ॥१५१॥

If the oil from the seed of *kusumbha* is applied over a place from where hair is removed, then there will be no further hair growth in that place.

सपद्मबीजा सितया भक्षिता पद्मचारिणी ।
प्रक्षालनं भगं नित्यं कृत्वामलकवल्कलैः ।
वृद्धापि कामिनी कामं वाले च कुरुते रतिम् ॥१५२॥

[There are errors in the text; hence left untranslated.]

सुरगोपकीटचूर्णमिलितं मूलं कारवेल्लस्य ।
स्मरमंदिरमभ्यंगात्संकोचयति प्रसूतायाः ॥१५३॥

The root of *kāravellaka* should be added with the powder of the insect called *indragopa*. Application of this contracts the genital tract of a woman after delivery.

मोचरसामलकी 'त्वक्[५] स्फटिकाकाकमाचीभिरतौ सुभगा ।
स्वभगे विधाय वर्त्तिं सुरते कान्तं सुखी कुरुते' ॥१५४॥

A *varti* (elongated pill) should be prepared of *mocarasa, āmalakī, tvak, sphaṭikā* and *kākamācī*. If the woman keeps this *varti* in her vagina during sexual intercourse, then this gives immence pleasure to her husband.

चूर्णं विधाय शम्बूक जलौका वाजिगन्धयोः (?)।
लेपोऽयं नवनीतेन विधेयो लिङ्गवृद्धये ॥१५५॥

*Śambūka, jalaukā* and *vājigandhā* should be reduced to a powder form. By adding butter, a paste should be prepared out of this powder. This paste should be applied externally for increasing the length of the penis.

भूमीकदंबकमूलं शशपित्तं माहिषं च नवनीतम् ।
दिनकरकिरणैस्तप्तं मुशलोपमं सेफ[६]सं कुरुते ॥१५६॥

Root of *bhūmī kadamba*, rabbit bile and butter of buffalo-milk should be mixed together and made hot by exposing to the sun rays. Application of this paste promotes hardness of the male genital organ.

'मायाफलवरटीधायौफुलयोनिप्रलेपेन[७] संकोचः ॥१५७॥

Application of the paste of *māyāphala, varaṭī* (wasp) and *dhātakī* flower in the vagina helps in the contraction of the female genital tract.

मायाफलवेरोजा कालाच्छडश्वेतखदिरपोटली भगे देयं संकोचः' ॥१५८॥

*Māyāphala, verojā, kālāchaḍa* and *śveta khadira* should be made to a paste and tied in the form of a *poṭṭalī* (tampoon). Keeping this in the vagina causes its contraction.

किमंत्र चित्रं यदि वज्रवल्ली वचाश्वगन्धा जलसूकरी च ।
बहिःप्रलेपो बृहतिरसेन क्षणेन कुर्यान्मुशलप्रमाणम् ॥१५९॥

*Vajravallī, vacā, aśvagandhā* and *jalasūkarī* should be triturated by adding the juice of *bṛhatī* and made to a paste. Application of this paste over the penis makes it very hard during sexual intercourse.

कासीसतुरगगन्धासावरगजपिप्पली विपक्वेन ।
तैलेन याति वृद्धिं स्तनकर्णवरांगलिंगानि' ॥१६०॥

Oil cooked with *kāsīsa, aśvagandhā, śāvara lodhra* and *gajapippalī*, if applied externally, helps in the increase in size of breasts, ears and female as well as male genital organs.

'दौर्बल्य'[८८] मुखशोषश्च पाण्डुत्वं सदनं भ्रमः ।
क्लैव्यं शुक्रविसर्गश्च क्षीणशुक्रस्य लक्षणम् ॥१६१॥

*Signs and Symptoms of Seminal Debility*

Weakness, dryness in mouth, pallor, prostration, giddiness, impotency and early as well as unnatural ejaculation of semen—these are signs and symptoms of seminal debility.

इति श्री'महाराजाधिराजश्रीटोडरमल्लविरचिते टोडरानन्दे आयुर्वेदसौख्ये वाजीकरणनिदानचिकित्साकथनं नामाष्टसप्ततितमो हर्षः' ॥

Thus, ends the 78th chapter dealing with diagnosis and treatment of sex disorders needing aphrodisiac therapy (*vājīkaraṇa*) in the *Āyurveda saukhya* of *Ṭoḍarānanda* composed by the great King Ṭoḍaramalla.

## NOTES AND REFERENCES

१. (क) This is the beginning of eighty second chapter of *Āyurveda saukhya* in *Ṭoḍarānanda* and invocation reads as follows :
'उलूखल निवद्धाय भुक्तिमुक्तिप्रदायिने ।
मंथानदधिचौराय नमोस्तु दनुजद्विषे' ।
(ख) 'उलूखल ...... द्विषे' पाठोऽयं चतुर्थषष्ठपुस्तकयोः नोपलभ्यते ।

२. अन्यैरम्लो. इति चतुर्थपुस्तके पाठः ।

३. सोमधातुक्षयो इति पंचमपुस्तके पाठः ।

४. 'क्लैव्यं ...... सहजं' पाठोऽयं चतुर्थपुस्तके नोपलभ्यते ।

५. यो इति आकरे पाठः ।

६. 'वचाकर्चूर ...... विचक्षणैः' पाठोऽयं षष्ठपुस्तके नोपलभ्यते ।
७. त्वचा इति चतुर्थपुस्तके पाठः ।
८. बाजीकरणमुच्यते इति षष्ठपुस्तके पाठः ।
९. 'सौमनस्यं ...... भवेत्' पाठोऽयं चतुर्थषष्ठपुस्तकयोः नोपलभ्यते ।
१०. बस्ताण्डयुग्मं इति षष्ठपुस्तके पाठः ।
११. भावितानि सकृत्तिलान् चतुर्थपुस्तके पाठः ।
१२. नरो इति आकरे पाठः ।
१३. 'सर्पिः ....... भावितम्' पाठोऽयं प्रथमपंचमपुस्तकयोः नोपलभ्यते ।
१४. कृत्वा इति आकरे पाठः ।
१५. (क) विदारीकन्दचूर्णं इति प्रथमचतुर्थपंचमपुस्तकेषु पाठः ।
(ख) विदारीकर्णचूर्णं इति षष्ठपुस्तके पाठः ।
१६. शृतेन इति प्रथमपंचमपुस्तकयोः पाठः ।
१७. सुखार्थिना इति आकरे पाठः ।
१८. माषं इति आकरे पाठः ।
१९. पेयातुपात यौ लिह्या नित्यवेगसमो भवेत् इति षष्ठपुस्तके पाठः ।
२०. शर्करासमैः इति षष्ठपुस्तके पाठः ।
२१. शृंगाटकफलयुगुलं इति पंचमपुस्तके पाठः ।
२२. पलं च इति चतुर्थपुस्तके पाठः ।
२३. (क) कामोद्वाधाकर्प्यास्तिदनु इति चतुर्थपुस्तके पाठः ।
(ख) कामोहोधायदनु इति षष्ठपुस्तके पाठः ।
२४. कामुकः इति षष्ठपुस्तके पाठः ।
२५. शुक्रवृद्धौ इति चतुर्थषष्ठपुस्तकयोः पाठः ।
२६. (क) रेतसौबुधिः इति चतुर्थपुस्तके पाठः ।
(ख) रेतसोः म्व्धिः इति षष्ठपुस्तके पाठः ।
२७. श्वेतार्द्धकार्द्धद्रकम् इति षष्ठपुस्तके पाठः ।
२८. पाठोऽयं प्रथमपंचमपुस्तकयोः नोपलभ्यते ।
२९. माषदापि इति चतुर्थषष्ठपुस्तकयोः पाठः ।
३०. नागफला. इति षष्ठपुस्तके पाठः ।
३१. प्रस्थं शतावरीचूर्णं इति आकरे पाठः ।
३२. दद्यात्सुचूर्णितम् इति आकरे पाठः ।
३३. तदर्धेन च वै इति आकरे पाठः ।
३४. पलार्द्धमुपभुञ्जीत इति चतुर्थपुस्तके पाठः ।

३५. चापि इति षष्ठपुस्तके पाठः ।

३६. (क) एतेषां इति षष्ठपुस्तके पाठः ।
(ख) एष इति आकरे पाठः ।

३७. (क) खालित्य मेहपाण्डवाढ्य पीनसान् इति भैषज्यरत्नावलीपाठः ।
(ख) प्लीहव्याधींश्च इति आकरे पाठः ।

३८. (क) अष्टादशैव इति भारतभैषज्यरत्नाकर पाठः ।
(ख) हन्त्यष्टादशकुष्ठानि इति भैषज्यरत्नावली पाठः ।

३९. सश्लिष्टान् इति चतुर्थषष्ठपुस्तकयोः पाठः ।

४०. सर्वानिर्शोगदान् इति आकरे पाठः ।

४१. (क) मृगराजविक्रमस्तुरङ्गवेगो जलदौघनिःस्वनः इति आकरे पाठः ।
(ख) .विक्रमस्तुरङ्गमञ्चाप्यनुयाति इति भैषज्यरत्नावली पाठः ।

४२. (क) सोऽतिरम्यः सरूपवान सत्ववतां वरिष्ठः इति आकरे पाठः ।
(ख) सातिरेकं प्रकृष्टपुष्टश्च यथा विहङ्गः इति भैषज्यरत्नावली पाठः ।

४३. पुत्रान् सञ्जनयेद्धीमान् नरसिंहनिभांस्तथा इति आकरे पाठः ।

४४. नारसिंहमिदं चूर्णं सर्वरोगहरं नृणाम् इति भैषज्यरत्नावली पाठः ।

४५. "पलं ...... कामदेवचूर्णम्" पाठोऽयं प्रथमपंचमपुस्तकयोः नोपलभ्यते ।

४६. गोक्षुरबीजं च इति आदर्शपुस्तकेषु पाठः ।

४७. नागबलाबीजं इति आकरे पाठः ।

४८. पलं त्रपुषबीजञ्च इति आकरे पाठः ।

४९. त्रिसुगन्धी इति आकरे पाठः ।

५०. वासा च तालमूली च इति आकरे पाठः ।

५१. बलाशाल्मलिमूलञ्च भवेदेकैका इति आकरे पाठः ।

५२. कुशकाशशिफासप्त शर्करा सप्तयोजितम् इति आकरे पाठः ।

५३. दुष्टशुक्रं वीर्यहानिं मूत्रकृच्छ्राणी यानि च ।
मूत्राघातं मूत्रदोषाञ्जयेच्छुक्रविवर्द्धनम् ।
दशकं गच्छति स्त्रीणां हयतुल्यपराक्रमः ।
कामदेवाभिधं चूर्णं धन्वन्तरिनिरूपितम् ॥ इति आकरे पाठः ॥

५४. 'विदारी चरामार्कटं वाजिगन्धंश्च दंष्टं क्षुरं क्रोडमौशल्य कोलम् ।
त्वचं केसरे स्नानता कोष्ठजातविरिव्योषमाषं सिता च होमं च ।
बलाभिर्युतं भावितं स्वस्वयूषैरिदं कामदेवाख्य चूर्णम् ।
त्रयांशं सखायोरसं मौक्तिकं हैमं रौप्यं सुवंगान्वितम् सेवयेत्माक्षिकेण

शतं क्षीरयोमाक्षिगोधूमभोजी सिता सर्पिषा मानीनां जयेद्धि क्रोडशब्देन वाराहीकन्दः ।

अत्र कोष्ठशब्देन चोपचीनी वाचकः । खश्च अयश्च रसश्च रवायोरसाः, रवायोरसैः सह वर्तमानं सरवायोरसं, ख शब्दोऽभ्रकवाचकः । अयः प्रसिद्धः । रसः रससिन्दूरः ।

॥ बृहत्कामदेवचूर्णम्' ॥

प्रमादपूर्णपाठोऽयं द्वितीयषष्ठपुस्तकयोः अधिकमुपलभ्यते ।

५५. "हरार्का. ......षण्मुखरसः" पाठोऽयं प्रथमपंचमपुस्तकयोः नोपलभ्यते ।

५६. गव्यदुग्धेक्षु. इति आकरे पाठः ।

५७. मालत्याः इति आकरे पाठः ।

५८. ससिद्धी रस उत्तमः इति आदर्शपुस्तके पाठः ।

५९. एतदनन्तरं चतुर्थषष्ठपुस्तकयोः पुष्पधन्वारसस्य बृहत्पुष्पधन्वारसस्य च पाठद्वयं विद्यते । अतिप्रमादपूर्णत्वात् नोद्धृतम् ।

६०. प्रलम्बं इति आकरे पाठः ।

६१. 'प्रमदासु ...... भिषग्जितम्' पाठोऽयं प्रथमपुस्तके नोपलभ्यते ।

६२. गुडकूष्माण्डवत् इति आकरे पाठः ।

६३. पाठोऽयं प्रथमपुस्तके नोपलभ्यते ।

६४. 'शतावरी ...... शतावर्याद्यं घृतम्' पाठोऽयं प्रथमपंचमषष्ठपुस्तकेषु नोपलभ्यते ।

६५. 'युवा ..... शतम्' पाठोऽयं आदर्शपुस्तकेषु नोपलभ्यते ।

६६. वञ्जुलः इति पंचमपुस्तके पाठः ।

६७. 'अथ संकोची करध्यं वरटीकगण्डूपदवृषगोपानाम् ।
चूर्णमेकैकं गव्यतक्रेण लेपात्संकोचयति स्मरापारम् ।
पाठोऽयं चतुर्थपुस्तके अधिकमुपलभ्यते ।

६८. सरूपालयौवन इति प्रथमपुस्तके पाठः ।

६९. नत्तेकेषोडशा. इति प्रथमपुस्तके पाठः ।

७०. ख्येस्य इति चतुर्थपुस्तके पाठः ।

७१. 'मुनिवर ..... तरुणीनाम्' पाठोऽयं चतुर्थषष्ठपुस्तकयोः नोपलभ्यते ।

७२. 'शशि ..... करम्' पाठोऽयं प्रथमपंचमपुस्तकयोः नोपलभ्यते ।

७३. स्पृशते इति चतुर्थषष्ठपुस्तकयोः पाठः ।

७४. 'नामा ..... संशयः' पाठोऽयं प्रथमपुस्तके नोपलभ्यते ।

७५. 'नागवल्ली ...... निरसगुटिका' पाठोऽयं प्रथमपंचमपुस्तकयोः नोपलभ्यते ।

७६. 'कण्टकारी ..... .योषितः' पाठोऽयं प्रथमपुस्तके नोपलभ्यते ।

७७. कर्पूर इति चतुर्थपुस्तके पाठः ।

७८. शिला च इति चतुर्थपुस्तके पाठः ।

७९. रोमापि इति चतुर्थपुस्तके पाठः ।

८०. 'सूर्यांशु. ...... .गन्धम्' पाठोऽयं चतुर्थपुस्तके अधिकमुपलभ्यते ।

८१. 'संयोजित. ..... .मधुकान्वितम्' पाठोऽयं चतुर्थपुस्तके अधिकमुपलभ्यते ।

८२. विनिष्ट इति चतुर्थपुस्तके पाठः ।

८३. चूर्णम् इति चतुर्थपुस्तके पाठः ।

८४. 'केतकी. ....... .भवः' इति चतुर्थपुस्तके अधिकः पाठः ।

८५. 'त्वक्. ....... कुरुते' पाठोऽयं पंचमपुस्तके नोपलभ्यते ।

८६. मेहनं इति चतुर्थपुस्तके पाठः ।

८७. 'मायाफल. ........ .संकोचः' पाठोऽयं प्रथमपुस्तके नोपलभ्यते ।

८८. 'दौर्बल्यं. ........ .हर्षः' पाठोऽयं चतुर्थपुस्तके नोपलभ्यते । अत्र ग्रन्थेऽस्मिन् बहवः बाजीकरणयोगाः उल्लिखिताः सन्ति । प्रमादबहुलत्वात् नोद्धृताः ।

८९. 'महाराजाधिराज. ...... सप्तं' पाठोऽयं षष्ठपुस्तके नोपलभ्यते ।

# CHAPTER XI

## ॥ अथ स्नेहपानविधिः ॥

*(Oleation Therapy)*

"यथादोषं यथाव्याधिं यथाकालं यथाबलम् ।
स्नेहं पक्वमपक्वं वा पातुं युञ्ज्यात् चिकित्सकः" ॥१॥

(वङ्गसेनसंहिता : स्नेहपानाधिकार : पृष्ठ ७७६)

A physician should administer cooked or uncooked *sneha* (oleation therapy) to a patient keeping in view the *doṣas* aggravated in his body, nature of the disease he is suffering from, season in which the therapy is to be administered and the physical strength as well as the power of digestion of the patient.

"केवलं पैत्तिके सर्पिर्वातिके लवणान्वितम्।
देयं बहुकफे चापि व्योषक्षारसमन्वितम्" ॥२॥

(सुश्रुत : चिकित्सा : ३१ : १९)

***Vehicles***

If the disease is caused by the aggravation of *pitta*, then only ghee (not mixed with any other drug) should be administered; if it is caused by the aggravation of *vāyu*, then ghee mixed with salt should be administered; and if it is caused by the aggravation of *kapha*, then ghee mixed with *śuṇṭhi*, *pippalī*, *marica* and alkali preparations (*kṣāra*) should be administered.

"स्नेहसात्म्यः क्लेशसहो दृढः काले च शीतले ।
अच्छमेव पिबेत्स्नेहमच्छपानं हि शोभनम्" ॥३॥
(सुश्रुत : चिकित्सा : ३१ : २१)

*Accha Sneha (Pure Fat)*

*Accha sneha* (pure fat not mixed with any drug) is very useful and it should be given to persons who are accustomed to regularly taking fat, who are capable of facing hardships and who are strong, and during cold seasons.

उत्तमस्य पलं मात्रा त्रिभिश्चाक्षैश्च मध्यमे ।
जघन्यस्य पलार्द्धेन स्नेहः क्वाथौषधेषु[३] च ॥४॥

*Dose*

The excellent dose of *sneha* (ghee, oil, etc.) is one *pala*, the medium dose is three *akṣas* and the inferior dose is half *pala*. In the dose ghee, oil, etc., should be added to decoctions and other drugs.

उष्णोदकानुपानं तु स्नेहानामथ शस्यते ।
"ऋते[४] भल्लातकस्नेहात्तत्र तोयं तु शीतलम्" ॥५॥
(वङ्गसेनसंहिता : स्नेहपानाधिकार : पृष्ठ ७७७)

*Post-Prandial Drink*

It is beneficial if the administration of *sneha* (ghee, oil, etc.) is followed by the *anupāna* (post-prandial drink) of hot water. But the only exception is the oil of *bhallātaka* after which only cold water should be given as *anupāna*.

"स्नेहपीतस्य तृष्णायां पिबेदुष्णोदकं नरः ।
एवं चानुपशाम्यन्त्यां स्नेहमुष्णाम्बुनोद्धरेत्" ॥६॥
(सुश्रुत : चिकित्सा : ३१ : २४)

### *Thirst After Sneha*

If the patient suffers from thirst after taking *sneha* (ghee, oil, etc.), then he should be given hot water to drink. If the thirst does not subside, then more of hot water should be given to him which will cause vomiting and thus, the fat will be taken out of the body.

"मिथ्याचाराद्बहुत्वाद्वा यस्य स्नेहो न जीर्यति ।
विष्टभ्य वापि जीर्ज्येत वारिणोष्णेन वामयेत् ॥७॥

### *Indigestion of Sneha*

If the *sneha* does not get digested or if there is flatulence and abdominal distension during the process of digestion of *sneha* because of wrong regimens or because of the intake of *sneha* in larger dose, then the patient should be administered emetic therapy with the help of hot water.

ततः स्नेहं पुनर्दद्याल्लघुकोष्ठाय देहिने ।
स्नेहाजीर्णविशंकायां पिबेदुष्णोदकं नरः ।
तेनोद्गारो भवेत् शुद्धो रुचिश्चान्नं भवेत् प्रति ॥८॥

If there is any doubt about the proper digestion of the administered *sneha*, then the patient should drink hot water. By this, he gets pure eructation and proper desire for taking food.

स्युः पच्यमाने तृट् दाहभ्रमसादारुचिक्लमाः ॥९॥
परिषिच्याद्भिरुष्णाभिः जीर्णे स्नेहे ततो नरम् ।
यवागूं पाययेदुष्णं कामं क्लिन्नाल्पतण्डुलाम्" ॥१०॥

(सुश्रुत : चिकित्सा : ३१ : ३१-३४)

If during the process of digestion, the patient suffers from thirst, burning sensation, giddiness, prostration, anorexia and fatigue, then his body should be sprinkled with warm water and he should be given adequate quantity of hot and sticky gruel containing less of rice.

"पिबेत्र्यहं चतुरहं पंचाहं षडहानि च ।
सप्तरात्रात्परं स्नेहः सात्मीभावाय[६] कल्पते" ॥११॥
(सुश्रुत : चिकित्सा : ३१ : ३६)

*Duration of Oleation Therapy*

Oleation therapy should be administered for three, four, five or six days. After the seventh day, the *sneha* (fat) becomes *sātmya* (gets assimilated into the body and therefore, does not work as a therapy).

शुद्ध्यार्थं पुनराहारे नैशे जीर्णे प्रयोजयेत् ।
पिबेत्संशमनीयार्थे[८] मात्रा काले प्रकांक्षितः ॥१२॥

*Sneha for Elimination & Alleviation Therapies*

As a prelude to *saṃśodhana* (purification or elimination) therapy, *sneha* (fat) should be administered at night after the food taken during the day time is digested. As a part of *saṃśamana* (alleviation of aggravated *doṣas*) therapy, *sneha* (fat) should be administered in appropriate dose during the prescribed time.

स्नेहद्विषः कृशान् वृद्धान्सुकुमारान् शिशूनपि ।
"तृष्णार्त्तानुष्णकाले[९] च सह भक्तेन पाययेत् ॥१३॥

*Sneha with Food*

*Sneha* (fat) should be administered along with food in the following circumstances :

(1) If the patient does not relish taking fat (separately);
(2) to emaciated and old persons, to persons of tender nature and to infants;
(3) if the patient is suffering from morbid thirst; and
(4) during summer season.

पिप्पल्यो लवणं स्नेहाश्चत्वारो दधिमस्तुकम् ।
पीतमैकध्यमेतद्धि[१०] सद्यः स्नेहनमुच्यते" ॥१४॥
(सुश्रुत : चिकित्सा : ३१ : ३७-३८)

***Instant Oleation Therapy***

Four types of *sneha* (fat, viz.; ghee, oil, *vasā* or muscle fat and bone-marrow) taken along with *pippalı*, salt and *dadhimastu* (cream of curd) cause oleation instantaneously.

"सर्पिष्मतीं बहुतिलां यवागूं स्वल्पतन्दुलाम्" ।

(सुश्रुत : चिकित्सा : ३१ : ४०)

पिबेत्सुखोष्णां मनुजः सद्यो रौक्षात्प्रमुच्यते ॥१५॥

*Yavāgū* (gruel) prepared of rice in small quantity and mixed with *tila* in large quantity should be added with *sneha* (fat) and taken by a person when it is luke warm. It causes instantaneous oleation and the person becomes free from ununctuousness.

"भृष्टमांसरसा[११] स्निग्धा यवागूः स्वल्पतन्दुला ।

सक्षौद्रा सेव्यमानस्तु सद्यः स्नेहनमुच्यते" ॥१६॥

(सुश्रुत : चिकित्सा : ३१ : ३९)

Gruel prepared with less of rice and added with fat as well as the soup of fried meat should be mixed with honey and taken. It causes oleation instantaneously.

शर्कराघृतसंसृष्टे दुग्धांगीकलशे[१२] पयः ।

पाययेद्रूक्षमेतद्धि सद्यः स्नेहनमुच्यते ॥१७॥

Milk kept in an earthen jar (which is regularly used for storing milk) should be added with sugar and ghee. By the intake of this potion, an ununctuous person gets oleated instantaneously.

"विवर्ज्जयेत्स्नेहपानमजीर्णी तरुणज्वरी ।

दुर्बलोऽरोचकी स्थूलो मूर्च्छार्त्तो मदपीडितः[१३] ॥१८॥

छर्द्यभिभूतस्तृषितः[१४-१५] श्रांतश्चापि क्लमान्वितः ।

बस्तिदत्तो विरिक्तो वा वांतो यश्चापि मानवः" ॥१९॥

(सुश्रुत : चिकित्सा : ३१ : ४६-४७)

"अकाले च प्रसूता स्त्री स्नेहपानं विवर्जयेत्" ॥२०॥

(सुश्रुत : चिकित्सा : ३१ : ४८)

*Prohibited Persons*

Oleation therapy should not be administered to the following persons :

(1) One suffering from indigestion or having the fever in its first stage;
(2) a weak person or a fatty person;
(3) one suffering from anorexia, fainting and intoxication;
(4) one suffering from vomiting, morbid thirst and physical and mental fatigue;
(5) one who is already administered enema, purgation or emetic therapy; and
(6) a woman who had untimely delivery.

"रूक्षं पुरीषं ग्रथितं कृच्छ्रादन्नं विपच्यते ।
उरो विदह्यते वायुः कोष्ठादुपरि धावति ।
दुर्वर्णो[६] दुर्बलश्चापि रूक्षो भवति मानवः" ॥२१॥

(सुश्रुत : चिकित्सा : ३१ : ५१-५२)

*Ununctuous Person*

A person who voids pieces of dry and hard stool, whose food gets digested with difficulty, who gets burning sensation in the chest, who gets quick movement of flatus in the gastro-intestinal tract, who is discoloured and who is weak, is called an ununctuous (*rūkṣa*) person.

"ग्लानिः सदनमङ्गानां अधस्तात्स्नेहदर्शनम् ।
सम्यक् स्निग्धस्य लिङ्गानि स्नेहद्वेषस्तथैव च ॥२२॥

*Appropriate Oleation*

Fatigue, prostration, appearance of fat in stool and urine and disliking for *sneha* (fat) — these are the signs and symptoms of a person who is properly oleated.

भुक्तद्वेषो मुखस्रावो गुदे पाकः प्रवाहिका ।
पुरीषातिप्रवृत्तिश्च भृशं स्निग्धस्य लक्षणम् ॥२३॥

*Excessive Oleation*

Disliking for food, excessive salivation, inflammation of the anus, tenesmus and voiding of stool in excess — these are the signs and symptoms of a person who is administered oleation therapy in excess.

रूक्षस्य स्नेहनं स्नेहैरतिस्निग्धस्य रूक्षणम् ।
श्यामाककोरदूषान्नतक्रपिण्याकशक्तुभिः" ॥२४॥

(सुश्रुत : चिकित्सा : ३१ : ५३-५५)

*Recipes*

An ununctuous person (or a person who has not taken oleation therapy in appropriate quantity) should be given oleation therapy with the help of fats. A person who is administered oleation therapy in excess should be administered drying (*rūkṣaṇa*) therapy with the help of *śyāmāka, koradūṣa*, butter-milk, oil-cake and *śaktu* (roasted corn-flour).

'टंकैकं'[१७] मरिचं प्रगे घृतपलं नित्यं पुमान्यः पिबेत्।
मासैकं नियतं बलाधिकतमः[१८] संजायते सर्वथा ॥२५॥
देहे शुक्रविवृद्धिता च बलता कर्णामयध्वंसता ।
मन्दाग्निक्षपता दृशोर्विमलता सर्वेंद्रियप्रौढता' ॥२६॥

If a person takes one *pala* of ghee along with one *taṅka* of *marica* at the day-break regularly for one month, he invariably gets endowed with excellence of physical strength; excess of good quality semen; he becomes free from ear-diseases and suppression of the power of digestion; his eyesight becomes clear; and all his sense organs function effectively.

"दीप्तांतराग्निः परिशुद्धकोष्ठः प्रत्यग्रधातुर्बलवर्णयुक्तः।
दृढेन्द्रियो मंदजरः शतायुः स्नेहोपसेवी पुरुषः प्रदिष्टः" ॥२७॥

(सुश्रुत : चिकित्सा : ३१ : ५६)

***Effect of Oleation Therapy***

If a person takes oleation therapy according to prescribed procedure, his power of digestion gets enhanced; his *koṣṭha* (visceras of the chest and abdomen) becomes clean; his tissue-elements remain in an excellent state; he becomes endowed with strength and complexion; his senses remain sharp; his aging process becomes slow and he lives for one hundred years.

स्नेहमेव परं विद्याद्दुर्बलानलदीपनम् ।
नालं स्नेहसमिद्धस्य[१९] शमायान्नं सुगुर्वपि ॥२८॥

***Sneha and Digestive Power***

Intake of *sneha* (fats) stimulates the weak digestive power. If the digestive enzymes are stimulated by the use of *sneha*, then even extremely heavy food becomes incapable of suppressing it.

"स्नेहमग्रे[२०] प्रयुञ्जीत ततः स्वेदं प्रयोजयेत् ।
स्नेहस्वेदोपपन्नस्य संशोधनमनन्तरम्" ॥२९॥

(चरक : सूत्रस्थान : १३ : ९९)

***Oleation and Elimination Therapy***

A person should first of all take oleation therapy which should be followed by fomentation therapy. After taking oleation and fomentation therapies, a person should take elimination (cleansing) therapies.

"स्नेही व्यायामशीतान्नवेगधारणजागरान् ।
दिवास्वप्नमभिष्यंदिरूक्षान्नं च विवर्जयेत्" ॥३०॥

(वङ्गसेनसंहिता : स्नेहपानाधिकार : पृष्ठ ७७९)

***Prohibitions***

A person taking oleation therapy should avoid exercise, cold-food, suppression of the manifested natural urges, remaining awake at night, sleep during the day time and intake of *abhiṣyandi* (which causes obstruction to the channels of circulation) and ununctuous food.

'अह्नोरात्रेण[21] महती जीर्यत्यह्निन तु मध्यमा ।
दिनार्द्धेन जीर्यत्यल्पा स्नेहमात्रा प्रमाणतः' ॥३१॥

(वङ्गसेनसंहिता : स्नेहपानाधिकार : पृष्ठ ७७७)

*Digestive Period*

If the fat is ingested in a heavy dose, then it gets digested in 24 hours; if it is ingested in a moderate dose, then it gets digested in 12 hours and if it is ingested in a small quantity, then it gets digested in six hours.

इति श्रीमहाराजाधिराजश्रीटोडरमल्लविरचिते टोडरानन्दे आयुर्वेदसौख्ये स्नेहपानविध्यधिकारकथन[22] नाम एकोनाशीतितमो हर्षः ॥

Thus, ends the 79th chapter dealing with the method of administering oleation therapy, in the *Āyurveda saukhya* of *Ṭodarananda* composed by the great King Ṭodaramalla.

## NOTES AND REFERENCES

१. (क) This is the beginning of the eighty third chapter of *Ayurveda saukhya* in *Ṭodarānanda* and invocation reads as follows :
"सजलांभोदनीलाय धात्रीहस्तावलंबिने ।
आनन्दांकुरकंदाय मुकुन्दाय नमो नमः" ।
संगृह्य विद्याः सकला सवेदैः गुरोर्विमृग्याखिलपद्धतिर्यः ।
गता सुपुत्रान् प्रददौ ददातु श्रीटोडरे पुत्रकलत्रभृत्यान् ॥

(ख) "सजलांभोदनीलाय ...... नमः" पाठोऽयं चतुर्थषष्ठपुस्तकयो नोपलभ्यते ।

२. देहं इति षष्ठपुस्तके पाठः ।

३. क्वाथौषधस्य इति षष्ठपुस्तके पाठः ।

४. शृते इति षष्ठपुस्तके आकरे च पाठः ।

५. तेन वेगो भवेच्छुद्धो हविश्चान्नं इति षष्ठपुस्तके पाठः ।

६. सात्म्य इति षष्ठपुस्तके पाठः ।

७. निशे इति षष्ठपुस्तके पाठः ।

८ .प्रंशमनीयाथ इति प्रथमपुस्तके पाठः ।

९. तृष्णाचोष्णकाले इति चतुर्थषष्ठपुस्तकयोः पाठः ।

१०. पीतमेकैकमेतद्धि इति षष्ठपुस्तके पाठः ।

११. (क) 'भृष्टमांसरसा ...... .मुच्यते' पाठोऽयं प्रथमपंचमपुस्तकयोः नोपलभ्यते ।
(ख) मृगमांसरसा इति षष्ठपुस्तके पाठः ।

१२. (क) स्वाहां इति चतुर्थपुस्तके पाठः ।
(ख) दुह्याङ्गं इति षष्ठपुस्तके पाठः ।

१३. विषपीडितः इति षष्ठपुस्तके पाठः ।

१४. मूर्छाभिभूतः इति चतुर्थषष्ठपुस्तकयोः पाठः ।

१५. पुरुषः इति षष्ठपुस्तके पाठः ।

१६. दुर्बलो इति षष्ठपुस्तके पाठः ।

१७. 'टंकैकं ...... प्रौढता' पाठोऽयं प्रथमपंचमपुस्तकयोः नोपलभ्यते ।

१८. बलाधिकमतः इति षष्ठपुस्तके पाठः ।

१९. स्नेहसमृद्धस्य इति चतुर्थपुस्तके पाठः ।

२०. "स्नेहमग्रे ..... विवर्जयेत्" पाठोऽयं प्रथमपंचमपुस्तकयोः नोपलभ्यते ।

२१. (क) 'अहो ...... प्रमाणतः' पाठोऽयं चतुर्थपुस्तके नोपलभ्यते ।
(ख) द्रष्टव्यन्-शार्ङ्गधरसंहिता : उत्तरखण्ड : १ : ९ ।

२२. स्नेहनिदानचिकित्साकथनं इति प्रथमपुस्तके पाठः ।

# CHAPTER XII

## ॥अथ स्वेद-नस्य-धूम्रपान-गण्डूष-कवल-प्रतिसारणाधिकारः॥

*(Fomentation, Inhalation, Smoking and Gargling Therapies)*

तप्तैः[1] सैकतपाणिकांस्यवसनैः स्वेदोथवांगारकैः ।
लेपैर्वातहरैः सहाम्ललवणैः स्नेहैः सुखोष्णैर्भवेत् ॥१॥
एवं तप्तपयोम्बुवातशमनक्वाथादिसेकादिभिः[2] ।
तप्तैस्तोयनिषेचनोद्गतमहावाष्पैः[3] शिलाद्यैः क्रमात् ॥२॥

*Modes of Administering Fomentation Therapy*

Fomentation therapy can be administered with the help of the following :

(1) Hot sand, hands, bronze vessels and cloth;
(2) hot charcoal;
(3) application of hot paste of drugs belonging to *Vātahara gaṇa* (group of drugs alleviating *vāyu*) prepared by triturating with sour juice and salt;
(4) application of luke warm fat (ghee, oil, etc.);
(5) sprinkling of warm milk, water or decoction of drugs alleviating *vāyu*; and

(6) hot steam which comes out when hot stone, etc., are gradually sprinkled with hot water.

तापोपनाहद्रववाष्पपूर्वाः स्वेदास्ततो स्यात् प्रथमौ कफे स्तः ।
वायौ द्वितीयः पवने कफे च पित्तोपसृष्टे विहितस्तृतीयः ॥३॥

*Fomentation for Different Doṣas*

*Tāpa* (heat of fire), *upanāha* (application of hot paste) and *vaṣpa* (hot steam) — these are the three methods of administering fomentation therapy. The first type is useful for treating aggravated *kapha*, the second type is useful for aggravated *vāyu* and simultaneous aggravation of *vāyu* and *kapha* and the third type is useful for treating aggravated *pitta*.

येषां नस्यं विधातव्यं बस्तिश्चापि हि देहिनाम् ।
शोधनीयाश्च ये केचित् पूर्वं स्वेद्यास्तु ते मताः ॥४॥

*Fomentation as Preparatory Therapy*

Persons who are to be given inhalation therapy, medicated enema or any other elimination therapy (viz., emetic, purgation or blood-letting therapy) should prior to them be given formentation therapy.

पश्चात्स्वेद्या हृते शल्ये मूढगर्भाऽनुपद्रवा ।
सम्यक् प्रजाता काले च पश्चात्स्वेद्यैवं जानता ॥५॥
स्वेद्यः पूर्वं च पश्चाच्च भगंदर्यर्शसस्तथा ॥६॥

*Other Indications*

To a woman of *mūḍha garbha* (having obstructed or malpresented foetus in the womb), fomentation therapy should be administered after the foetus is removed provided the enceint is not suffering from any complication. If the enceinte has normal delivery, then also fomentation therapy should be administered. If a person is suffering from fistula-in-ano or piles, then fomentation therapy should be administered both before and after the treatment (surgical operation).

"स्नेहक्लिन्ना धातुसंस्थाश्च दोषा
स्वस्थानस्था ये च मार्गेषु लीनाः ।
सम्यक् स्वेदैर्योजितास्ते द्रवत्वम्
नीताः कोष्ठं शोधनैर्याति शान्तिम्"[५] ॥७॥

(सुश्रुत : चिकित्सा : ३२ : २१)

*Mode of Action*

The aggravated *doṣas* in the tissue elements, either located in their own sites or adhered to the channels of circulation in the body, become sticky [and detached] by the administration of oleation therapy. By the administration of fomentation therapy, these sticky *doṣas* get dissolved (become liquified) and come down to the *koṣṭha* (gastro-intestinal tract). Thereafter, by the administration of elimination therapies, these aggravated *doṣas* are removed from the body resulting in their alleviation.

अग्नेर्दीप्तिं मार्द्दवं त्वक्प्रसादम्
भक्तश्रद्धां स्रोतसां निर्मलत्वम् ।
कुर्यात् स्वेदस्तंद्रिनिद्रेव हन्यात्
सन्धीन् स्तब्धान्[६] चेष्टयेदाशु युक्तः ॥८॥

(सुश्रुत : चिकित्सा : ३२ : २२)

*Benefits of Fomentation*

Fomentation therapy endows a person with the following benefits

(1) His power of digestion becomes strong;
(2) his skin becomes soft and of good complexion;
(3) he relishes food;
(4) his channels of circulation become clean;
(5) he becomes free from drowsiness and excess of sleep; and
(6) his stiff joints start moving immediately.

सर्वान् स्वेदान्निवाते तु जीर्णेन्नेनावचारयेत् ॥९॥
स्नेहाभ्यक्तशरीरस्य[७] शीतैराच्छाद्य चक्षुषी ।
हृदयं वृषणौ दृष्टिः स्वेदयेत् मृदुनाऽग्निना[८] ॥१०॥

*How to Administer Fomentation*

For the administration of fomentation therapy, the following points should be kept in view :

(1) Fomentation should be given in a room which is free from wind;
(2) it should be administered after the food taken by the patient is digested;
(3) the body of the patient should be smeared with oil before fomentation;
(4) eyes of the patient should be covered with cold-pack; and
(5) heart, testicles and eyes of the patient should be fomented with very mild heat [or fomentation of such places should be avoided].

"शीतशूलव्युपरमे तन्द्रागौरवनिग्रहे ।
संजाते मार्दवे देहे[१] स्वेदनाद्विरतिर्मता" ॥११॥

(चरक : सूत्रस्थान : १४ : १३)

*When to Stop Fomentation*

Fomentation therapy should be discontinued after the chill (feeling of cold) and pain have disappeared; after the patient is free from drowsiness and heaviness of the body and after the body has become soft.

स्वेदास्रावो व्याधिहानिर्लघुत्वं,
शीतार्थित्वमार्दवं चातुरस्य ।
सम्यक् स्विन्ने लक्षणं प्राहुरेतत्
मिथ्यास्विन्ने व्यत्ययेनैतदेव ॥१२॥

*Signs of Proper Fomentation*

The following are the signs and symptoms of proper fomentation :

(1) The patient perspires profusely;
(2) the disease of the patient disappears;
(3) the patient feels lightness of the body;
(4) he desires to have cooling regimens; and
(5) his body becomes soft.

In the case of improper fomentation, opposite signs and symptoms appear in the patient.

स्फोटोत्पत्तिः पित्तरक्तप्रकोपो
मदो मूर्च्छा भ्रमदाहौ[10] क्लमश्च ।
अतिस्विन्ने संधिपीडा तृषा च
शीताः क्रियास्तत्र कुर्याद् विधिज्ञः ॥१३॥

*Excessive Fomentation*

Excess administration of fomentation therapy gives rise to the following complications :

(1) Appearance of pustular eruptions;
(2) vitiation of *pitta* and *rakta*;
(3) feeling of intoxication, fainting, giddiness, burning sensation and fatigue; and
(4) pain in joints and excessive thirst.

If the above signs and symptoms appear, then the patient should be administered cooling therapies.

अतिस्विन्नमथाश्वास्य शीताम्बु प्राशनं हितम् ।
स्नानमुष्णाम्बुना चापि निर्वातं चालयं नयेत् ॥१४॥
भोजयेच्चानभिष्यन्दि सर्वं स्वाचारमाचरेत्[11] ॥१५॥

*Management of Complications*

In the event of complications arising out of excessive fomentation, the patient should be consoled and given cold water to drink. He should take bath in warm water and stay in a room without wind. He should eat such food and drinks as are not *abhiṣyandi* (which obstruct channels of circulation) and should resort to wholesome regimens.

नाभ्यक्ते नापि चास्निग्धदेहे
स्वेदो योज्यः स्वेदविद्भिः कथंचित् ।
दृष्टं लोके काष्ठमस्निग्धमाशु
यायाद् भंगं स्वेदयोगैर्गृहीतम् ॥१६॥

A person should never be given fomentation therapy unless his body is fully massaged with oil and unless he is oleated. If a piece of wood is fomented without application of oil, then it immediately breaks. [Similarly a person taking fomentation therapy without oleation suffers.]

पाण्डुर्मेही रक्तपित्ती तृषार्तः क्षतक्षीणो दुर्बलोऽजीर्णभक्तः ।
दकोदरी गर्भिणी पानासक्तो नैते स्वेद्या यश्च मर्त्योऽतिसारी ।
'स्वेदादेषां याति देहो विनाशं असाध्यत्वं याति चैषां विकारः ॥१७॥
॥ इति स्वेदाधिकारः' ॥

*Unsuitable Patients*

Patients suffering from anemia, *meha* (obstinate urinary disorders including diabetes), *rakta pitta* (a disease characterised by bleeding from different parts of the body), morbid thirst, phthisis, weakness, indigestion, ascites, pregnancy, alcoholism and diarrhoea should not be administered fomentation therapy.

Thus, ends the description of fomentation therapy.

अथ नस्यविधिः

"नस्यं तत्कथ्यते[१२] धीरैर्नासाग्राह्यं यदौषधम् ।
नावनं नस्यकर्मेति तस्य नामद्वयं मतम् ॥१८॥

## INHALATION THERAPY

*Definition*

The therapy which is administered through the nose (*nāsā*) is called *nasya* (inhalation therapy). *Nāvana* and *nasya karma* — these are its two synonyms.

नस्यभेदो द्विधा प्रोक्तो रेचनं स्नेहनं पृथक्[१३] ।
रेचनं कर्षणं प्रोक्तं स्नेहनं बृंहणं मतम् ॥१९॥

*Varieties*

*Nasya* (inhalation therapy) is of two types, viz., *recana* (which causes elimination of *doṣas* from the head) and *snehana* (which produces oleating effect). The former is also called *karṣaṇa* (which causes drying or depleting effect) and the latter is also called *bṛṃhaṇa* (which produces nourishing effect).

कफपित्तानिलध्वंसे[१४] पूर्वमध्यापराह्णके ।
दिनस्य गृह्यते नस्यं रात्रावप्युत्कटे गदे[१५] ॥२०॥

*Time of Administration*

For the alleviation of *kapha, pitta* and *vāyu,* inhalation therapy should be administered during the forenoon, midday and afternoon respectively. However, if the patient is suffering from a serious disease, then inhalation therapy can be administered at night also.

नस्यं त्यजेद् भोजनांते दुर्दिने चापतर्पितः[१६] ।
तथा नवप्रतिश्यायी[१७] गर्भिणी गरदूषितः ॥२१॥
अजीर्णी दत्तबस्तिश्च पीतस्नेहोदकासवः ।
क्रुद्धः शोकाभिभूतश्च[१८] तृष्णार्त्तो वृद्धबालकौ ।
वेगावरोधी स्नातश्च स्नातुं कामश्च[१९] वर्ज्जयेत् ॥२२॥

***Contra-Indications***

One should avoid the administration of inhalation therapy in the following situations :

(1) After food;
(2) during a rainy day;
(3) if the patient is fasting;
(4) if the patient is suffering from freshly occuring *Pratiśyāya*, (coryza);
(5) if the lady is pregnant;
(6) if the patient is suffering from afflictions by *gara* (artificial poison) and indigestion;
(7) if the patient is already under enema therapy or oleation therapy;
(8) if the patient has consumed excess of water or alcoholic drinks.
(9) if the patient is angry or sorrowful;
(10) if the patient is suffering from morbid thirst;

(11) if the patient is an infant or an old person;
(12) if the patient has suppressed his manifested natural urges; and
(13) after the patient has taken bath or if he wants to take bath soon.

अष्टवर्षस्य बालस्य नस्यकर्म समाचरेत्[20] ।
अशीतिवर्षादूर्ध्वं च नावनं नैव दीयते ॥२३॥

*Age of Patient*

One can administer inhalation therapy if the patient is above eight years old. To a person above eighty years of age, this therapy should not be administered.

अथ वैरेचनं नस्यं ग्राह्यं तैलैः सुतीक्ष्णकैः।
तीक्ष्णभेषजसिद्धार्थस्नेहैः क्वाथै रसैस्तथा ॥२४॥

*Vairecana Nasya*

*Vairecana* type of *nasya* (inhalation therapy for the elimination of *doṣas* from the head) should be administered with the help of medicated oil having *tīkṣṇa* (pungent or sharp) effects. This should be prepared by cooking mustard oil with the decoction and juice of pungent (sharp) drugs.

नासिकारंध्रयोरष्टौ षट्चत्वारश्च विंदवः ।
प्रत्येकं रेचनं योज्यं मुख्यमध्याल्पमात्रया ॥२५॥

*Dose*

For *recana nasya*, the dose of the medicated oil should be either eight drops (excellent dose) or six drops (medium dose) or four drops (small dose) to be poured into each nostril for deep inhalation.

नस्यकर्मणि दातव्यं शाणैकं तीक्ष्णमौषधम् ।
हिंगु स्याद् यवमात्रं तु माषैकं सैन्धवं मतम् ॥२६॥
क्षीरं चैवाष्टशाणं स्यात्पानीयं[21] च त्रिकार्षिकम् ।
कार्षिकं मधुरं द्रव्यं नस्यकर्म्मणि योजयेत् ॥२७॥

### *Quantity of Ingredients in Recipe*

For the preparation of a recipe for inhalation therapy, *tīkṣṇa* (pungent or sharp) drugs should be added in the quantity of one *śāṇa, hiṅgu* of one *yava, saindhava* of one *māṣa*, milk of eight *śāṇas*, water of three *karṣas* and sweet-drugs should be added in the quantity of one *karṣa*.

अवपीडः प्रधमनं द्वौ भेदावपरौ स्मृतौ[२२] ।
शिरोविरेके[२३] नस्यार्थं तौ तु देयौ यथायथम् ॥२८॥

### *Two Varieties of Recana Nasya*

*Avapīḍa* (which is administered through pressure) and *pradhamana* (which is administered by blowing powdered drugs into the nostrils)—these are the two varieties of *virecana nasya* (inhalation therapy for the elimination of *doṣas* from the head). These are to be administered appropriately for the elimination of *doṣas* from the head.

कल्कीकृतादौषधिभ्यः पीडितो निःसृतो रसः ।
सोऽवपीडः[२४] समुद्दिष्टः तीक्ष्णद्रव्यसमुद्भवः ॥२९॥

### *Avapīḍa Nasya*

Pungent drugs should be made to a paste. The juice should be squeezed out of this paste and poured into the nostril. This is called *avapīḍa nasya*.

षडंगुला द्विवक्त्रा या नाडी चूर्णं तथा धमेत् ।
तीक्ष्णं कोलमितं प्रोक्तं[२५] वाते प्रधमनं हितम् ॥३०॥

### *Pradhamana Nasya*

Through a tube of six *aṅgulas* (finger breadth) in length and having two openings, one *kola* of the powder of sharp drugs should be blown into the nostrils. This is called *pradhamana nasya* and it is useful in the treatment of *vātika* diseases.

उर्द्ध्वजत्रुगते रोगे कफजे स्वरसंक्षये ।
अरोचके प्रतिश्याये शिरःशूले च पीनसे ।
शोफापस्मारकुष्ठेषु नस्यं वैरेचनं हितम्[२६] ॥३१॥

### *Indications for Virecaka Nasya*

*Virecaka* type of *nasya* (inhalation therapy used for the elimination of *doṣas* from the head) should be administered for curing diseases of the head and neck caused by aggravated *kapha*, aphasia, anorexia, coryza, headache, chronic rhinitis, oedema, epilepsy and *kuṣṭha* (obstinate skin diseases including leprosy).

भीरुस्त्रीकृशबालानां नस्यं स्नैहिकमिष्यते ॥३२॥

### *Indications for Snaihika Nasya*

*Snaihika* type of *nasya* (inhalation therapy producing oleation effect) should be administered to patients who are afraid of such therapies, to women to emaciated persons and to patients of tender age.

गलरोगे सन्निपाते निद्रायां[१२] सविषे ज्वरे ।
मनोविकारे कृमिषु युज्यते चावपीडनम् ॥३३॥

### *Indications for Avapīḍa Nasya*

*Avapīḍa* type of *nasya* (inhalation therapy which is administered by applying pressure) is useful in throat diseases, diseases caused by the simultaneous vitiation of all the three *doṣas* (*sannipata*), excessive sleep, poisoning, fever, mental disorders and parasitic infestations.

अत्यन्तोत्कटदोषेषु विसंज्ञेषु[२८] च दीयते ।
चूर्णं प्रधमनं धीरैस्तद्धि तीक्ष्णतरं यतः ॥३४॥

### *Indications for Pradhamana Nasya*

If, in a patient, *doṣas* are aggravated seriously much in excess and if he is unconscious, then an expert physician should administer powdered drugs by blowing into the nostrils (*pradhamana*). It is a sharply acting therapy.

नस्यवैरेचनं यथा

नस्यं स्याद्गुडशुण्ठीभ्यां पिप्पल्या सैन्धवेन च ।
जलपिष्टेन तेनाक्षिकर्णनासाशिरोगदाः ।
मन्याहनुगलोद्भूता नश्यन्ति भुजपृष्ठजाः ॥३५॥

*Recipes*

*Guḍa* and *śuṇṭhī* or *pippalī* and *saindhava* are to be made to a paste by triturating with water. Use of these recipes for inhalation therapy cures diseases of eyes, ears, nose, head, *manyā* (sterno-mastoid region), jaws, throat, arms and back.

मधूकसारकृष्णाभ्यां वचामरिचसैन्धवैः ।
नस्यं कोष्णजलैः पिष्टं दद्यात्संज्ञाप्रबोधनम्[२९] ।
अपस्मारे तथोन्मादे सन्निपातेऽपतन्त्रके[३०] ॥३६॥

*Madhūkasāra* and *pippalī* or *vacā, marica* and *saindhava* should be made to a paste by triturating with luke warm water. Use of these recipes for inhalation therapy stimulates consciousness, and these recipes are useful for epilepsy, insanity, diseases caused by the simultaneous vitiation of all the three *doṣas* and *apatantraka* (convulsions).

सैन्धवं श्वेतमरिचं सर्षपाः कुष्ठमेव च ।
बस्तमूत्रेण पिष्टानि नस्यं तन्द्रानिवारणम् ॥३७॥

*Saindhava, śveta marica, sarṣapa* and *kuṣṭha* should be made to a paste by triturating with goat's urine. Using this recipe for inhalation therapy cures drowsiness.

रोहितकमत्स्यपित्तैर्भावयेन्मरिचं[३१] वचा ।
कट्फलं चेति तच्चूर्णं देयं प्रधमनं बुधैः ॥३८॥

*Marica, vacā* and *kaṭphala* should be impregnated with the bile of *rohita* fish and made to a powder. This recipe should be used for *pradhamana nasya* (a type of inhalation therapy in which the powdered recipe is blown into the nostrils).

अथ बृंहणनस्यस्य कल्पना कथ्यतेऽधुना ।
'मर्शश्च[३२] प्रतिमर्शश्च द्वौ भेदौ स्नेहने मतौ ॥३९॥

### *Varieties of Snehana Nasya*

Now, *snehana* or *bṛṃhaṇa* type of *nasya* (inhalation therapy) will be described. It is of two types, viz., *marśa* and *pratimarśa*. [According to *Aṣṭāṅgahṛdaya* : *Sūtra* 20 : 9, the difference between these two varieties is only in the dose of the therapy].

मर्शस्य तर्प्पणी मात्रा मुख्या शाणैः स्मृताष्टभिः ।
मध्यमा च चतुःशाणैर्हीना शाणमिता स्मृता ॥४०॥

### *Dose*

For the purpose of producing nourishing effect, *marśa* type of *nasya* should be used in the dose of eight *śāṇas* which is the excellent dose. Otherwise, its medium dose is four *śāṇas* and the inferior dose is one *śāṇa*.

एकैकस्मिन् तु मात्रेयं देया नासापुटे बुधैः' ।
मर्शश्च द्वित्रिवेलं वा वीक्ष्य दोषबलाबलम्[33] ॥४१॥

In the above mentioned dose, the recipe should be used in each of the nostrils and depending upon the strength of vitiated *doṣas*, it can be administered two or three times per day.

एकान्तरं द्व्यन्तरं वा नस्यं दद्याद्विचक्षणः ।
त्र्यहं पंचाहमथवा सप्ताहं वा सुयंत्रितः ॥४२॥

### *Frequency of Therapy*

*Marśa* (*snehana*) type of *nasya* (inhalation therapy) should be administered when the patient has maintained proper pose. This therapy can be repeated after a gap of one, two, three, five or seven days.

मर्शो शिरोविरेके च व्यापदो विविधा स्मृताः ।
'दोषोत्क्लेशात्[34] क्षयाच्चैव विज्ञेयस्ता यथाक्रमम्' ॥४३॥
दोषोत्क्लेशनिमित्तासु युंज्या'द्वमनशोधनम्[35-36] ।
अथ क्षयनिमित्तासु पयसा[37] बृंहणं हितम् ॥४४॥

### *Complications*

Several complications may arise because of the administration of *snehana* and *recana* types of *nasya*. It can be because of the stimulation (*utkleśa*) of *doṣas* or because of the decrease in the quantity of *doṣas*. In the former case, the patient should be given emetic type of elimination therapy and in the latter case, he should be treated by nourishing therapies containing milk.

शिरोनासाक्षिरोगेषु सूर्यावर्त्तार्द्धभेदके ।
दंतरोगे बले हीने मन्याबाह्वंसजे गदे ॥४५॥
मुखशोषे कर्णनादे वातपित्तगदे तथा ।
अकालपलिते चैव केशश्मश्रुप्रपातने ।
युज्यते बृंहणं नस्यं स्नेहैर्वा मधुरद्रवैः ॥४६॥

### *Indications of Snehana Nasya*

*Snehana* (*bṛṃhaṇa*) type of *nasya* (inhalation therapy) prepared of oil and (or) drugs belonging to *Madhura gaṇa* (group of sweet drugs) is useful for the following ailments :

(1) Diseases of head, nose and eyes;
(2) *sūryavartta* (a type of headache which increases as per the movement of sun in the sky) and *arddhavabhedaka* (hemicrania);
(3) diseases of teeth;
(4) lack of strength;
(5) diseases of *manyā* (sterno-mastoid region), arms and *aṃsa* (shoulders);
(6) dryness in the mouth and tinnitus;
(7) diseases caused by aggravated *vāyu* and *pitta*; and
(8) premature graying of hair and fall of hair from the head and beard.

बृंहणं नस्यं यथा

सशर्करः पयःपिष्टं भृष्टमाज्येन कुंकुमम् ।
नस्यप्रयोगतो हन्याद्वातरक्तभवा रुजः ।
भ्रूशंखाक्षिशिरःकर्णसूर्यावर्त्तार्द्धभेदकाः[३८] ॥४७॥

*Recipes of Snehana Nasya*
*[Kuṅkuma Nasya]*

*Kuṅkuma* should be fried in ghee and triturated by adding sugar and milk to make a paste. Use of this paste for inhalation therapy cures the following ailments :

(1) Pain caused by the aggravated *vāyu* and *rakta*;
(2) pain in eyebrows, temples, eyes, head and ears; and
(3) *sūryāvarta* (a type of headache which increases as per the movement of the sun in the sky) and *ardhāvabhedaka* (hemicrania).

नस्यं स्यादणुतैलेन तथा नारायणेन च ।
माषादिना वा सर्पिर्भिस्तत्तद्भेषजसाधितैः ॥४८॥

*Nasya* (inhalation therapy) can be given with *Aṇu taila, Nārāyaṇa taila, Māṣa ghṛta* or any other recipe of fat prepared by boiling with appropriate medicines.

तैलं कफे सवाते च केवले पवने वसा।
दद्यात्सर्पिः सदा[३९] पित्ते मज्जानं च समारुते ॥४९॥

Oil should be used for inhalation therapy if the disease is caused by *kapha* along with *vāyu* and if it is caused by only *vāyu*, then inhalation therapy should be given by *vasā* (muscle fat). Inhalation therapy with ghee is always useful in the diseases caused by *pitta*. If, however, the disease is caused by *pitta* along with *vāyu*, then the inhalation therapy with *majjā* (bone-marrow) is useful.

माषात्मगुप्ताराष्णाभिर्बलापुष्कररोहिषैः ।
कृतोश्वगन्धाक्वाथैस्तु हिंगुसैन्धवसंयुतः ॥५०॥
कोष्णनस्यप्रयोगेन पक्षाघातं सकम्पनम् ।
जयेदर्दितवातांश्च[४०] मन्यास्तम्भावबाहुकौ ॥५१॥

*[Māṣādi Nasya]*

The decoction of *māṣa, ātmaguptā, rāsnā, balā, puṣkara, rohiṣa* and *aśvagandhā* should be added with the powders of *hiṅgu* and *saindhava*. Use of this recipe for inhalation therapy, when it is luke warm, cures paralysis associated with trembling, facial paralysis, torticolis and *avabāhuka* (pain in the root of arms).

प्रतिमर्शस्य मात्रा तु द्वि द्वि बिंदुमिता मता ।
प्रत्येकशो नासिकयोः स्नेहेनेति विनिश्चितम् ॥५२॥

### *Pratimarśa Type of Nasya*

For the *pratimarśa* type of oleating inhalation therapy, the medicated oil should be inhaled in the dose of two drops in each nostril. This certainly causes oleation.

स्नेहे ग्रन्थिद्वयं यावन्निमानं[४१] चोद्धृतं ततः ।
तर्ज्जनीयं स्रवेद्बिंदुं सा मात्रा बिंदुसंज्ञिता[४२] ॥५३॥
एवंविधैर्बिन्दुसंज्ञैरष्टभिः[४३] शाण उच्यते ।
स देयो मर्शनस्येषु प्रतिमर्शो द्विबिंदुकः ॥५४॥

### *Measurement of Drop*

If two phalanges of the index finger are immersed into the fat and taken out, then the drop that falls down should be treated as one *bindu* (drop). Eight such drops constitute one *śāṇa*. In *marśa* type of *snehana nasya*, the medicated oil should be administered in the dose of one *śāṇa* and in the *pratimarśa* type of *snehana nasya*, the dose should be two drops in each nostril.

समयाः प्रतिमर्शस्य बुधैः प्रोक्ता चतुर्द्दश ।
प्रभाते दन्तकाष्ठान्ते गृहान्निर्गमने तथा ॥५५॥
व्यायामाध्वव्यवायान्ते विण्मूत्रान्तेंजने[४४] कृते ।
कवलान्ते भोजनान्ते दिवास्वप्नोत्थिते तथा ।
वमनान्ते तथा सायं प्रतिमर्शः प्रयुज्यते ॥५६॥

### *When to Use Pratimarśa Nasya ?*

*Pratimarśa* type of inhalation therapy can be used in 14 different times as follows :

(1) During early morning;
(2) after brushing teeth;
(3) while moving out of the house;
(4) at the end of exercise;
(5) at the end of walk;
(6) after sexual intercourse;
(7) after passing stool;
(8) after passing urine;
(9) after applying collyrium;
(10) after taking *kavala* (keeping mouthful of drugs in paste form);
(11) after meals;
(12) after getting up from sleep during daytime;
(13) after emetic therapy; and
(14) during the evening.

ईषदुच्छिं[४५]दनात्स्नेहो यदा वक्त्रं प्रपद्यते ।
नस्ये[४६] निषिक्तं तं विद्यात्प्रतिमर्शप्रमाणतः ।
उच्छिंघ्य[४७] न पिबेच्चैतन्निष्ठीवेन्मुखमागतम् ॥५७॥

*Mode of Administration*

When the medicated oil is dropped into the nostrils and deeply inhalated, it will come to the mouth (through the nasopharynx). This should be determined as the appropriate dose and mode of taking this therapy. While deeply inhaling, the oil that will come into the mouth should not be swallowed but it should be spitted out.

क्षीणे तृष्णास्यशोषार्त्ते बालवृद्धेषु युज्यते ।
प्रतिमर्शेन शाम्यन्ति रोगाश्चैवोर्द्ध्वजत्रुजाः ।
बलीपलितनाशश्च बलमिन्द्रियजं भवेत् ॥५८॥

*Indications of Pratimarśa Nasya*

*Pratimarśa* type of *snehana nasya* should be administered to the following types of persons :

(1) Those who are emaciated;
(2) those suffering from morbid thirst and dryness of the mouth;
(3) infants and old persons;

(4) for the cure of the diseases of the head and neck;
(5) to cure wrinkling of the skin and graying of hair; and
(6) to promote the functions of the sense organs.

बिभीतनिम्बकम्भारी शिवा शेलुश्च काकिनी ।
एकैकं तैलनस्येन पलितं नस्यति ध्रुवम् ॥५९॥

***Inhalation Therapy for Gray Hair***

Inhalation of the oil of either *bibhītaka, nimba, gambhārī, harītakī, śelu* or *kākinī* certainly cures graying of hair.

अथ नस्यविधिं वक्ष्ये नस्याद् ग्रहणहेतवे ।
देशे वातरजोमुक्ते कृतदन्तप्रघर्षणे ॥
विशुद्धं धूमपानेन स्विन्नं[४८] तालुगलं तथा ॥६०॥
उत्तानशायिनं किंचित्प्रलंबशिरसं नरम् ।
आस्तीर्णं हस्तपादं च वस्त्राच्छादितलोचनम् ।
समुन्नमितनासाग्र[४९] वैद्यो नस्येन योजयेत् ॥६१॥

***Method of Administration***

Now the method of administration of inhalation therapy through the nostrils will be described. Inhalation therapy should be administered in a place free from wind and dust. Before that, the patient should have completed tooth brushing followed by smoking for the fomentation of palate and throat.

He should lie down on his back with his head slightly elongated and his hands as well as legs spread out. His eyes should be covered with cloth. The nose-tip of the patient should be pulled up and the physician should pour the medicated recipe into the nostrils

कोष्णमच्छिन्नधारं च हेमतारादिशुक्तिभिः[५०] ।
शुक्त्या वा पत्रशुक्त्या[५१] वा प्लोतैर्वा नस्यमाचरेत् ॥६२॥

The medicated oil to be used for the inhalation therapy should be lukewarm and it should be poured uninterruptedly with the help of droppers prepared of gold, silver or snail. In addition to *śukti* (snail) and *patraśukti*, cotton pads can also be used for pouring this oil into the nostrils.

नस्यैश्च[१२] सिंच्यमानेषु शिरो नैव प्रकम्पयेत् ।
न प्रकुप्येन्न भाषेत् नोच्छिन्द्येन्न हसेत्तथा ॥६३॥
एतैर्हि विहितस्नेहो नैवान्तः सम्प्रपद्यते ।
ततः कासप्रतिश्यायशिरोक्षिगदसंभवः[५३] ॥६४॥

While sprinkling the nasal drop, the patient should not shake his head. He should not get angry, should not speak, should not sneeze and should not laugh. If these precautions are taken, then oil does not go to the pharynx or larynx. If such precautionary measures are not observed, then the patient suffers from cough, cold and other diseases of the head and eyes.

शृंगाटकमभिप्लाव्य स्थापयेन्न गिले द्रवम् ॥६५॥
'पंचसप्तदशैव'[१४] स्युर्मात्रा नस्यस्य धारणे ।
उपविश्याथ निष्ठीवेन्नासावक्त्रगतं द्रवम्' ।
वामदक्षिणपाश्वर्भ्यां निष्ठीवेत्स सुखेन[५५] हि ॥६६॥

After the oil has flooded the *śṛṅgāṭaka* (upper part of the nasal passage), it should not thereafter be retained in the throat. The oil can be retained in the nasal passage only for a brief period till one counts five, seven or ten. Thereafter, he should throw out the liquid in the nose and the mouth by spitting. He should spit out either through the left side or through the right side as he finds it easy.

नीते नस्ये मनस्तापं रजः क्रोधञ्च संत्यजेत् ।
शयीत निद्रां त्यक्त्वा च प्रोत्तानो वाक्शतं नरः ।
तथा पिबेच्च[१६] नस्यान्ते धूमो वा कवलो हितः ॥६७॥

While using the inhalation therapy, the patient should avoid worry, dust and anger. Thereafter, he should continue to lie down on his back, but should not sleep, till the counting of one hundred. After the inhalation therapy is over, the patient should use smoking (therapy) and *kavala* (keeping mouthful of drugs).

नस्ये त्रीण्युपदिष्टानि लक्षणानि प्रयोगतः[५७] ।
शुद्धहीनातियोगानि विशेषाच्छास्त्रचिन्तकैः ॥६८॥

According to the experts in this therapy, three types of signs may appear by the administration of oleation therapy, viz., (1) those of appropriate administration, (2) those of less administration, and (3) those of excessive administration.

लाघवं मनसः शुद्धिः स्रोतसां व्याधिसंक्षयः ।
चित्तेन्द्रियप्रसादश्च शिरसः शुद्धिलक्षणम् ॥६९॥

*Signs of Appropriate Administration*

If there is appropriate administration of the inhalation therapy, following signs and symptoms will appear :

(1) Feeling of lightness in the mind;
(2) clearance (non-obstruction) of the channels of circulation;
(3) alleviation of the disease; and
(4) happiness of the mind and feeling of comfort in the sense organs.

कण्डूपदेहो गुरुता स्रोतसां कफसंस्रवः ।
मूर्ध्नि हीनविशुद्धे वा[५८] लक्षणं परिकीर्त्तितम् ॥७०॥

*Signs of Less Administration*

If the inhalation therapy is administered in less quantity, then the following signs and symptoms will appear :

(1) Itching sensation;
(2) feeling of stickiness over the body;
(3) feeling of heaviness in the channels of circulation; and
(4) excessive exudation of excreta from the head (nose and mouth).

मस्तुलुंगागमो वातवृद्धिरिंद्रियविभ्रमः ।
शून्यता शिरसश्चापि मूर्ध्नि गाढं विरेचिते ॥७१॥

### *Signs of Excessive Administration*

If the inhalation therapy is administered in excess quantity then the following signs and symptoms will appear :

(1) Coming out of *mastulunga* (brain matter);
(2) aggravation of *vāyu*;
(3) malfunctioning of senses; and
(4) feeling of emptiness in the head.

हीनातिशुद्धे शिरसि कफवातघ्नमाचरेत् ।
सम्यग्विशुद्धे शिरसि सर्पिर्नस्ये निषेचयेत्[१] ॥७२॥

### *Management*

If the therapy is administered in less quantity, then treatment for the alleviation of *kapha* should be initiated. If the therapy is administered in excess, then the treatment for the alleviation of *vāyu* should be initiated. If the therapy is properly administered, then ghee should be sprinkled over the nostrils.

कफप्रसेकः शिरसो गुरुतेन्द्रियविभ्रमः ।
लक्षणं तदतिस्निग्धे तत्र रूक्षं प्रदापयेत् ।
भोजयेच्चानभिष्यन्दी नस्याचारिकमादिशेत् ॥७३॥

### *Excessive Oleation*

Excessive oleation causes salivation, heaviness of the head an malfunctioning of senses. In such an event, ununctuous therapies shoul be administered. The patient should be given such food and drinks whic are not *abhiṣyandī* (which obstruct the channels of circulation).

वमनं रेचनं नस्यं निरूहश्चानुवासनम् ।
एतानि पंचकर्माणि कथितानि मुनीश्वरैः" ॥७४॥

(शार्ङ्गधर : उत्तरखण्ड : ८ : १-६४)

### *Pañca Karma (Five Specialised Therapies)*

*Vamana* (emesis), *recana* (purgation), *nasya* (inhalation therap *nirūha* (enema with decoctions, etc.) and *anuvāsana* (enema with c etc.)—these therapies taken together are called *Pañcakarma* (five specialised therapies).

अथ धूमपानविधिः

"धूमस्तु षड्विधः प्रोक्तः शमनो बृंहणस्तथा ।
रेचनः कासहा चैव वामनो व्रणधूपनः ॥७५॥

## SMOKING THERAPY

### Varieties

Smoking therapy is of six types as follows :

(1) *Śamana* which causes alleviation of *doṣas*;
(2) *bṛṃhaṇa*-which produces nourishing effect;
(3) *recana* which causes elimination of *doṣas* from the body;
(4) *kāsahā* which alleviates coughing;
(5) *vāmana* which causes emesis; and
(6) *vraṇa dhūpana* which is used for the fumigation of ulcers.

शमनस्य तु पर्यायौ मध्यः प्रायोगिकस्तथा ।
बृंहणस्यापि पर्यायौ स्नेहनो मृदुरेव च ।
रेचनस्यापि पर्यायौ शोधनस्तीक्ष्ण एव च ॥७६॥

### Synonyms

*Madhya* (medium) and *prāyogika*, these are the synonyms of *śamana dhūma*; *snehana* (oleation) and *mṛdu* (mild), these are the synonyms of *bṛṃhaṇa dhūma*; and *śodhana* (cleansing) and *tīkṣṇa* (sharp), these are the synonyms of *recana dhūma*.

अधूमार्हश्च खल्वेते श्रांतो भीतश्च दुःखितः ।
दत्तबस्तिविरिक्तश्च रात्रौ जागरितश्च यः ॥७७॥
पिपासितश्च दाहार्त्तस्तालुशोषी[60] तथोदरी ।
शिरोऽभितापी तिमिरी छर्द्याध्मानप्रपीडितः ॥७८॥
क्षतोरस्कः प्रमेहार्त्तः पाण्डुरोगी च गर्भिणी ।

रूक्षः क्षीणोऽभ्यवहित[61] क्षीरक्षौद्रघृतासवः ।
भुक्तान्नदधिमत्स्याश्च बालो वृद्धः कृशस्तथा ॥७९॥

*Unsuitable Persons*

Following categories of patients are not suitable for the administration of smoking therapy :

(1) Those who are tired, afraid and sorrowful;
(2) those who have administered enema and purgation therapies;
(3) those who have remained awake at night;
(4) those suffering from morbid thirst, burning sensation, dryness of the mouth and *udara* (obstinate abdominal disorders including ascites);
(5) those suffering from burning sensation in the head, cataract, vomiting, flatulence, consumption, *prameha* (obstinate urinary disorders including diabetes) and anemia;
(6) pregnant women;
(7) those who are ununctuous and emaciated;
(8) those who have consumed milk, honey, ghee, alcoholic drinks, food, curd and fish; and
(9) infants, old persons and thin persons.

अकाले चातिपीतश्च धूमः कुर्यादुपद्रवान् ।
तत्रेष्टं सर्पिषा[62] पानं नावनांजनतर्पणम् ॥८०॥
सर्पिरिक्षुरसं द्राक्षा पयो वा शर्कराम्बु वा ।
मधुराम्लौ रसौ वापि वमनाय प्रदापयेत् ॥८१॥

*Complications and Their Management*

If smoking therapy is taken in excess and untimely, then this gives rise to several complications. For their cure, the patient should be given ghee to drink, *nāvana* (inhalation therapy), collyrium and *tarpaṇa* (nourishing therapy).

The patient should be given ghee, sugar-cane juice, grapes, milk or water mixed with sugar. He should also be given sweet and sour juice for emesis.

धूमस्तु द्वादशाद् वर्षाद् गृह्यतेऽशीतिकान्न च ॥८२॥

कासश्वासप्रतिश्यायान् मन्याहनुशिरोरुजः ।
वातश्लेष्मविकारांश्च हन्याद्धूमः सुयोजितः ॥८३॥

### *Suitable Persons for Smoking*

Smoking therapy should be administered to a person who is above 12 years and below 80 years of age. When appropriately administered, it cures cough, asthma, coryza, pain in the sterno-mastoid region, jaw and head and diseases caused by *vāyu* and *kapha*.

धूमोपयोगात्पुरुषः प्रसन्नेन्द्रियवाङ्मनः ।
दृढकेशद्विजश्मश्रुसुगंधिवदनो भवेत् ॥८४॥

### *Smoking for a Healthy Person*

Smoking therapy endows a healthy person with the following benefits :

(1) His senses, speech and mind become refreshed;
(2) his hair, teeth and beard become strong; and
(3) his mouth becomes aromatic.

धूमनाडीभवेत्तत्र त्रिखण्डा च त्रिपर्विका ।
कनिष्ठिकापरीणाहा राजमाषागमांतरा ॥८५॥

### *Smoking Pipe*

Smoking pipe should be made of three pieces having three joints. It should be of the diameter of the little finger. The hole inside the pipe should allow a seed of *rājamāṣa* to pass.

धूमनाडीभवेद्दीर्घा शमने रोगिणोंगुलैः ।
चत्वारिंशोन्मितैस्तद्वद्द्वात्रिंशद्भिर्मृदौ मता[६३] ॥८६॥
तीक्ष्णे[६४] चतुर्विंशतिभिः कासघ्ने षोडशोन्मितैः ।
दशाङ्गुलैर्वामनीये तथा स्याद् व्रणनाडिके[६५] ॥८७॥

The length of smoking pipe for different types of smoking therapy should be as follows :

| | *Type* | *Length* |
|---|---|---|
| 1. | *Śamana* | 40 *aṅgulas* |
| 2. | *Mṛdu (bṛṃhaṇa)* | 32 *aṅgulas* |
| 3. | *Tīkṣṇa (recana)* | 24 *aṅgulas* |
| 4. | *Kāsaghna* | 16 *aṅgulas* |
| 5. | *Vāmanīya* | 10 *aṅgulas* |
| 6. | *Vraṇa nāḍī* | 10 *aṅgulas* |

In the above measurement, the term *aṅgula* means the breadth of the patient's own middle finger.

कलायमण्डलस्थूला कुलत्थागमरंध्रिका ।
अथेषिकां प्रलिंपेत् सुश्लक्ष्णं द्वादशाङ्गुलम् ॥८८॥
धूमद्रव्यस्य कल्केन लेपश्चाष्टाङ्गुलः स्मृतः ।
कल्कं कर्षमितं लिप्त्वा छायाशुष्कं च कारयेत् ।
इषीकामपनीयाथ स्नेहाक्तां वर्तिमादरात् ॥८९॥

*Preparation of Cigar*

A reed having the thickness of a pea and a hole in the pith to allow a seed of *kulattha* to pass through should be collected. It should be smooth outside and of 12 *aṅgulas* in length. Over that, the paste of drugs (to be used for smoking) should be smeared and it should be dried in the shade. Then the reed should be taken out and the cigar should be smeared with fat (ghee or oil) and stored carefully.

अंगारे दीपितां कृत्वा धृत्वा नेत्रस्य रंध्रके।
वदनेन पिबेद्धूमं वदनेनैव संत्यजेत् ॥९०॥
नासिकाभ्यां ततः पीत्वा मुखेनैव वमेत्सुधीः ।
'विलोमगोह्याशु धूमः कुर्याद्दृर्शनविभ्रमम्' ॥९१॥

*Mode of Administration*

The cigar, then should be pushed into the hole of the pipe and the outer end should be ignited with fire. The smoking should be performed through the mouth and the residual smoke should be blown out through the mouth. One can inhale the smoke through the nostril and the residual smoke may then be thrown out through the mouth. If the opposite method, i.e. taking in the smoke through the mouth and throwing out the residual smoke through the nostrils, is followed then this immediately causes impairment of the functioning of the eyes.

शरावसम्पुटे क्षिप्त्वा कल्कमङ्गारदीपितम् ।
छिद्रे नेत्र[66] निवेश्याथ व्रणं तेनैव धूपयेत् ॥९२॥

### *Method of Vraṇa Dhūpana*

For fumigating an ulcer, the paste of the drugs should be kept between two earthen plates with a hole at the top and the borders of these two jars should be sealed [with mud smeared cloth]. This should then be placed over burning charcoal. The smoke of the drugs inside the plates will come out through the hole in the upper plate. The ulcer should then be fumigated with this smoke.

एलादिकल्कं शमने स्निग्धं सर्ज्जरसं[67] मृदौ ।
रेचने तीक्ष्णकल्कं च कासघ्ने[68] क्षुद्रिकोषणम् ॥९३॥
वामने स्नायुचर्माद्यं दद्याद्धूमस्य पानकम् ।
व्रणे वा निम्बपंचाद्यं[69] धूपने सम्प्रशस्यते ॥९४॥

### *Recipes for Different Types of Smoking*

For *śamana* type of smoking therapy, the paste of drugs belonging to *Elādi* group should be used; for *mṛdu* (*snehana*) type, *sarja rasa* mixed with ghee or oil should be used; for *recana* type, the paste of *tīkṣṇa* (*marica*) should be used; for *kāsaghna* type, *kaṇṭakārī* and *marica* should be used; for *vāmana* type, ligaments, skin, etc., of animals should be used and for *vraṇa dhūpana* type of smoking therapy, leaves of *nimba*, etc., are useful.

यथा

मयूरपिच्छं निम्बस्य पत्राणि बृहतीफलम् ।
मरिचं हिंगुमांसी च बीजं कार्प्पाससंभवम् ॥९५॥
छागरोमाहिनिर्मोकं विष्ठां वैडालिकीं तथा ।
गजदन्तश्च तच्चूर्णं किंचित् घृतविमिश्रितम् ॥९६॥

गृहेषु[७०] धूपनं दत्वा सर्वान्बालग्रहान् जयेत् ।
पिशाचान् राक्षसान् जित्वा सर्वज्वरहरं भवेत् ॥९७॥
॥ अपराजितो धूपः ॥

*Aparājita Dhūpa*

Peacock feather, leaves of *nimba*, fruit of *bṛhatī, marica, hiṅgu, jaṭāmāṃsī*, seed of *kārpāsa*, hair of goat, slough of snake, stool of cat and tusk of elephant should be made to a powder and added with ghee. Fumigation of the house with this recipe cures afflictions by all the types of *bālagrahas* (evil spirits possessing a child), *piśācas* (a class of demons fond of flesh) and *rākṣasas* (a class of demons = goblins). It also cures all types of fever.

परिहारस्तु धूमेषु कार्यो रेचननस्यवत् ।
नेत्राणि धातुजान्याहुर्नलवंशादिजान्यपि'' ॥९८॥
॥ इति धूमपानविधिः[७१] ॥
(शार्ङ्गधर : उत्तरखण्ड : १० : १-२५)

*Prohibitions*

Prohibitions prescribed for the *recana* type of inhalation therapy are to be followed in the case of smoking therapy also. For the preparation of smoking-pipes, metals, *nala* and bamboo can also be used.

Thus, ends the description of smoking therapy.

अथ गण्डूषकवलप्रतिसारणविधिरुच्यते

गण्डूषस्तु चतुर्द्धा स्यात्स्नैहिकः शमनस्तथा ।
शोधनो रोपणश्चैव कवलश्चापि तद्विधः ॥९९॥

## *GAṆḌŪSSA, KAVALA AND PRATISĀRAṆA*

***Gaṇḍūṣa (Rinsing the Mouth With Mouthful of Decoction): Varieties***

*Gaṇḍūṣa* is of four types as follows :

(1) *Snaihika* (oleating);
(2) *śamana* (alleviating *doṣas*);

(3) *śodhana* (eliminating *doṣas*); and
(4) *ropaṇa* (healing ulcers).

*Kavala* (rinsing the mouth with mouthful of paste of drugs) is similarly of four types.

स्निग्धोष्णैः स्नैहिको वाते स्वादुशीतप्रसादनः[७२] ।
पित्ते कट्वम्ललवणैरुष्णैः संशोधनः कफे ॥१००॥
कषायतिक्तमधुरैः गण्डूषो[७३] रोपणो व्रणे ।
चतुः प्रकारो गण्डूषकवलश्चापि कीर्त्तितः ॥१०१॥

### Preparation of Different Types of Gaṇḍūṣa

*Snaihika* type of *gaṇḍūṣa* alleviates *vāyu* and it is prepared of unctuous and hot drugs. *Śamana* type of *gaṇḍūṣa* is used for the alleviation of *pitta* and it is prepared of sweet and cooling drugs. *Saṃśodhana* type of *gaṇḍūṣa* alleviates *kapha* and it is prepared of pungent, sour, saline and hot drugs. *Ropaṇa* type of *gaṇḍūṣa* is used for healing of ulcers and it is prepared of astringent, bitter and sweet drugs.

Similarly, four types of *kavala* are also prepared.

असंचारि मुखे पूर्णे गण्डूषः कवलश्च[७४] सः ।
तत्र द्रवेण गण्डूषः कल्केन[७५] कवलस्मृतः ॥१०२॥
दद्याद् द्रवेषु[७६] चूर्णं च गंडूषे कोलमात्रकम् ।
कर्षप्रमाण[७७] कल्कस्तु कवले दीयते बुधैः ॥१०३॥

### Gaṇḍūṣa and Kavala

In both the *gaṇḍūṣa* and *kavala*, the mouth is filled with decoction (in the case of *gaṇḍūṣa*) or paste (in the case of *kavala*) of drugs and a little space is left in the mouth for the movement of these preparations. In *gaṇḍūṣa*, the mouth is filled with liquids, and in *kavala*, the mouth is filled with the paste of drugs. In *gaṇḍūṣa*, one *kola* of the powdered medicine is added to the liquid and in *kavala*, the powdered medicine should be added in the dose of one *karṣa* to the paste. [There appears to be an error in the text].

धार्यते[७८] पंचमाद्वर्षाद् गण्डूषकवलादयः ॥१०४॥

### *Age of Patient*

The patient should be above five years old for administering *gaṇḍūṣa, kavala*, etc.

गण्डूषस्तु स्थितः कुर्यात्स्विन्नः भालगलादिकः ।
मनुष्यस्त्रीं तथा पंच सप्त वा दोषनाशनात् ॥१०५॥

### *Duration of Holding Gaṇḍūṣa in Mouth*

*Gaṇḍūṣa*, kept in the mouth, causes fomentation of the forehead and the throat. It should be administered for three, five or seven times or till the aggravated *doṣas* get alleviated.

कफपूर्णास्यता यावत्छेदो दोषस्य वा भवेत् ।
नेत्रघ्राणस्रुतिर्यावत्तावद् गण्डूषधारणम् ॥१०६॥

One should hold *gaṇḍūṣa* till such time as the mouth becomes full of phlegm or till the aggravated *doṣas* are alleviated or till there is excretion of water from the eyes and nose.

तिलकल्कोदकं क्षीरं स्नेहो वा स्नैहिकं मतम्[१] ॥१०७॥

### *Recipes for Gaṇḍūṣa*

*Gaṇḍūṣa* prepared of the paste of *tila*, water, milk and ghee or oil produces oleating effect.

तिलं नीलोत्पलं सर्पिः शर्करा क्षीरमेव च ।
सक्षौद्रो हनुवक्त्रस्थो गण्डूषो दोषनाशनः ॥१०८॥

*Gaṇḍūṣa* prepared of *tila, nīlotpala*, ghee, sugar and milk along with honey cures diseases of the mandibles and mouth.

वैशद्यं जनयत्यास्ये संदधाति मुखे व्रणान् ।
दाहतृष्णाप्रशमनं मधुगण्डूषधारणम् ॥१०९॥

*Gaṇḍūṣa* of honey produces clarity of mouth and cures ulcers in the mouth, burning sensation and morbid thirst.

विषक्षाराग्निदग्धे च सर्पिर्धार्यं पयोऽथवा ।
तैलसैन्धवगण्डूषो दन्तचाले प्रशस्यते ॥११०॥

For curing afflictions by poisons, alkalies and burns by fire, one should use ghee or milk for *gaṇḍūṣa*. *Gaṇḍūṣa* of oil and *saindhava* helps in the settling of loose teeth.

शोषं मुखस्य वैरस्यं गण्डूषात्कांजिको जयेत् ।
सिंधुत्रिकटुराजीभिः आर्द्रकेण कफे हितः ॥१११॥

Dryness and distaste in the mouth is corrected by *gaṇḍūṣa* with *kāñji* (a sour preparation). *Gaṇḍūṣa* with *saindhava, śuṇṭhī, pippalī, marica, rājikā* and *ārdraka* helps in the alleviation of *kapha*.

त्रिफलामधुगण्डूषः कफासृक्पित्तनाशनः ॥११२॥

*Gaṇḍūṣa* prepared of *harītakī, bibhītaka, āmalakī* and honey cures aggravation of *kapha, rakta* and *pitta*.

दार्वीगुडूचीत्रिफलाद्राक्षाजात्याश्च पल्लवाः ।
यवासश्चेति तत्क्वाथः यष्टीक्षौद्रेण संयुतः ।
शीतो मुखे धृतो हन्यान्मुखपाकं त्रिदोषजम् ॥११३॥

*Gaṇḍūṣa* with the cold decoction of *dāru haridrā, guḍūcī, harītakī, bibhītaka, āmalakī, drākṣā,* leaves of *jātī* and *yavāsa* mixed with the powder of *yaṣṭimadhu* and honey cures stomatitis caused by the simultaneous vitiation of all the three *doṣas*.

यस्यौषधस्य गण्डूषस्तथैव[60] प्रतिसारणम् ।
कवलश्चापि तस्यैव ज्ञेयोऽत्र कुशलैनरैः ॥११४॥

Drugs, described above for *gaṇḍūṣa* can also be used for *pratisāraṇa* (rubbing) and *kavala* for the respective diseases.

कवलो यथा

केशरं मातुलुंगस्य सैन्धवोषणसंयुतम् ।
हन्यात्कवलतो जाड्यमरुचिं कफवातजम् ॥११५॥

*Recipes for Kavala*

*Kavala* (keeping mouthful of paste in the mouth) prepared of the stamens of *mātuluṅga* added with *saindhava* and *marica* cures *jāḍya* (aphasia) and anorexia caused by *kapha* and *vāta*.

कल्कोऽवलेहोऽथ चूर्णं[८१] त्रिविधं प्रतिसारणम् ।
अङ्गुल्यग्रप्रणीतं च यथास्वं मुखरोगिणाम् ॥११६॥

*Pratisāraṇa (Rubbing of Drugs)*

*Pratisāraṇa* is of three types, viz., (1) which is rubbed in the form of paste, (2) which is rubbed in the form of linctus, and (3) which is rubbed in the form of powder. These drug preparations should be taken on the tip of finger and rubbed in the affected part of the mouth.

प्रतिसारणं चूर्णं यथा

कुष्ठं दार्वी लोध्रमब्दं समंगा पाठा तिक्ता च तेजनी पीतिका ।
'एषां[८२] चूर्णं घृष्टमाशु द्विजानां रक्तस्रावं हन्ति कण्डूं रुजं च' ॥११७॥

*Recipes for Pratisāraṇa*

*Pratisāraṇa* (rubbing) with the powder of *kuṣṭha, dārvī, lodhra, abda, samaṅgā, pāṭhā, tiktā, tejanī* and *pītikā* instantaneously cures bleeding from gums (teeth), itching and pain.

'तेजिनी[८३] मुस्तलोध्रं च चूर्णं स्यात्प्रतिसारणम् ।
रक्तस्रुतिं दन्तपीडां शोथं दाहं विनाशयेत्'[८४] ॥११८॥

*Pratisāraṇa* (rubbing) with the powder of *tejanī, mustā* and *lodhra* cures pain, oedema and burning sensation in the gums (teeth).

हीनयोगात्कफोत्क्लेशो रसाज्ञानारुचिं तथा ।
अतियोगान्मुखे पाकः शोषस्तृष्णाक्लमो भवेत् ॥११९॥
व्याधेरचयस्तुष्टिर्वैशद्यं वक्त्रलाघवम् ।
इन्द्रियाणां प्रसादश्च गण्डूषैः शुद्धिलक्षणम्' ॥१२०॥
(शार्ङ्गधर : उत्तरखण्ड : १० : १-२०)

*Improper and Proper Administration*

If *gaṇḍūṣa* (including *kavala* and *pratisāraṇa*) is administered in less quantity, then this leads to excessive salivation, inability to appreciate taste and anorexia. If it is administered in excess, then the patient suffers from stomatitis, dryness, morbid thirst and fatigue. Properly administered *gaṇḍūṣa* causes alleviation of the disease, produces the sense of satisfaction, clarity and lightness of the mouth and sharpness in the perception of senses.

इति श्रीमहाराजाधिराजटोडरमल्लविरचिते टोडरानन्दे आयुर्वेदसौख्ये (स्वेद)-नस्य-धूमपान-गण्डूष-(कवल)-प्रतिसारण(विधिवर्णन)नामाशीतितिमो हर्षः ॥

Thus, ends the 80th chapter dealing with the description of fomentation, inhalation, smoking, *gaṇḍūṣa, kavala* and *pratisāraṇa* therapies in the *Āyurveda saukhya* of *Ṭoḍarānanda* composed by the great King Ṭoḍaramalla.

## NOTES AND REFERENCES

१. (क) This is the beginning of the eighty fourth chapter of *Āyurveda saukhya* in *Ṭoḍarānanda* and invocation reads as follows :

'सुरन्न (स्न) वासांसि महावनानि नन्द यदा त्वा विनयं चकार ।
प्रेम्ना स्वपित्ते सकृपां नरेन्द्रे करोतु, श्री टोडरमल्लसंज्ञे' ॥

(ख) 'सुरन्न. ...... संज्ञे' पाठोऽयं चतुर्थषष्ठपुस्तकयोः नोपलभ्यते ।

२. तप्तपयोनुवातशमनं इति षष्ठपुस्तके पाठः ।

३. .निषवनो. इति षष्ठपुस्तके पाठः ।

४. .स्वेद्या विजानता इति चतुर्थषष्ठपुस्तकयोः पाठः ।

५. (क) सद्यः इति षष्ठपुस्तके पाठः ।
(ख) शोधनैर्यान्त्यशेषम् इति आकरे पाठः ।

६. स्वचा इति षष्ठपुस्तके पाठः ।

७. स्नेहात्पक्वः इति षष्ठपुस्तके पाठः ।

८. मृदुना नवा इति प्रथमपुस्तके पाठः ।

९. चैव इति प्रथमपुस्तके पाठः ।

१०. भ्रान्ति इति षष्ठपुस्तके पाठः ।

११. स्वाचारमादिशेत् इति षष्ठपुस्तके पाठः ।

१२. कथितं इति षष्ठपुस्तके पाठः ।

१३. तथा इति आकरे पाठः ।

१४. ध्वंसं इति षष्ठपुस्तके पाठः ।

१५. गदौ इति षष्ठपुस्तके पाठः ।

१६. चापतर्पिते इति षष्ठपुस्तके पाठः ।

१७. वृद्धः प्रतिश्यायी इति षष्ठपुस्तके पाठः ।

१८. शोकार्दितः श्रातस्त्रिदोषी द्रवपीडितः इति षष्ठपुस्तके पाठः ।

१९. कासश्च इति प्रथमपुस्तके पाठः ।

२०. स्नातुकर्मसमाचरेत् इति प्रथमपुस्तके पाठः ।

२१. स्यात्पाणीयं च कार्षिकम् इति प्रथमपुस्तके पाठः ।

२२. मतौ इति चतुर्थपुस्तके पाठः ।

२३. विरेकनस्यार्द्धं इति प्रथमपुस्तके पाठः ।

२४. सोऽवपीडा इति पंचमपुस्तके पाठः ।

२५. (क) वक्रं इति पंचमपुस्तके पाठः ।
(ख) प्राक्तं चान्ने प्रधमनं मतम् इति षष्ठपुस्तके पाठः ।

२६. स्मृतम् इति चतुर्थपुस्तके पाठः ।

२७. निशायां इति षष्ठपुस्तके पाठः ।

२८ विषगेषु इति पंचमपुस्तके पाठः ।

२९. .प्रवाहनम् इति षष्ठपुस्तके पाठः ।

३०. च शस्यते इति षष्ठपुस्तके पाठः ।

३१. .माहिषैः इति प्रथमपुस्तके पाठः ।

३२. 'मर्शश्च ...... बुधैः' पाठोऽयं प्रथमपुस्तके नोपलभ्यते ।

३३. दोषचलाचलम् इति षष्ठपुस्तके पाठः ।

३४. 'दोषोत्क्लेशात् ..... क्रमम्' पाठोऽयं चतुर्थषष्ठपुस्तकयोः नोपलभ्यते ।

३५. 'द्वमनशोधनम् ....... हीने' पाठोऽयं चतुर्थपुस्तके नोपलभ्यते ।

३६. शोधकाम् इति षष्ठपुस्तके पाठः ।

३७. यथास्त्वं इति प्रथमपुस्तके आकरे च पाठः ।

३८. (क) भेदकम् इति चतुर्थषष्ठपुस्तकयोः पाठः ।
(ख) भेदकान् इति पंचमपुस्तके पाठः ।

३९. तथा इति षष्ठपुस्तके पाठः ।

४०. जयेदर्बुद. इति षष्ठपुस्तके पाठः ।

४१. यावन्निममां चो धृतां ततः इति प्रथमपुस्तके पाठः ।

४२. विंदुसंमिता इति षष्ठपुस्तके पाठः ।

४३. .संघैरष्टभिः इति षष्ठपुस्तके पाठः ।

४४. कृते इति षष्ठपुस्तके पाठः ।

४५. ईषदुच्छिंदनात्स्नेहो इति प्रथमपुस्तके पाठः ।

४६. नश्ये निषक्तंनं इति षष्ठपुस्तके पाठः ।

४७. उच्छिन्दन्न इति आकरे पाठः ।

४८. (क) विशुद्धधूमपानेन खिन्नतामागतं तथा इति षष्ठपुस्तके पाठः ।
(ख) स्विन्नभालगलं इति आकरे पाठः ।

४९. सुमुन्नमितनासाग्रं वैद्यो नस्यो न योजयेत् इति चतुर्थपुस्तके पाठः ।

५०. हेमधारादि इति षष्ठपुस्तके पाठः ।

५१. यत्र युक्त्या इति आकरे पाठः ।

५२. नस्येष्व इति प्रथमपुस्तके पाठः ।

५३. .पीडिताः इति चतुर्थषष्ठपुस्तकयोः पाठः ।

५४. 'पंच. ...... द्रवम्' पाठोयं चतुर्थषष्ठपुस्तकयोः नोपलभ्यते ।

५५. निष्ठीवेत्संमुखे न हि इति आकरे पाठः ।

५६. वैरेचनश्चान्ते धूमो इति आकरे पाठः ।

५७. समासतः इति आकरे पाठः ।

५८. तु इति आकरे पाठः ।

५९. नियोजयेत् इति चतुर्थषष्ठपुस्तकयोः पाठः ।

६०. श्वासार्त्तः इति षष्ठपुस्तके पाठः ।

६१. .वह्नत. इति आकरे पाठः ।

६२. सर्पिषः इति आकरे पाठः ।

६३. स्मृता इति आकरे पाठः ।

६४. तीक्ष्णै इति पंचमपुस्तके पाठः ।

६५ .नाडिका इति चतुर्थषष्ठपुस्तकयोः आकरे च पाठः ।

६६ पिबेद्धूमं मुखेनैव व्रणं इति चतुर्थषष्ठपुस्तकयोः पाठः ।

६७. सरसं इति षष्ठपुस्तके पाठः ।

६८. श्वसने इति षष्ठपुस्तके पाठः ।

६९. निम्बवचाद्यं धूपनं संप्रचक्षते इति पंचमपुस्तके पाठः ।

७०. अन्येऽपि धूमा गेहेषु कर्तव्या रोगशान्तये इति आकरे पाठः ।

७१. पाठोऽयं प्रथमचतुर्थपंचमपुस्तकेषु नोपलभ्यते ।

७२. (क) .शीतैः प्रसादनः इति चतुर्थपुस्तके आकरे च पाठः ।
(ख) प्रसाधनः इति षष्ठपुस्तके पाठः ।

७३. कटुष्णो इति आकरे पाठः ।

७४. (क) कवलोन्यथा इति चतुर्थपुस्तके पाठः ।
(ख) कवलश्चरः इति पंचमपुस्तके आकरे च पाठः ।

७५. 'गण्डूषमुष्णै संशोधन कफे । कषायतिक्तमुधरैः कटुष्णो रोपणे व्रणः । द्रवेन तत्र गण्डूष' पाठोऽयं षष्ठपुस्तके अधिकमुपलभ्यते ।

७६. द्रव्येषु इति षष्ठपुस्तके पाठः ।

७७. .प्रमाणतः कल्कः इति चतुर्थषष्ठपुस्तकयोः पाठः ।

७८. धार्यन्ते इति आकरे पाठः ।

७९. स्नैहिके हितम् इति चतुर्थषष्ठपुस्तकयोः आकरे च पाठः ।

८०. गण्डूषस्तस्यैव प्रतिसारणम् इति षष्ठपुस्तके पाठः ।

८१. कल्कोवलेहश्चूर्णं इति षष्ठपुस्तके आकरे च पाठः ।

८२. 'एषां ...... रुजं च' पाठोऽयं प्रथमपुस्तके नोपलभ्यते ।

८३. 'तेजिनी ...... विनाशयेत्' पाठोऽयं चतुर्थषष्ठपुस्तकयोः नोपलभ्यते ।

८४. च नाशयेत् इति आकरे पाठः ।

# CHAPTER XIII

## ।। वमनविरेचनविधिः ।।

## *(Emetic and Purgation Therapies)*

'दोषा' कदाचित्कुप्यन्ति जिताः लंघनपाचनैः ।
ये तु संशोधनैः शुद्धाः न तेषां पुनरुद्भवः' ।।१ ।।

*Importance*

If the aggravated *doṣas* are subdued by alleviation therapies like *laṅghana* (fasting) and *pācana* (therapy for the metabolic transformation), they may reappear. But if these are corrected by *saṃśodhana* (elimination) therapies, then there is no possibility of their reappearance (getting aggravated or vitiated again).

### अथ वननविधिरुच्यते

(वमन-विरेचनकालः)

''शरत्काले वसन्ते च प्रावृट्काले च देहिनाम् ।
वमनं रेचनं चैव कारयेत् कुशलो भिषक् ।।२ ।।

## *EMETIC THERAPY*

### *Seasons for Administration*

A wise physician should administer emetic and purgation therapies during autumn, spring and *prāvṛt* (beginning of the rainy season).

(वाम्याः)

बलवन्तं कफव्याप्तं हृल्लासादिनिपीडितम्[2] ।
तथा वमनसात्म्यं च धीरचित्तं च वामयेत् ॥३॥
विषदोषे स्तन्यरोगे मन्देऽग्नौ श्लीपदेऽर्बुदे ।
हृद्रोगकुष्ठवीसर्पमेहाजीर्णभ्रमेषु च ॥४॥
विदारिकाऽपचीकासश्वासपीनसवृद्धिषु ।
अपस्मारे ज्वरोन्मादे तथा रक्तातिसारिषु ॥५॥
नासाताल्वोष्ठपाकेषु कर्णस्रावेऽधिजिह्वके[3] ।
गलशुण्ड्यामतीसारे[4] पित्तश्लेष्मगदे तथा ।
मेदोगदेऽरुचौ वापि वमनं कारयेद्भिषक् ॥६॥

### *Suitable Persons for Emetic Therapy*

Emetic therapy should be administered to the following types of persons (patients) :

(1) Those who are strong and whose bodies are pervaded with [aggravated] *kapha*;
(2) those suffering from nausea, etc.;
(3) those who are accustomed to taking emetic therapy, i.e. who do not adversely react to such therapy;
(4) those having patience;
(5) in the case of poisoning;
(6) those afflicted with the vitiation of breast-milk;
(7) those having suppressed power of digestion;
(8) those suffering from filariasis, tumour, heart disease, *kuṣṭha* (obstinate skin diseases including leprosy), erysipelas, *meha* (obstinate urinary disorders including diabetes), indigestion, giddiness, *vidārikā* (a type of diabetic carbuncle), tubercular lymphadenitis, cough, asthma, chronic rhinitis, hydrocele, epilepsy, fever, insanity and blood-diarrhoea;

(9) those suffering from the suppuration of the nose, palate and lips, otitis media, *adhijihvā* (enlarged adenoid glands), *galaśuṇḍı* (tonsillitis) and diarrhoea;
(10) those suffering from diseases caused by the aggravation of *pitta* and *kapha*; and
(11) those suffering from vitiated fat tissue and anorexia.

(अवाम्याः)

न वामनीयस्तिमिरी न गुल्मी नोदरी कृशः ।
नातिवृद्धो गर्भिणी च न स्थूलो न क्षतातुरः ॥७॥
मदार्त्तो बालको रूक्षः क्षुधितश्च निरूहितः ।
उदावर्त्यूर्ध्वरक्ती च दुश्च्छर्दः केवलानिली ॥८॥
नेत्ररोगी चक्षुरंधः चक्षुपीडायुस्तु वा ।
पाण्डुरोगी कृमिव्याप्तः पठनात् स्वरघातकः[५] ॥९॥

### *Persons Unsuitable for Emetic Therapy*

The following types of persons are not suitable for the administration of emetic therapy :

(1) Those suffering from cataract, *gulma* (phantom tumour) and *udara* (obstinate abdominal disorders including ascites);
(2) emaciated persons;
(3) very old persons and pregnant women;
(4) those suffering from adiposity, tuberculosis and alcoholism;
(5) infants, ununctuous persons and those who are hungry;
(6) those who are given *nirūha* type of medicated enema;
(7) those suffering from *udāvarta* (upward movement of flatus in the abdomen) and *ūrdhvaga rakta pitta* (bleeding through upward tracts);
(8) those who get vomiting with difficulty;
(9) those suffering from diseases caused by the vitiation of *vāyu* exclusively;
(10) those suffering from eye diseases including blindness and pain in eyes; and
(11) those suffering from anemia, excessive parasitic infestation and hoarseness of voice caused by reading in loud voice.

एतेऽप्यजीर्णव्यथिता वाऽन्ये ये विषपीडिताः ।
कफव्याप्ताश्च ते वाम्या मधुकक्वाथपानतः ।
सुकुमारं कृशं बालं वृद्धं भीरुं न वामयेत् ॥१०॥

*Exceptions*

If the above mentioned persons suffer from excessive of indigestion, if they have consumed poison and if their body is pervaded with the excessive of aggravated *kapha*, then they may be given [mild] emetic therapy with the help of the decoction of *yaṣṭimadhu*. However, tender and emaciated persons, infants, old persons and those who are afraid of taking emetics should not be administered such therapy.

(पूर्वकर्म)

पीत्वा यवागूमाकण्ठं क्षीरतक्रदधीनि च ।
असात्म्यैः श्लेष्मलैर्भोज्यैर्दोषानुत्क्लेश्य देहिनाम् ।
स्निग्धस्विन्नाय वमनं दत्तं सम्यक् प्रवर्त्तते ॥११॥

*Preparatory Treatment*

Before administering emetic therapy, the patient should be given bellyful of gruel, milk, butter-milk, curd and such other food which are unwholesome and which cause aggravation of *kapha*. This causes *utkleśa* (excitement) of *doṣas*. The patient should be given oleation and fomentation therapies prior to the administration of emetic therapy which facilitates easy removal of the vitiated *doṣas*.

(वमनद्रव्यम्)

वमनेषु च सर्वेषु सैन्धवं मधुना हितम् ।
बीभत्सं वमनं दद्याद्विपरीतं विरेचनम् ॥१२॥

*Nature of Ingredients*

In all the recipes of emetic therapy, addition of rock-salt and honey is useful. The ingredients for emesis should be unpalatable (despisable). On the other hand, palatable ingredients should be used for purgation therapy.

क्वाथ्यद्रव्यस्य कुडवं श्रपयित्वा जलाढके ।
अर्द्धभागावशिष्टं च वमनेष्वचारयेत्[९] ॥१३॥

*Preparation of Decoction*

For the purpose of emetic therapy, one *kuḍava* of pounded drugs should be boiled with one *āḍhaka* of water and reduced to half. This decoction should be used for emetic therapy.

(वमनमात्रा)

क्वाथपाने नवप्रस्थ[१०] ज्येष्ठा मात्रा प्रकीर्त्तिता ।
मध्यमा षण्मिता प्रोक्ता द्विप्रस्थ[११] च कनीयसी' ॥१४॥

(भावप्रकाश : पञ्चविधिप्रकरण ५ : १-१५)

कल्कश्चूर्णावलेह्यानां त्रिपलं ज्येष्ठमात्रया[१२] ।
मध्यमं द्विपलं विद्यात्कनीयस्तु पलं भवेत् ॥१५॥

*Dose*

For the emetic therapy, intake of decoction in the quantity of nine *prasthas* constitutes the excellent dose, in the quantity of six *prasthas* constitutes the medium dose and in the quantity of two *prasthas* constitutes inferior (small) dose.

Similarly, intake of paste, powder and linctus in the quantity of three *palas* constitutes the excellent dose, in the quantity of two *palas* constitutes the medium dose and in the quantity of one *pala* constitutes the inferior (small) dose.

(वमनवेगाः)

'वमने[१३] चापि वेगाः स्युरष्टौ पित्तान्त उत्तमः ।
षड्वेगैः मध्यमो वेगाश्चत्वारस्त्ववरो मतः' ॥१६॥

(भावप्रकाश : पञ्चविधिप्रकरण ५ : १७-१८)

*Bouts of Vomiting*

If by the administration of the therapy, the patient gets eight bouts of vomiting and bile comes out at the end, then it is excellent; if he gets six bouts of vomiting, then it is medium; and if he gets only four bouts of vomiting, then it is inferior.

(मानपरिभाषा)

"वमने च विरेके तथा शोणितमोक्षणे ।
सार्द्धत्रयोदशपलं प्रस्थमाहुर्मनीषिणः" ॥१७॥

(भावप्रकाश : पञ्चविधिप्रकरण ५ : १६)

*Measurement*

For the purpose of preparing recipes for emetic, purgation and blood-letting therapies, thirteen and half *palas* constitute one *prastha.* [This is an exception to the general rule.]

(दोषानुसारं वमनद्रव्यम्)

"कफं कटुकतीक्ष्णोष्णैः पित्तं स्वादुहिमैर्जयेत् ।
सस्वादुलवणाम्लोष्णैः[१४] संस्पृष्टं[१५] वायुना कफम् ॥१८॥

*Ingredients for Different Doṣas*

For aggravated *kapha*, pungent, sharp and hot ingredients should be used. For aggravated *pitta*, sweet and cooling ingredients should be used. If aggravated *vāyu* is associated with aggravated *kapha*, then drugs which are sweet, saline, sour and hot should be used for the preparation of emetic recipes.

कृष्णाराठफलं[१६] सिन्धुं कफे कोष्णजलैः पिबेत् ।
पटोलवासानिंबैश्च[१७] पित्ते शीतं[१८] जलं पिबेत् ॥१९॥
सश्लेष्मवातपीडायां सक्षीरं मदनं पिबेत् ।
अजीर्णे कोष्णं पानीयं सिन्धुं पीत्वा वमेत्सुधीः ॥२०॥

If *kapha* is aggravated, then the patient should take *pippalī, madana phala* and rock-salt along with hot water. If *pitta* is aggravated, then the patient should take *paṭola, vāsā* and *nimba* along with cold water. If aggravated *vāyu* is associated with aggravated *kapha*, then the patient should take *madana phala* along with milk. If the patient is having indigestion, then intake of *saindhava* along with hot water facilitates emesis.

(प्रयोगविधिः)

वमनं पाययित्वा च जानुमात्रासने स्थितम् ।
कण्ठमेरण्डनालेन स्पृशन् तं वामयेद्भिषक् ॥२१॥

*Method of Administration*

After administering emetic recipe, the patient should be made to squate with folded knees kept upwards. Then his throat should be tingled with a castor stalk which gives rise to emesis.

(असम्यक् प्रयोगे लक्षणम्)

प्रसेको हृद्ग्रहः कोठकण्डूर्दुश्छर्दिते भवेत् ।
अतिवान्ते भवेत्तृष्णा हिक्कोद्गारो विसंज्ञता[१९] ॥२२॥
जिह्वानिःसर्पण[२०] चाक्ष्णोः[२१] व्यावृत्तिर्हनुसंगतिः ।
रक्तच्छर्दिष्ठीवनं च[२२] कण्ठपीडा च जायते ॥२३॥

*Signs of Improper Emesis*

If the emesis does not take place properly, then the patient suffers from salivation, stiffness in the cardiac region, urticaria and itching. If there is emesis in excess, then following signs and symptoms will appear :

(1) Morbid thirst, hiccup, eructation and unconsciousness;
(2) his tongue protrudes out of the mouth;
(3) his eyeballs remain open and fixed;
(4) his jaw bones get dislocated;
(5) he vomits blood and spits in excess; and
(6) there will be pain in his throat.

(उपद्रवचिकित्सा)

वमनस्यातियोगे च मृदु कुर्याद्विरेचनम् ॥२४॥

### Management of Complications

If complications arise because of excessive vomiting, then in general the patient should be given a mild purgative.

वमनान्तःप्रविष्टायां[२३] जिह्वायां कवलग्रहः[२४] ।
स्निग्धाम्ललवणैर्हृद्यैर्घृतक्षीररसैर्हितः[२५] ।
फलान्यम्लानि खादेयुस्तस्य चान्येऽग्रतो नरः ॥२५॥

### Shrinking of the Tongue

If the tongue gets shrunk inside the mouth, then the patient should be given *kavala* therapy with the help of unctuous, sour and saline drugs, which are cardiac tonics, along with ghee, milk and meat soup. The patient should take sour fruits.

निःसृतां तु तिलद्राक्षाकल्कलिप्तां[२६] प्रवेशयेत् ॥२६॥

### Protrusion of Tongue

If the tongue gets protruded, then after being smeared with the paste of *tila* and *drākṣā*, it should be inserted inside the mouth.

व्यावृत्तेऽक्षिण घृताभ्यक्ते पीडयेच्च[२७] शनैः शनैः ॥२७॥

### Opened Eyes

If the eyes remain open and fixed, then the eyelids should be smeared with ghee and then gently and gradually pressed for their closure.

हनुमोक्षे स्मृतः स्वेदो नस्यं च श्लेष्मवातहृत् ॥२८॥

### Dislocation of Mandibular Joint

If the mandibular joint gets dislocated because of excessive vomiting, then it should be set right after the administration of fomentation therapy. Thereafter, the patient should be given inhalation therapy for the alleviation of *kapha* and *vāyu*.

रक्तपित्तविधानेन रक्तछर्दिं[२८] ह्युपाचरेत् ॥२९॥

### *Blood-Vomiting*

If the patient vomits blood because of excessive emetic therapy, then he should be treated on the line suggested for *rakta pitta* (an ailment characterised by bleeding from different parts of the body).

धात्रीरसांजनोशीरलाजाचन्दनवारिभिः ।
मन्थं कृत्वा पाययेच्च सघृतक्षौद्रशर्करम्[२९] ।
शाम्यन्त्यनेन तृष्णाद्याः पीडाश्छर्दिसमुद्भवाः[३०-३१] ॥३०॥

### *Morbid Thirst, etc.*

The patient getting morbid thirst, pain etc., because of excessive vomiting should be given *mantha* (thin gruel) prepared with the decoction of *āmalakī, rasāñjana, uśīra, lājā* and *candana,* and mixed with ghee, honey and sugar.

(सम्यक्वान्तलक्षणम्)

हृत्कण्ठशिरसां शुद्धिर्दीप्ताग्नित्वं च लाघवम् ।
कफपित्तविनाशश्च सम्यग्वान्तस्य लक्षणम् ॥३१॥

### *Signs of Proper Emesis*

If the patient gets proper emesis, then the following signs and symptoms are manifested :

(1) There will be feeling of clarity in the heart, throat and head;
(2) the digestive power will get stimulated;
(3) there will be the feeling of lightness in the body; and
(4) there will be alleviation of *kapha* and *pitta.*

(संसर्जनक्रमः)

ततोऽपराह्ने दीप्ताग्निर्मुद्गषष्टिकशालिभिः[३२] ।
हृद्यैश्च जांगलरसैः कृत्वा यूषं च भक्षयेत्[३३] ॥३२॥

### *Post-Therapeutic Measures*

After the emetic therapy, in the afternoon, when the patient is hungry, he should be given *mudga, ṣaṣṭika* and *śāli* along with delicious meat soup of animals living in arid land and vegetable soup to eat.

तन्द्रानिद्रास्यदौर्गन्ध्यकण्डूनिग्रहणी[३४] विषम् ।
सुवान्तस्य न पीडायै भवन्त्येते कदाचन ॥३३॥

*Therapeutic Effects of Emesis*

A person who has taken emetic therapy never suffers from excessive sleep, drowsiness, foul smell coming out of the mouth, itches, *grahaṇī* (spruc syndrome) and poisoning.

(अपथ्यम्)
अजीर्णं शीतपानीयं व्यायामं मैथुनं तथा ।
स्नेहाभ्यङ्गं प्रकोप[३५] च दिनैकं[३६] वर्जयेत्सुधी[३७]" ॥३४॥

(भावप्रकाश : पञ्चकर्मविधिप्रकरणम् ५ : १९-३३)
(शार्ङ्गधर : उत्तरखण्ड : ३ : १-३३)

*Prohibitions*

A wise person taking emetic therapy should avoid indigestion (ingestion of heavy food), cold drinks, exercise, sexual intercourse, massage with fat and anger for one day after the therapy.

अगस्त्यसिन्धुमदनतालीकटुपटोलिकम् ।
कज्जलीबीजमुष्णाम्बुसहितं वमनं हितम् ॥३५॥

Emetic therapy along with *agastya, saindhava, madana, tālīśapatra,* bitter variety of *paṭola, kajjalī* (black collyrium of mercury and sulphur), *bīja* (?) and hot water is useful. [There are errors in this text.]

अथ विरेचनविधिरुच्यते[३८]

(कदा विरेचनं देयम्)
"स्निग्धस्विन्नस्य वांतस्य दद्यात् सम्यग्विरेचनम् ।

अवान्तस्य त्वधःस्रसतो ग्रहणीं स्थापयेत्कफः[39] ।
मन्दाग्निं गौरवं कुर्याज्जनयेद्वा प्रवाहिकाम् ॥३६॥
अथवा पाचनैरामं बलासं च विपाचयेत्[40] ।
स्निग्धस्य स्वेदनं कार्यं स्वेदैः स्विन्नस्य रेचनम् ॥३७॥

## PURGATION THERAPY

### Time of Administration

After oleation, fomentation and emetic therapies, a person should be given purgation therapy appropriately. If a person is given purgation therapy without prior administration of emetic therapy, then the *kapha* of the stomach while coming downwards obstructs the *grahaṇī* (duodenum including small intestine). As a result of this, the patient suffers from reduced power of digestion, heaviness and *pravāhikā* (dysentery). Alternatively, the patient should be given carminative drugs for the metabolic transformation of *āma* (uncooked material) and *kapha*. Thereafter, he should be given oleation and fomentation therapies to be followed by purgation therapy.

शरदृतौ वसन्ते च देहशुद्ध्यै[41] विरेचयेत् ।
अन्यदात्ययिके[42] कार्यं शोधनं शीलयेद् बुधः ॥३८॥

### Suitable Seasons for Purgation

Purgation therapy should be administered during autumn and spring seasons regularly for cleansing the body. In the advent of any acute disease, this therapy can be administered in other seasons also.

(विरेच्याः)
पित्ते विरेचनं युञ्ज्यादामोद्भूतगदे[43] तथा ।
आध्मानकुष्ठयोश्चैव[44] देहशुद्धौ विशेषतः ॥३९॥

### Indications

Purgation therapy should be administered to a patient suffering from aggravated *pitta*, diseases caused by *āma* (product of improper digestion and metabolism), flatulence and *kuṣṭha* (obstinate skin diseases including leprosy). It is specially useful for cleansing the body.

(अविरेच्याः)

बालवृद्धावतिस्निग्धः[४५] क्षतक्षीणो भयान्वितः ।
कामार्तो मार्गविश्रान्तः कृशोऽतिसुकुमारकः ॥४०॥
श्रान्तस्तृडार्तः[४६] स्थूलश्च गर्भिणी च नवज्वरी ।
नवप्रसूता नारी च मंदाग्निश्च मदात्ययी ।
शल्यार्दितश्च रूक्षश्च न विरेच्या विजानता ॥४१॥

*Unsuitable Persons*

Following types of persons are not suitable for the administration of purgation therapy :

(1) Infants and old persons;
(2) those who are excessively oleated;
(3) those suffering from consumption;
(4) those scared of taking purgation therapy;
(5) those indulging in excess of sex and fatigued by walk for a long distance;
(6) those who are emaciated and who are of very tender nature;
(7) those suffering from fatigue, morbid thirst, obesity and freshly occuring fever;
(8) pregnant women and those who have recently delivered;
(9) those suffering from suppressed power of digestion, alcoholism and injury by weapons; and
(10) those who are ununctuous (having dry and rough body).

(विरेच्याः)

जीर्णज्वरी गरव्याप्तो वातरोगी भगन्दरी ।
अर्शःपाण्डूदरग्रन्थिहृद्रोगारुचिपीडिताः ॥४२॥
योनिरोगप्रमेहार्त्ता गुल्मरोगी व्रणार्दिताः[४७] ।
विद्रधिश्छर्दिविस्फोटविसूचीकुष्ठसंयुताः ॥४३॥
कर्णनासाशिरोवक्त्रगुदमेढ्रामयान्विताः ।

प्लीहशोथाक्षिरोगार्त्ताः कृमिक्षारानिलरान्विताः[४८] ।
शूलिनो मूत्रघातार्त्ता नाविरेच्या[४९] नरा मताः ॥४४॥

*Suitable Patients*

Patients suffering from chronic fever, excessive poisoning, diseases caused by *vāyu*, anal fistula, piles, anemia, *udara* (obstinate abdominal diseases including ascites), lymphadenitis, heart disease, anorexia, diseases of genital tract (females), *prameha* (obstinate urinary disorders including diabetes), *gulma* (phantom tumour), ulcers, abscess, vomiting, pustular eruptions, cholera, *kuṣṭha* (obstinate skin diseases including leprosy), diseases of ears, nose, head, mouth, anus and male genital organ, splenic disorders, oedema, eye diseases, parasitic infestation, affliction by alkalies and wind, colic-pain and urinary obstruction are not prohibited from taking purgation therapy.

(कोष्ठभेदः)

बहुपित्तो मृदुः प्रोक्तो[५०] बहुश्लेष्मा च मध्यमः ।
बहुवातः क्रूरकोष्ठो दुर्विरेच्यः स कथ्यते ॥४५॥

*Nature of Koṣṭha (Colon)*

If the *koṣṭha* (colon) is dominated by excess of *pitta*, then it is called *mṛdu koṣṭha* (tender colon). If it is dominated by aggravated *kapha*, then it is called *madhyama koṣṭha* (moderate bowel). If it is dominated by aggravated *vāyu*, then it is called *krūra koṣṭha* (costive bowel). In this third category, purgation takes place with difficulty.

तीक्ष्णा[५१] क्रूरे मता द्रव्यैर्मृदुमध्यमतीक्ष्णकैः ॥४६॥
मृदुर्द्राक्षापयश्चाम्बुतैलैरपि विरिच्यते ।
मध्यमस्त्रिवृतातिक्ताराजवृक्षैर्विरिच्यते ।
क्रूरः स्नुक्पयसा हेमक्षीरीदन्तीफलादिभिः[५२] ॥४७॥

***Dose and Drugs for Different Koṣṭhas***

In *mṛdu koṣṭha* (soft or tender bowel), the purgation therapy should be administered only in small dose. In the *madhyama koṣṭha* (moderate bowel), the purgation therapy should be administered only in moderate dose. For the patients having *krūra koṣṭha* (costive bowel), sharp acting (strong) recipes should be used for purgation therapy.

The patient belonging to the first category gets purgation even by the intake of *drākṣā*, milk, water or oil. In the patient of the second category, recipes containing *trivṛt, tiktā* and *rājavṛkṣa* should be administered for purgation. For the patient of third category, milky-latex of *snuhī, hemakṣīrī* and fruits of *dantī* should be used in purgation therapy.

(विरेचनवेगः)

मात्रोत्तमा विरेकस्य त्रिंशद्वेगैः कफान्तिका ।
वेगैर्विंशतिभिर्मध्या हीनोक्ता दशवेगकैः[५३] ॥४८॥

### *Bouts of Purgation*

If the patient purges for 30 times and *kapha* comes out at the end, then the dose of purgative recipe is to be considered as excellent. If he purges for 20 times, then the dose is medium; and if he purges for 10 times then the dose is inferior.

(विरेचनमात्रा)

द्विपलं श्रेष्ठमाख्यातं मध्यमं च पलं भवेत् ।
पलार्धं तु कषायाणां कनीयस्तु विरेचनम् ॥४९॥

### *Dose of Decoction*

Decoction in the dose of two *palas* is excellent; in the dose of one *pala* is moderate; and in the dose of half *pala* is small for purgation therapy.

कल्कमोदकचूर्णानां कर्षमध्वाज्यलेहृतः ।
कर्षद्वयं पलं वापि वयोरोगाद्यपेक्षया ॥५०॥

### *Other Ingredients*

Depending upon the age of the patient and nature of the disease, pastes, *modakas* (large size pills) and powders, mixed with honey and ghee should be given in the dose of one or two *karṣas* or one *pala*.

(दोषभेदेन विरेचनद्रव्यम्)

पित्तोत्तरे त्रिवृच्चूर्णं द्राक्षाक्वाथादिभिः पिबेत् ।
त्रिफलाक्वाथगोमूत्रैः पिबेद् व्योषं कफार्दितः ॥५१॥
त्रिवृत्सैन्धवशुण्ठीनां चूर्णमम्लैः पिबेन्नरः ।
वातार्दितो विरेकाय जांगलानां रसेन च[14] ॥५२॥
एरण्डतैलं त्रिफलाक्वाथेन मधुनापि[15] वा ।
युक्तं पीतं पयोभिर्वा न चिरेण विरिच्यते ॥५३॥

***Recipes for Different Doṣas***

If there is aggravation of *pitta*, then the patient should be given the powder of *trivṛt* along with the decoction of *drākṣā*. If there is aggravation of *kapha*, then the patient should be given the powder of *trikaṭu* (*śuṇṭhī, pippalī* and *marica*) along with the decoction of *triphalā* (*harītakī, bibhītaka* and *āmalakī*) and cow's urine. If there is aggravation of *vāyu*, then the patient should be given the powders of *trivṛt, saindhava* and *śuṇṭhī* along with sour drinks and soup of meat of animals inhabiting arid zone. Such a patient may be given castor oil along with the decoction of *triphalā* or honey or milk for quick purgation.

(ऋतुभेदेन विरेचनद्रव्यम्)

त्रिवृता कौटजं बीजं पिप्पली विश्वभेषजम् ।
समृद्वीकं[16] रसं क्षौद्रं वर्षाकाले विरेचनम् ॥५४॥
त्रिवृद्दुरालभामुस्ताशर्करोदीच्यचन्दनम् ।
द्राक्षाम्बुना सयष्ट्याह्वं शीतलं च घनात्यये ॥५५॥
पिप्पलीं नागरं सिन्धुं श्यामात्रिवृतया सह ।
लिह्यात् क्षौद्रेण शिशिरे वसन्ते च विरेचनम्" ॥५६॥

(शार्ङ्गधर : उत्तरखण्ड : ४ : १-२५)

***Recipes for Different Seasons***

In [beginning of] rainy season, the recipe containing *trivṛt*, seeds of *kuṭaja, pippalī, śuṇṭhī*, grape-juice and honey should be administered for purgation. In the autumn season, the rcipe containing *trivṛt, durālabhā, mustā*, sugar, *udīcya, candana*, grape-juice and *yaṣṭi madhu* should be administered for purgation. This recipe should be cooled and then given to the patient. In both the winter and spring seasons, the recipe containing *pippalī, nāgara, saindhava* and *śyāmā trivṛt* should be made to a paste by adding honey and given as a linctus for purgation.

(अभयामोदकः)

“अभया मरिचं शुण्ठी विडङ्गामलकानि च ।
पिप्पली पिप्पलीमूलं त्वक्पत्रं मुस्तमेव च ॥५७॥
एतानि समभागानि दन्ती च द्विगुणा[५७] भवेत् ।
त्रिवृदष्टगुणा ज्ञेया[५८] षड्गुणा चात्र शर्करा ॥५८॥
मधुना मोदकं कृत्वा कर्षमात्रं[५९] प्रमाणवत् ।
एकैकं भक्षयेत्प्रातः शीतं चानु पिबेज्जलम् ॥५९॥
तावद्विरिच्यते जन्तुर्यावदुष्णं न सेवते ।
पानाहारविहारेषु भवेन्निर्यन्त्रणः पुमान् ॥६०॥
विषमज्वरमन्दाग्निपाण्डुकासभगन्दरान् ।
दुर्नामकुष्ठगुल्मार्शोगलगण्डभ्रमोदरान्[६०] ॥६१॥
विदाहप्लीहमेहांश्च यक्ष्माणं नयनामयान् ।
वातरोगांस्तथाध्मान[६१] मूत्रकृच्छ्राणि[६२] चाश्मरी[६३] ॥६२॥
पृष्ठपार्श्वोरुजघनजङ्घोदररुजां जयेत् ।
सततं शीलनादेव पलितानि प्रणाशयेत् ।
अभया मोदका ह्येते रसायनवराः स्मृताः” ॥६३॥

॥ अभयामोदकः[६४] ॥

(भावप्रकाश : पञ्चकर्मविधिप्रकरणम् : ५ : ३४-६६)

(शार्ङ्गधर : उत्तरखण्ड : ४ : २७-३४)

*Abhayā Modaka*

One part of each of *abhayā, marica, śuṇṭhī, viḍaṅga, āmalaka, pippalī,*

*pippalī mūla, tvak, patra* and *mustā*, two parts of *dantī*, eight parts of *trivṛt* and six parts of sugar should be added with honey. From out of this, *modakas* of one *karṣa* each should be prepared. One such *modaka* should be taken every day in the morning and cold water should be taken thereafter. By the intake of this recipe, a person starts purging till he takes hot water (when the purging stops). While taking this recipe, the patient is free to take any drink, diet or regimen. It cures *viṣama jvara* (irregular fever), suppressed power of digestion, anemia, cough, anal fistula, anal piles, *kuṣṭha* (obstinate skin diseases including leprosy), *gulma* (phantom tumour), *arśas* (polyps), enlarged thyroid gland, giddiness, *udara* (obstinate abdominal diseases including ascites), burning sensation, splenic disorder, *meha* (obstinate urinary disorders including diabetes), tuberculosis, eye diseases, diseases caused by *vāyu*, flatulence, dysuria, stone in urinary tract and pain in the back, sides of the chest, chest, thighs, calf region and abdomen. Regular use of this recipe cures graying of hair. It is called *Abhayā modaka* and it is an excellent rejuvenating recipe.

नीलिनी-शंखिनी-दन्ती-त्रिवृदारग्वधं गवाम् ।
मूत्रेण भाव्यं सप्ताहं स्नुहीक्षीरे ततः परम् ॥६४॥
कीर्णं तेनैव चूर्णेन माल्यं वसनमेव वा ।
आघ्रायावृत्य वा सम्यक् मृदुकोष्ठो विरिच्यते ॥६५॥

*Recipe*

*Nīlinī, śaṅkhinī, dantī, trivṛt* and *āragvadha* should be impregnated with cow's urine for one week. Thereafter, it should be impregnated with the milky-latex of *snuhī* and made to a powder. Smelling of the garland and wearing of cloth sprinkled with this powder causes purgation in a person having *mṛdu koṣṭha* (soft bowel).

"पीत्वा विरेचनं शीतजलैः संसिक्तचक्षुषी[६५] ।
सुगन्धं[६६] किञ्चिदाघ्राय ताम्बूलं शीलयेद्वरम्[६७]" ॥६६॥

(भावप्रकाश : पञ्चकर्मविधिप्रकरणम् ५ : ६७)

(शार्ङ्गधर : उत्तरखण्ड : ४ : ३४-३५)

कुङ्कुमं चन्दनं चोचं कस्तूरी मृगसंमदा ।
कर्पूरं सर्वगात्रेषु लेपयेदगरादिकम् ॥६७॥

After taking purgation therapy, the patient should wash his eyes with cold water, inhale aromatics and thereafter, take betel-leaf. His entire body should be smeared with the paste of *kuṅkuma, candana, coca,* musk, camphor, *agaru,* etc.

“निवातस्थो[६८] न वेगांश्च धारयेन्न स्वपेत्तथा[६९] ।
शीताम्बुं न स्पृशेत् क्वापि कोष्णनीरं पिबेन्मुहः ॥६८॥

*Precautions*

While taking the purgation therapy, the patient should observe the following precautionary measures :

(1) He should reside in a room free from wind;
(2) he should not suppress the manifested natural urges;
(3) he should not sleep [during the day time];
(4) he should not touch cold water; and
(5) he should drink luke warm water frequently.

बलासौषधपित्तानि[७०] वायुर्वान्ते तथा व्रजेत् ।
रेकात्तथा मलं पित्तं भेषजं च कफो व्रजेत् ॥६९॥

*Emetic and Purgation Therapies*

In emetic therapy, the patient vomits out *kapha* (phlegm), medicines, *pitta* (bile) and *vāyu* (flatus) seriatum. Similarly, by the administration of purgation therapy, the patient voids stool, *pitta* (bile), medicines and *kapha* (phlegm) one after the other.

(दुर्विरिक्तलक्षणम्)
दुर्विरिक्तस्य नाभेस्तु स्तब्धत्वं[७१] कुक्षिशूलता ।
पुरीषवातसङ्गश्च कण्डूमण्डलगौरवम् ॥७०॥

*Improper (Less of) Purgation Therapy*

Improper purgation therapy will give rise to the following signs and symptoms :

(1) Stiffness in the umbilical region;
(2) pain in the pelvic region;

(3) arrest of the stool and flatus; and
(4) appearance of itches, urticaria and heaviness.

(दुर्विरिक्तचिकित्सा)

तं पुनः पाचनैः स्नेहैः पक्त्वा[७२] संस्नेह्य रेचयेत् ।
तेनास्योपद्रवा यान्ति दीप्तोऽग्निर्लघुता भवेत् ॥७१॥

### Management

If the purgation therapy is not properly administered, then the patient should be administered *pācana* (therapy for the metabolic transformation of uncooked material) and oleation therapy. Then he should be given oily purgation therapy. This subsides the likely complications, in proves the digestive power of the patient and brings about lightness of the body.

(अतियोगलक्षणम्)

विरेकस्यातियोगेन मूर्च्छा भ्रंशो गुदस्य च ।
शूलं कफातियोगः स्यान्मांसधावनसन्निभम् ।
मेदोनिभं जलाभासं रक्तं चापि विरिच्यते ॥७२॥

### Excessive Purgation

Excessive purgation gives rise to the following signs and symptoms :
(1) Fainting and prolapse of rectum;
(2) colic pain, excess voiding of *kapha* (phlegm);
(3) the stool looks like water washed with flesh, fat or water; and
(4) the patient may also void blood.

(चिकित्सा)

तस्य शीताम्बुभिः सिक्त्वा शरीरं तण्डुलाम्बुभिः ।
मधुमिश्रैस्तथा शीतैः कारयेद् वमनं मृदुः ॥७३॥
सहकारत्वचः कल्को दध्ना सौवीरकेण वा ।
पिष्ट्वा नाभिप्रलेपेन हन्त्यतीसारमुल्वणम् ॥७४॥

*Management*

The patient having excess of purgation should be treated as follows :

(1) His body should be smeared with cold water;

(2) he should be given rice-wash mixed with honey and cooled for light emesis; and

(3) the paste of the bark of *āmra* prepared by triturating with curd or *sauvīraka* (vinegar) should be applied over the umbilical region.

These recipes cure excessive loose motions.

(संसर्जनक्रम)

आजं क्षीरं रसं वापि[७३] वैष्किरं हारिणं तथा ।
शालिभिः षष्टिकैः[७४] स्वल्पं मसूरैश्चापि भोजयेत्' ॥७५॥

(भावप्रकाश : पञ्चकर्मविधिप्रकरणम् ५ : ६८-७६)

"शीतैः संग्राहिभिर्द्रव्यैः कुर्यात्संग्रहणं भिषक् ।
लाघवे[७५] मनसस्तुष्टिरनुलोमं गतेऽनिले ।
सुविरिक्तं नरं ज्ञात्वा पाचनं पाययेन्निशि ॥७६॥

*Post-Therapeutic Regimens*

After purgation therapy, the patient should take the following food and drinks :

(1) Goat's milk or the soup of the meat of goat, *viṣkira* (gallinacious birds) and deer; and

(2) *śāli* and *ṣaṣṭika* types of rice added with *masūra* in small quantity;

(3) loose motions of the patient should be corrected by the administration of cooling and constipative drugs; and

(4) after the patient is appropriately purged, his body has become light, he feels satisfied and there is downward movement of flatus, the patient should be given *pācana* (drugs for the metabolic transformation of uncooked product of digestion) at night.

(रेचनगुणाः)

इन्द्रियाणां बलं बुद्धिप्रसादो[७६] वह्निदीपनम्[७७] ।
धातुस्थैर्यं बलस्थैर्यं[७८] भवेद्रेचनसेवनात् ॥७७॥

### *Effects of Purgation Therapy*

Purgation therapy makes a person endowed with the following benefits :

(1) Strength of sense organs;
(2) clarity of wisdom;
(3) promotion of digestive power; and
(4) stability of tissue elements and physical strength.

(अपथ्य:)

प्रवातसेवां शीताम्बु स्नेहाभ्यङ्गमजीर्णताम् ।
व्यायामं मैथुनं चैव न सेवेत विरेचितः ॥७८॥

### *Prohibitions*

The patient taking purgation therapy should avoid the following :

(1) Exposure to excessive wind;
(2) cold water;
(3) massage with ghee, oil, etc.;
(4) indigestion;
(5) physical exercise; and
(6) sexual intercourse.

(पथ्य:)

शालिषष्टिकमुद्गाद्यैर्यवागूं भोजयेत्कृताम् ।
जाङ्गलविष्किराणां वा रसैः शाल्योदनं हितम् ॥७९॥

(भावप्रकाश : पञ्चकर्मविधिप्रकरणम् ५ : ७७-८१)

(शार्ङ्गधर : उत्तरखण्ड : ४ : ३५-४८)

॥ इति विरेचनविधिः ॥

### *Wholesome Food*

For a patient who has taken purgation therapy, following types of food are wholesome :

(1) Sizzled gruel prepared of *śāli* and *ṣaṣṭika* types of rice, *mudga* etc.; and
(2) *śāli* rice with the soup of the meat of *jāṅgala* (animals inhabiting arid land) and *viṣkira* (gallinacious birds).

Thus, ends the description of purgation therapy.

## इति श्रीमहाराजाधिराजटोडरमल्लविरचिते[१] टोडरानन्दे आयुर्वेदसौख्ये द्रव्यगुणवमनविरेचनकथनं नामाष्टमो हर्षः ॥

Thus, ends the 8th chapter dealing with materia medica (see Foot Note) and emetic as well as purgation therapies in *Āyurveda saukhya* in *Ṭoḍarānanda* composed by the great King Ṭoḍaramalla.

### NOTES AND REFERENCES

१. (क) In the mss., this forms a part of the eighth chapter which deals with materia medica (a portion of it) and includes emetic as well as purgation therapies. Materia medica portion is already included in Volume I of this series; and for convenience, the remaining part is taken separately here; hence there is no invocation.

(ख) 'दोषा ...... पुनरुद्भवः' पाठोऽयं प्रथमपंचमपुस्तकयोः नोपलभ्यते ।

२. हृल्लासार्ति. इति आकरे पाठः ।

३. द्विजिह्वके इति आकरे पाठः ।

४. गलगण्ड. इति द्वितीयपुस्तके पाठः ।

५. पवनात्स्वरघातवान् इति आकरे पाठः ।

६. वाम्या इति आकरे पाठः ।

७. 'पाययित्वा यवागूं वा क्षीरतक्रदधीनि च' इति आकरे पाठः ।

८. देहिनः इति प्रथमद्वितीयपंचमपुस्तकेषु पाठः ।

९. वमनेष्ववतारयेत् इति प्रथमद्वितीयपंचमपुस्तकेषु पाठः ।

१०. नवप्रस्था इति आकरे पाठः ।

११. त्रिप्रस्था इति आकरे पाठः ।

१२. (क) मात्रयोत्तमम् इति आकरे पाठः ।

(ख) श्रेष्ठमात्रया इति शार्ङ्गधरे पाठः ।

१३. वमने चाष्टवेगाः स्युः पित्तान्ता उत्तमास्तु ते । षड्वेगा मध्यमा वेगाश्चत्वारस्त्वपरे मताः । इति आकरे पाठः ।

१४. सुस्वादुलवणाम्लोष्णैः इति आकरे पाठः ।

१५. संसृष्टं इति आकरे पाठः ।

१६. कृष्णा राट्फलं इति आकरे पाठः ।
१७. पटोलवासानिम्बांश्च इति आकरे पाठः ।
१८. शीतजलैः इति आकरे पाठः ।
१९. विसंज्ञिता इति आकरे पाठः ।
२०. जिह्वानिः सरागं इति आकरे पाठः ।
२१. चाक्ष्योः इति आकरे पाठः ।
२२. तु इति आकरे पाठः ।
२३. वमनेन इति आकरे पाठः ।
२४. कवलग्रहाः इति आकरे पाठः ।
२५. र्हिताः इति आकरे पाठः ।
२६. कल्कं लिप्त्वा इति आकरे पाठः ।
२७. पीडनञ्च इति आकरे पाठः ।
२८. रक्तष्ठीवमुपाचरेत् इति आकरे पाठः ।
२९. सघृतं इति आकरे पाठः ।
३०. रोगाश्छर्दिसमुद्भवा इति आकरे पाठः ।
३१. एतदनन्तरं चतुर्थपुस्तके बहवो वामकयोगाः वर्णिताः सन्ति; प्रमादबहुलात् नोद्धृताः ।
३२. दीप्ताग्निं इति आकरे पाठः ।
३३. भोजयेत् इति आकरे पाठः ।
३४. तन्द्रानिद्रास्यदौर्गन्ध्यं कण्डूश्च ग्रहणी इति आकरे पाठः ।
३५. रोषञ्च इति आकरे पाठः ।
३६. दिनमेकं इति आकरे पाठः ।
३७. सुधीरत्यजेत् इति आकरे पाठः ।
३८. विरेचनविधिः इति द्वितीयपुस्तके पाठः ।
३९. छादयेत्कफः इति आकरे पाठः ।
४०. परिपाचयेत् इति आकरे पाठः ।
४१. देहशुद्धौ इति प्रथमपुस्तके आकरे च पाठः ।
४२. अन्यदाऽऽत्ययिके इति आकरे पाठः ।
४३. युञ्ज्यादामोद्भूते गदे इति आकरे पाठः ।
४४. उदरे च तथाऽऽध्माने कोष्ठशुद्धौ विशेषतः इति आकरे पाठः ।
४५. बालो वृद्धो भृशं स्निग्धः इति आकरे पाठः ।
४६. श्रान्तस्तृषाऽऽर्त्तः इति आकरे पाठः ।

४७. गुल्मप्लीहव्रणार्दिताः इति पंचमपुस्तके आकरे च पाठः ।

४८. कृमिक्षारानिलार्दिताः इति आकरे पाठः ।

४९. विरेकार्हा इति आकरे पाठः ।

५०. कोष्ठो इति आकरे पाठः ।

५१. क्रूरे तीक्ष्णा इति आकरे पाठः ।

५२. हेमक्षीरीदन्ती इति आकरे पाठः ।

५३. दशवेगिका इति आकरे पाठः ।

५४. वा इति आकरे पाठः ।

५५. द्विगुणेन इति आकरे पाठः ।

५६. समृद्वीकारसं इति आकरे पाठः ।

५७. त्रिगुणा इति आकरे पाठः ।

५८. त्रिवृताऽष्टगुणा इति आकरे पाठः ।

५९. कर्षमात्रान्प्रमाणवत् इति आकरे पाठः ।

६०. दुर्नामिकुष्ठगुल्मार्शोगलगण्डोदरभ्रमान् इति आकरे पाठः ।

६१. वातरोगांस्तथाऽऽध्मानं इति आकरे पाठः ।

६२. मूत्रकृच्छ्रादि इति आकरे पाठः ।

६३. चाश्मरीम् इति आकरे पाठः ।

६४. एतदनन्तरं चतुर्थपुस्तके बहवो विरेचनयोगाः लिखिताः सन्ति । प्रमादबाहुल्यान्नात्रोद्धृतम् ।

६५. संसिच्य इति आकरे पाठः ।

६६. सुगन्धि इति आकरे पाठः ।

६७. शीलयेद् बुधः इति आकरे पाठः ।

६८. निर्वातस्थो इति आकरे पाठः ।

६९. शयीत च इति आकरे पाठः ।

७०. बलासोषधपित्तानि इति आकरे पाठः ।

७१. स्तब्धता कुक्षिशूलरुक् इति आकरे पाठः ।

७२. पक्त्वा स्निग्धं तु रेचयेत् इति आकरे पाठः ।

७३. चापि इति आकरे पाठः ।

७४. षष्टिकैस्तुल्यैर्मसूरैर्वाऽपि भोजयेत् इति आकरे पाठः ।

७५. लाघवे मनसस्तुष्टावनुलोमं इति आकरे पाठः ।

७६. बुद्धे इति आकरे पाठः ।

७७. वह्निदीप्तता इति आकरे पाठः ।

७८. वयः स्थैर्यं इति आकरे पाठः ।

७९. In the first and fifth mss., description of materia medica (only a portion), emetic therapy and purgation therapy are all included in the eighth chapter. The materia medica portion is already included in Volume I of this series. Because of their relevance, portion dealing with emetic and purgation therapies is described here separately.

# CHAPTER XIV

## ।। अथ बस्तिविधिः ।।

*(Medicated Enema)*

अथ[1] बस्तिविधिरुच्यते

"बस्तिर्द्विधानुवासानाख्यो निरूहश्च ततः परम् ।
यः स्नेहैर्दीयते स स्यादनुवासनसंज्ञकः[2] ।
कषायक्षीरतैलैर्यो निरूह स निगद्यते ॥१॥

***Varieties***

*Basti* (medicated enema) is of two types, viz., *anuvāsana* and *nirūha*. The medicated enema in which recipes containing only fat (oil, ghee, etc.) is used is called *anuvāsana basti*. If decoction, milk and oil are used in the recipe, then it is called *nirūha basti*.

तत्रानुवासनाख्यो हि बस्तिर्यः सोऽत्र कथ्यते ।
पूर्वमेव, ततो बस्ति निरूहाख्यो भविष्यति ।
निरूहादुत्तरश्चैव बस्ति स्यादुत्तराभिधः ॥२॥

### *Order of Description*

In the beginning, *anuvāsana* type of *basti* will be described. Thereafter will be the description of *nirūha* type of *basti*. This will be followed by the description of *uttara basti* (urethral and vaginal douche).

अनुवासनभेदश्च मात्राबस्तिरुदाहृता ।
पलद्वयं तस्य मात्रा तस्मादर्द्धापि भावयेत् ॥३॥

### *Mātrā Basti*

A variety of *anuvāsana* is called *mātrā basti*. It is administered in the dose of two *palas* or half of it, i.e. one *pala*.

अनुवास्यस्तु रूक्षः स्यात्तीक्ष्णाग्निः केवलानिली ।
नानुवास्यस्तु कुष्ठीस्यान्मेही स्थूलस्तथोदरी ॥४॥
नास्थाप्याः नानुवास्याः स्युरजीर्णोन्मादतृड्युताः ।
शोषमूर्च्छारुचिभयश्वासकासक्षयातुराः[३] ॥५॥

### *Suitable and Unsuitable Patients*

Persons who are ununctuous, who have sharp power of digestion and who suffer from diseases caused by the aggravated *vāyu* alone, are suitable for the administration of *anuvāsana* type of medicated enema. Patients suffering from *kuṣṭha* (obstinate skin diseases including leprosy), *meha* (obstinate urinary disorders including diabetes), obesity and *udara* (obstinate abdominal diseases including ascites) should not be given *anuvāsana* type of medicated enema.

Both *nirūha* and *anuvāsana* types of enema are contra-indicated in indigestion, insanity, morbid thirst, consumption, fainting, anorexia, fear complex, asthma, cough and tuberculosis.

नेत्रकार्यं सुवर्णादिधातुभिर्वृक्षवेणुभिः ।
नलैर्दन्तैर्विषाणाग्रैर्मणिभिर्वा विधीयते ॥६॥

### *Nozzle for Enema*

The nozzle for enema should be prepared of metals like gold, wood, bamboo, *nala*, tooth tip of horn or gems.

एकवर्षानु षट्वर्षं यावन्मानं षडंगुलम् ।
ततो द्वादशकं यावन्मानं स्यादष्टसंज्ञितम् ॥७॥
ततः परं द्वादशभिरङ्गुलैर्नेत्रदीर्घता ।
मुद्गछिद्रं कलायाभं छिद्रं कोलास्थिसन्निभम् ॥८॥
यथासंख्यं भवेन्नेत्रं श्लक्ष्णं गोपुच्छसन्निभम् ।
आतुरांगुष्ठमानं[४] तु मूलं स्थूलं विधीयते ॥९॥
कनिष्ठिकापरीनाहमग्रे च गुटिकामुखम् ।
तन्मूले कर्णिकि द्वे च कार्यं भागचतुर्थकात् ।
योजयेत्तत्र[५] बस्तिं च बंधद्वयविधानतः ॥१०॥

### *Size and Shape of Nozzle*

For a patient of one to six years of age, the length of the nozzle should be six *angulas*; for a patient of six to twelve years of age, the length should be eight *angulas*; and for a patient above twelve years of age, the length of the nozzle should be twelve *angulas*. The hole inside the first type of nozzle should be of the size of *mudga*, the hole inside the second type should be of the size of a pea and the hole inside the third type of nozzle should be of the size of the *kola* seed.

The nozzle should be smooth and of the shape of a cow's tail. The thickness at the root of the nozzle should be like that of the thumb of the patient and at the top, the thickness should be like that of the little finger of the patient. There should be round bud at the top of the nozzle. In the last one fourth part of the nozzle, there should be two rings between which the *basti* (urinary bladder of animals) should be tied with two knots.

मृगाजशूकरगवां महिषस्यापि वा भवेत् ।
मूत्रकोशस्य बस्तिस्तु तदलाभेन चर्मजः ।
कषायरक्तः समृदुः बस्तिस्निग्धो दृढो हितः[६] ॥११॥

### *Selection of Urinary Bladder for Basti*

For preparing *basti* (enema can), the urinary bladder of deer, goat, pig, cattle or buffalo should be selected. If such a bladder is not available, then a sac should be prepared of leather and used as enema can. this sac should be *kaṣāya* (reddish brown) or red, soft, unctuous and strong.

व्रणबस्तेस्तु नेत्रं स्यात् श्लक्ष्णमष्टाङ्गुलोन्मितम् ।
मुद्गच्छिद्रं गृध्रपक्षनलिकापरिणाहि च ॥१२॥

*Vraṇa Basti*

The nozzle of *vraṇa basti* (douche for cleansing ulcers) should be smooth and eight *aṅgulas* in length. It should have a hole in the centre which should allow a seed of *mudga* to pass through. In diameter, it should be like the tube (stalk) of a vulture's feather.

शरीरोपचयं वर्णं बलमारोग्यमायुषः ।
कुरुते परिवृद्धिं च बस्तिः सम्यगुपासितः ॥१३॥

*Effects of Basti*

*Basti* (medicated enema), when appropriately taken, causes plumpness of the body, refreshes complexion and promotes strength, health and longevity.

'दिवा' शीते वसन्ते च स्नेहबस्तिः प्रदीयते ।
ग्रीष्मे वर्षाशरत्काले रात्रौ स्यादनुवासनम् ॥१४॥

*When to Administer Anuvāsana Basti*

*Anuvāsana* type of enema should be administered during the day time in winter and spring seasons. In summer, rainy and autumn seasons, it should be given at night.

न चातिस्निग्धमशनं भोजयित्वानुवासयेत् ।
मदमूर्च्छां च जनयेत् द्विधा स्नेहप्रयोजितः ॥१५॥
'रूक्षं' भुक्तवतोत्यन्तं बलं वर्णं च हीयते ।
युक्तस्नेहमतो जन्तुं भोजयित्वानुवासयेत् ॥१६॥

*Food Before Basti*

*Anuvāsana basti* should not be administered after the patient has consumed excessively fatty food because the fat taken in double quantity (once with food and second time with enema) gives rise to *mada* (intoxicating effect) and fainting. Before *anuvāsana basti*, the patient should also avoid the intake of excessively ununctuous food because it causes depletion of strength and complexion. Therefore, the patient should be given appropriate (neither too fatty nor too ununctuous) food before *anuvāsana* type of enema.

हीनमात्रादुभौ बस्तिर्नातिकार्यकरौ स्मृतौ ।
अतिमात्रं तथानाहक्लमातीसारकारकौ[9] ॥१७॥
उत्तमस्य पलैः षड्भिर्मध्यमस्य पलैस्त्रिभिः ।
पलैकार्द्धेन[10] हीनस्य युक्ता मात्रानुवासने ॥१८॥

*Dose*

Both *anuvāsana* and *nirūha* types of *basti*, if taken in small dose do not produce the desired effect. If administered in a large dose, they cause flatulence, mental fatigue and diarrhoea. *Anuvāsana basti* should be administered in a dose of six *palas* to a person having excellent power of digestion and strength; in a dose of three *palas* to the person having moderate power of digestion and strength and in a dose of one and half *pala* to the person having less power of digestion and strength.

'शताह्वा'[11]सैन्धवाभ्यां च देयं स्नेहे च चूर्णकम् ।
तन्मात्रोत्तममध्यान्तः षट्चतुर्द्वयमाषकैः ॥१९॥

Along with *sneha* (oil, etc.), the powder of *śatāhvā* and *saindhava* should be given in the dose of six, four or two *māṣas* to a patient having excellent, moderate or inferior strength respectively.

विरेचनात्सप्तरात्रे गते जाते च[12] लाघवे ।
भुक्तान्नायानुवास्याय बस्तिर्देयोनुवासनः ॥२०॥

Seven days after the purgation therapy, when the body has become light, the patient should be given food, and thereafter, he should be administered *anuvāsana* type of enema.

अथानुवास्यं स्वभ्यक्तमुष्णांबुस्वेदितं शनैः ।
भोजयित्वा यथाशास्त्रं कृतं चंक्रमणं ततः ॥२१॥
उत्सृष्टानिलविण्मूत्रं योजयेत्स्नेहबस्तिना ।
सुप्तस्य वामपार्श्वेन[१३] वामजङ्घाप्रसारिणः ॥२२॥
कुंचितापरजंघस्य नेत्रं स्निग्धे गुदे न्यसेत् ।
बध्वा बस्तिमुखं तत्र वामहस्तेन धारयेत् ॥२३॥
'पीडयेद्दक्षिणेनैव मध्यवेगेन धीरधीः ।
जृम्भाकासक्षवादींश्च बस्तिकाले न कारयेत्'[१४] ॥२४॥

*Method of Administration*

The patient, selected for *anuvāsana basti*, should first of all be given massage and fomentation therapy gradually with warm water. Then he should be given prescribed food and made to walk. After he has voided flatus, stool and urine, he should be given *anuvāsana* type of enema.

The patient should be made to lie in the left side, his left thigh should be streched, the calf region of the right leg should be flexed and then the nozzle should be administered into the anus. The mouth (opening) of the sac (bladder containing drugs) should be tied to the nozzle and supported by left hand. With moderate pressure, the sac should then be pressed with the help of the right hand. While taking medicated enema, the patient should not yawn, cough or sneeze.

त्रिंशन्मात्रामितं कालः प्रोक्तो बस्तेस्तु[१५] पीडने ।
ततः प्रणिहितस्नेह[१६] उत्तानो वाक्शतं भवेत् ॥२५॥

***Duration***

Pressure should be applied over the sac for a duration of 30 *mātrās* (length of time required to pronounce one short vowel—also see explanation below). Thereafter, the patient should be made to lie on his back till the count of one hundred numbers.

जानुमण्डलमावेष्ट्य कुर्यात्छोटिकया युतं ।
एकमात्रा भवेदेषा सर्वत्रैष विनिश्चयः ॥२६॥

*Mātrā*

A person should squat with folded knee and surround his knees with the hand. Then he should produce sound with the help of thumb and middle finger by strongly pressing and then immediately releasing. This process is called *śoṭikā*. One such sound constitute one *mātrā* and this general rule should be followed in accounting for the duration of time.

प्रसारितैः सर्वगात्रैर्यथा वीर्यं विसर्पति ।
ताडयेत्तलयोरेनं त्रिंस्त्रीन्वारान् शनैः शनैः ॥२७॥
स्फिजश्चैव ततः श्रोणीं शय्यां चैव क्षिपेत्ततः[१७] ।
जाते[१८] विधाने तु ततः कुर्या निद्रां यथासुखम् ॥२८॥

After the *anuvāsana* type of enema is thus administered, the patient should be made to strech all his limbs so that the effect of the *basti* spreads to all the parts of the body. The palms and soles of the patient should be slowly knocked for three times in each. Then his hips, lumber region and the bed should be raised. Thereafter, the patient should made to sleep comfortably.

सानिलः सपुरीषश्च स्नेहः प्रत्येति यस्य तु ।
उपद्रवं विना चैव[१९] स सम्यगनुवासितः ॥२९॥

*Signs of Appropriately Administered Anuvāsana*

If *anuvāsana* type of enema is properly administered, then patient voids flatus along with stool and fat (administered as enema) without any complication.

जीर्णान्नमथ सायाह्ने स्नेहे प्रत्यागते पुनः ।
लघ्वन्नं भोजयेत्कामं दीप्ताग्निस्तु नरो यदि ॥३०॥

### After Care

In the evening, after the food is digested and after the complete elimination of the administered oil, the patient should be given light diet in sufficient quantity to eat if he has a strong power of digestion.

अनुवासिताय दातव्यमितरोह्नि सुखोदकम् ।
धान्यशुण्ठीकषायं वा स्नेहव्यापत्तिनाशनम् ॥३१॥

On the next day, after *anuvāsana basti*, the patient should be given either luke warm water or the decoction of *dhānyaka* and *śuṇṭhī* to drink. This will prevent future complications.

अनेन विधिना षट् च सप्त चाष्टौ नवापि वा ।
विधेया बस्तयस्तेषां मन्ते चैव निरूहणम्" ॥३२॥
(शार्ङ्गधर : उत्तरखण्ड : ५ : १-३४)

### Course of Anuvāsana Basti

Following the above mentioned procedure, the patient should be given six, seven, eight or nine such enemata. After that, *nirūha* type of enema should be administered.

"अथवा यस्य तत्कालं स्नेहो निर्याति केवलः ।
तस्यान्योल्पतरो देयो न हि स्निह्यत्यतिष्ठति ॥३३॥

If the oil comes out through the anus immediately after the administration of *anuvāsana basti*, then another enema containing less of oil should be administered, because the patient does not get oleated without the retention of oil in the rectum during the therapy.

अशुद्धस्य मलोन्मिश्रः स्नेहो नैति यदा पुनः ।
तदाङ्गशैथिल्याध्मान[२०] शूलं श्वासश्च जायते ॥३४॥
'पक्वाशये[२१] गुरुत्वं च तत्र दद्यान्निरूहणम् ।
तीक्ष्णं, तीक्ष्णौषधैर्युक्ता फलवर्तिर्हिताथवा ॥३५॥

यथानुलोमनं वायुर्मलं स्नेहं च जायते ।
तथा विरेचनं दद्यात्तीक्ष्णं नस्यं च शस्यते ॥३६॥

If the patient is not cleansed [by the prior administration of purgation therapy], then the oil along with stool will not come out after the administration of the therapy and the patient will feel prostration in the limbs, flatulence, colic pain, dyspnoea and heaviness in the colon. To such a patient, strong type of *nirūḥa basti* should be administered. For such patients, *phalavarti* (suppository) prepared of *tīkṣṇa* (sharp) drugs is useful. This helps in the downward movement of flatus, stool and oil (given through the therapy earlier). Alternatively, purgative or inhalation therapy prepared of *tīkṣṇa* (sharp) drugs should be administered for the benefit of such patients.

यस्य नोपद्रवं कुर्यात्स्नेहबस्तिरनिसृतः ।
सर्वोऽल्पो वावृतो रौक्ष्यादुपेक्ष्यः स विजानता ॥३७॥

If, because of ununctuousness (*raukṣya*), the oil of enema gets covered and does not come out or comes out only in small quantity but does not cause any complication, then a wise physician should discard such a patient, i.e. he is incurable.

आनायात[22] त्वहोरात्रे स्नेहः संशोधनैर्हरेत् ।
'स्नेहबस्तावनायाते नान्यः[23] स्नेहो विधीयते' ॥३८॥

(सुश्रुत : चिकित्सा : ३७ : ९९)

If the oil administered through enema does not come out within twenty four hours, then the patient should be given a cleansing therapy (purgation or *nirūha basti*). If the oil of *anuvāsana basti* does not come out, then another *anuvāsana basti* should not be administered to such a patient.

गुडूच्यैरण्डपूतीकभार्गीवृषकरोहिषम् ।
शतावरीसहचरं काकनासा पलोन्मितम् ॥३९॥

यवमाषातसीकोलकुलत्थान्प्रसृतोन्मितान् ।
चतुर्द्रोणेंभसः पक्त्वा द्रोणशेषेन तेन च ॥४०॥
पचेत्तैलाढकं पेष्यैः जीवनीयैः पलोन्मितैः ।
अनुवासनमेतद्धि सर्ववातविकारनुत्" ॥४१॥
(शार्ङ्गधर : उत्तरखण्ड : ५ : ४१-५०)

*Guḍūcyādi Taiḷa*

One *pala* of each of *guḍūcī, eraṇḍa, pūtīka, bhārṅgī, vṛṣaka, rohiṣa, śatāvarī, sahacara* and *kākanāsā* and one *prasṛta* of each of *yava, māṣa, atasī, kola* and *kulattha* should be added with four *droṇas* of water and cooked till one fourth remains. Along with this decoction, one *āḍhaka* of oil should be cooked by adding one *pala* of the paste of drugs belonging to *Jīvanīya* group. Using this medicated oil for *anuvāsana* type of *basti* cures all types of *vātika* diseases.

"षट्सप्तति व्यापदस्तु जायन्ते बस्तिकर्मणः ।
दर्शिता समुदायेन ते चिकित्स्यास्तु सुश्रुतात् ॥४२॥

***Complications***

By the administration of *anuvāsana basti*, 76 types of complications are likely to occur. Details of these complications and their treatment are described in the *Suśruta saṃhitā* (*Suśruta : Cikitsā* 36: 3-50) which should be followed.

पानाहारविहाराश्च परिहार्याश्च[24] कृत्स्नशः ।
स्नेहपानसमा कार्या नात्र कार्या विचारणा" ॥४३॥
(शार्ङ्गधर : उत्तरखण्ड : ५ : ५७-५९)

***Regimens***

Diet, drinks and other regimens to be followed and to be avoided by the patient taking *anuvāsana basti* are the same as those prescribed and proscribed for oleation therapy.

अथ निरूहणबस्तिविधि

"निरूहबस्तिर्बहुधा भिद्यते कारणान्तरैः ।
तैरेव तस्य नामानि कृतानि मुनिपुंगवैः ॥४४॥

## *NIRŪHA BASTI*

### *Varieites*

*Nirūha basti* is of different types depending upon several factors. On the basis of these factors, different names are given to these varieties of *nirūha* by the expert sages.

निरूहस्यापरं नाम प्रोक्तमास्थापनं बुधैः।
स्वस्थानस्थापनाद्दोषधातूनां स्थापनं मतम् ॥४५॥

### *Synonym*

*Āsthāpana* is the synonym of *nirūha basti.* It is called *āsthāpana* because it helps in maintaining the homeostasis (*sthāpana*) of *doṣas* and *dhātus* (tissue elements).

निरूहस्य प्रमाणं च प्रस्थः पादोत्तरं परम्।
मध्यमं प्रस्थमुद्दिष्टं हीनं च कुडवस्त्रयः[२५] ॥४६॥

### *Dose*

For *nirūha* (enema), $1^1/_4$ *prastha* constitutes the excellent dose, one *prastha* the moderate dose, and three *kuḍavas* constitute the inferior dose.

अतिस्निग्धोत्क्लिष्टदोषक्षतोरस्कः कृशस्तथा ।
आध्मानच्छर्दिहिक्कार्शकासश्वासप्रपीडितः ॥४७॥
गुदशोथोतिसारार्त्तो विसूचीकुष्ठसंयुतः ।
गर्भिणी मधुमेही च नास्थाप्यश्च जलोदरी ॥४८॥

### *Unsuitable Persons*

The following types of patients are not suitable for the administration of *nirūha basti* :

(1) Those who are excessively oleated:
(2) whose *doṣas* are excited (*utkliṣṭa*);
(3) those suffering from phthisis, emaciation, flatulence, vomiting, hiccup, piles, cough, asthma, swelling in the anal region,

diarrhoea, cholera and *kuṣṭha* (obstinate skin diseases including leprosy);

(4) pregnant woman;

(5) those suffering from diabetes mellitus; and

(6) those suffering from ascites.

वातव्याधावुदावर्त्ते वातासृग्विषमज्वरे ।
मूर्च्छातृष्णोदरानाहमूत्रकृच्छ्राश्मरीषु[२६] च ॥४९॥
वृद्धचसृग्दरमन्दाग्निप्रमेहेषु[२७] निरूहणम् ।
शूलाम्लपित्तहृद्रोगे योजयेद्विधिवद्बुधः ॥५०॥

### *Suitable Persons for Nirūha*

*Nirūha* type of enema should be appropriately administered to those suffering from *vātika* diseases, *udāvarta* (upward movement of the flatus in the abdomen), *vāta raka* (gout), *viṣama jvara* (irregular fever), fainting, morbid thirst, *udara* (obstinate abdominal diseases), flatulence, dysuria, stone in the urinary tract, hydrocele, menorrhagia, suppressed power of digestion, *prameha* (obstinate urinary disorders), colic pain, hyper acidity and heart diseases.

उत्सृष्टानिलविण्मूत्रं स्निग्धं स्विन्नमभोजितम् ।
मध्याह्ने गृहमध्ये च यथायोग्यं निरूहयेत् ॥५१॥
स्नेहबस्तिविधानेन बुधः कुर्यान्निरूहणम् ।
जाते निरूहे च ततो भवेदुत्कटुकासनः ॥५२॥
तिष्ठेन्मुहूर्त्तमात्रं तु निरूहागमनेच्छया ।
अनायातं मुहूर्त्तात्तु निरूहं शोधनैर्हरेत् ।
निरूहैरेव मतिमान् क्षारमूत्राम्लसैंधवैः[२८] ॥५३॥

### *Method of Administration*

To the patient who has passed flatus, stool and urine, who is unctuous, who has taken fomentation therapy and who has not taken food, *nirūha* type of enema should be appropriately administered inside a house during the noon time. The procedure prescribed for *anuvāsana basti* should also be followed in the case of *nirūha basti.* After the administration of enema, the patient should be made to sit in a squatting posture and remain like that for one *muhūrtta* (48 minutes) with a view to facilitate the elimination of administered drugs. If this does not take place, then the cleansing type of *nirūha* containing alkalis, urine, vinegar and rock-salt should be given to the patient.

यस्य क्रमेण गच्छन्ति विट् पित्तकफवायवः ।
लाघवं चोपजायेत सुनिरूहं तमादिशेत् ॥५४॥

*Signs of Appropriately Administered Nirūha*

If by the *nirūha* therapy, stool, *pitta* (bile), *kapha* (phlegm or mucus) and flatus are voided one after the other and the patient feels lightness in his body, then it is to be considered as appropriately administered therapy.

'यस्य[२१] स्याद्बस्तिरल्पाल्पवेगो हीनमलानिलः ।
मूर्च्छार्त्तिजाड्यरुचिमान् दुर्निरूहं तमादिशेत्' ॥५५॥

*Signs of Improper Nirūha*

If by the administration of *nirūha basti*, the patient gets much less urge for voiding and he voids less of stool and flatus as a result of which he suffers from fainting, pain, stiffness and anorexia, then this is to be considered as a case of improper *nirūha*.

विविक्तता मनस्तुष्टि स्निग्धता व्याधिनिग्रहः ।
आस्थापनस्नेहबस्त्योः सम्यग्दाने तु लक्षणम् ॥५६॥

*Signs of Proper Nirūha and Anuvāsana*

Signs and symptoms of proper administration of *nirūha* and *anuvāsana* are as follows :

(1) The patient feels like remaining alone or he feels lightness in his body;
(2) he gets mental satisfaction;
(3) he gets oleated; and
(4) he gets cured of his disease.

अनेन विधिना[30] युंज्यान्निरूहं बस्तिदानवित् ।
द्वितीयं वा तृतीयं वा चतुर्थं वा यथोचितम् ॥५७॥

*Course of Nirūha*

Following the above mentioned procedure, an expert physician should administer *nirūha basti* for the second, third or fourth time as found appropriate for the patient.

सस्नेह[31] एकः पवने पित्ते द्वौ पयसा सह ।
कषायकटुमूत्राद्याः कफे चोष्णत्रयो हिताः ॥५८॥

*Nirūha for Different Doṣas*

If *vāyu* is aggravated in the patient, then only one *niruha basti* should be given and it should be mixed with *sncha* (fat or oil). In the case of aggravated *pitta*, the patient should be given *nirūha basti* mixed with milk for two times. If *kapha* is aggravated, then *nirūha basti* should be given for three times and the recipe should be prepared of astringent and pungent drugs, cow's urine, etc. which are hot in potency.

पित्तश्लेष्मानिलाविष्टं क्षीरयूषरसैः क्रमात् ।
निरूहं भोजयित्वा च ततस्तदनुवासयेत् ॥५९॥

*After Care*

Patient suffering from diseases caused by aggravated *pitta, kapha* and *vāyu* should be given milk, vegetable soup and meat soup respectively after the *nirūha basti*. Thereafter, *anuvāsana basti* should be administered.

सुकुमारस्य वृद्धस्य बालस्य च मृदुर्हितः ।
बस्तिस्तीक्ष्णः प्रयुक्तस्तु तेषां हन्याद्बलायुषम् ॥६०॥

*Mild Nirūha*

To a tender person, to an old person and to an infant, it is useful to give *nirūha basti* with recipes containing mild drugs. If such persons are given strong *nirūha basti*, then this causes depletion of their strength and longevity.

दद्यादुत्क्लेशनं पूर्वं मध्यदोषहरं ततः ।
पश्चात् संशमनीयं च दद्याद्बस्तिं विचक्षणः" ॥६१॥
(शार्ङ्गधर : उत्तरखण्ड : ६ : १-१९)

*Three Types of Basti*

In the beginning, *nirūha basti* should be given with such recipe as would excite (*utkleśana*) the adhered *doṣas*. Thereafter, *basti* should contain recipe for the elimination (*doṣahara*) of *doṣas*. At the end, the wise physician should give *basti* with such drugs as would alleviate (*saṃśamana*) the *doṣas*.

[32]'पलशुक्तिकर्षकुडवैरम्लीकाहिंगुसिन्धुजगोमूत्रैः ।
ईषत्तैलयुतो बस्तिः शूलानाहामवातहरः ॥६२॥
भोजयित्वाथ सायमह्ने सर्वस्यायं प्रयुज्यते ।
अथ चेद्बलवान् जन्तुरभुक्त्वा तु तदा क्वचित् ॥६३॥
॥ वैतरणा बस्तिः' ॥

*Vaitaraṇā Basti*

*Amlikā* (one *pala*), *hiṅgu* (one *śukti*), *saindhava* (one *karṣa*) and cow's urine (one *kuḍava*) should be added with small quantity of oil. This recipe should be used for *basti* (enema) which cures colic pain, flatulence and *āmavāta* (rheumatism). All types of patients should be given this *basti* after food in the evening. If, however, the patient is strong enough, then this *basti* can occasionally be given on empty stomach.

"एरण्डबीजं मधुकं पिप्पली सैन्धवं वचा ।
हपुषा फलकल्कैश्च बस्तिरुत्क्लेशन स्मृतः" ॥६४॥
(शार्ङ्गधर : उत्तरखण्ड : ६ : १९-२०)

*Utklesana Basti (Exciting Enema)*

Enema administered with the recipe containing the paste of the seeds of *eraṇḍa, madhuka, pippalī, saindhava* and fruits of *hapuṣā* causes excitation (*utkleśana*) of *doṣas*.

त्रिदोषहारिणो बस्तिरगस्त्याः बीजतैलतः ।
"प्रियंगुर्मधुकं मुस्ता तथैव च रसाञ्जनम् ॥६५॥

*Doṣahara Basti (Doṣa-Eliminating Enema)*

Enema administered with the recipe containing the oil of the seed of *agasti, priyaṅgu, madhuka, mustā* and *rasāñjana* causes alleviation of all the three *doṣas.*

सक्षीरः शस्यते बस्तिस्त्रिदोषशमने परम् ॥६६॥
॥ शोधनबस्तयः[33] ॥

*Śodhana or Śamana Basti (Alleviating Enema)*

Enemas administered with the recipes containing milk, among others, alleviate (*śamana*) all the three *doṣas.*

त्रिफलाक्वाथगोमूत्रैः क्षौद्रक्षारसमायुतः ।
उषकादि प्रतीवापाः बस्तयो लेखना स्मृता ॥६७॥
॥ लेखनबस्तयः[34] ॥

*Lekhana Basti (Depleting Enema)*

Enemas administered with the recipes containing the decoction of *triphalā*, cow's urine, honey and alkalies and sprinkled with the powder of drugs belonging to *Uṣakādi* group cause *lekhana* (depletion of tissues).

बृंहणद्रव्यनिःक्वाथाः कल्कैर्मधुरकैर्युताः ।
सर्पिर्मांसरसोपेताः बस्तयो बृंहणा स्मृताः ॥६८॥
॥ बृंहणबस्तयः[35] ॥

*Bṛṃhaṇa Basti (Nourishing Enema)*

Enemas administered with the recipes containing the decoctions and pastes of nourishing drugs and mixed with sweet drugs, ghee and meat-soup cause nourishment (*bṛṃhaṇa*).

बदर्यैरावतीशेलुशाल्मलीधान्यनागराः ।
क्षीरसिद्धा क्षौद्रयुक्ता नाम्ना पिच्छिलसंज्ञिता ॥६९॥
अजोरभ्रेणरुधिरैर्युक्ता देया विचक्षणैः ।
मात्रा पिच्छिलबस्तीनां पलैर्द्वादशभिर्मता ॥७०॥
॥ पिच्छिलबस्तयः[३६] ॥

*Picchila Basti (Slimy Enema)*

*Badarī, erāvatī (nāgabalā), śelu, śālmalī, dhānya* and *nāgara* should be boiled with milk. To this medicated milk, honey should be added. This is called the recipe of *Picchila basti*. It should be administered with the blood of goat and sheep and given for enema by a wise physician. Recipes for *Picchila basti* should be administered in the dose of twelve *palas*.

दत्वादौ सैन्धवस्याक्षमधुनः प्रसृतिद्वयम् ।
विनिर्मथ्य ततो दद्यात्स्नेहस्य प्रसृतित्रयम् ॥७१॥
एकीभूते ततः स्नेहे कल्कस्य प्रसृतिं क्षिपेत् ।
संमूर्च्छितं कषायं तु चतुःप्रसृतिसंमितम् ।
क्षिप्त्वा विमथ्य दद्याच्च निरूहं कुशलो भिषक् ॥७२॥

*Quantity of Drugs in Enema*

One *akṣa* of *saindhava* and two *prasṛtis* of honey should be mixed together. To this, three *prasṛtis* of oil should be added and triturated till it becomes homogenous. To this, one *prasṛti* of the paste of drugs should be added and mixed well. Then four *prasṛtis* of the decoction should be added and triturated well. This recipe should then be used for the *nirūha* type of *basti*.

वाते चतुष्पलं क्षौद्रं दद्यात्स्नेहस्य षट्पलम् ।
पित्ते चतुष्पलं क्षौद्रं स्नेहं दद्यात्पलत्रयम् ।
कफे[३७] च षट्पलं क्षौद्रं क्षिपेत्स्नेहं चतुष्पलम् ॥७३॥
॥ इति निरूहणे मात्राविधिः ॥

### *Quantity of Drugs for Different Doṣas*

For *vātika* diseases, the recipe of enema should contain four *palas* of honey and six *palas* of oil. For *paittika* diseases, the recipe should contain four *palas* of honey and three *palas* of oil. For *kaphaja* diseases, six *palas* of honey and four *palas* of oil should be added to the recipe of *basti* (enema).

एरण्डक्वाथतुल्यांशं मधुतैलपलाष्टकम् ।
शतपुष्पा पलार्द्धेन सैन्धवार्द्धेन संयुतम् ॥७४॥
माधुतैलिकसंज्ञोयं बस्तिः खजविलोडितः ।
मेदो गुल्मकृमिप्लीहमदोदावर्त्तनाशनः ।
बलवर्णकरश्चैव वृष्यो बृंहणदीपनः ॥७५॥
॥ माधुतैलिकबस्तिः ॥

### *Mādhu Tailika Basti*

Decoction of *eraṇḍa* (eight *palas*), *madhu* (eight *palas*), oil (eight *palas*) *śatapuṣpā* (half *pala*) and *saindhava* ($^1/_4$th *pala*) should be mixed together. This is called *Mādhu tailika basti*. This should be well mixed by triturating (churning) with a rod. Use of this recipe for enema cures fat-diseases, *gulma* (phantom tumour), parasitic infestation, splenic disorders, *mada* (intoxication) and *udāvarta* (upward movement of flatus in the abdomen). It promotes strength, complexion, virility, nourishment and the power of digestion.

क्षौद्राज्यक्षीरतैलानां प्रसृतं प्रसृतं भवेत् ।
हपुषासैन्धवक्षारैर्बस्ति स्याद् दीपनः परः ॥७६॥
॥ दीपनबस्तिः ॥

### *Dīpana Basti (Digestive-Stimulant Enema)*

One *prasṛta* of each of honey, ghee, milk and oil should be added with *hapuṣā*, *saindhava* and alkalies. Administration of the enema containing this recipe causes stimulation of the digestive power.

एरण्डमूलनिःक्वाथो मधुतैलं ससैन्धवम् ।
एष युक्तरसो[३८] बस्तिः सवचापिप्पलीयुतः ॥७७॥
॥ युक्तरसबस्तिः[३९] ॥

*Yuktarasa Basti*

Decoction of the root of *eraṇḍa*, honey, oil, *saindhava, vacā* and *pippalī* should be mixed together and used for *basti* (enema). This is called *Yuktaras(th)a basti.*

पंचमूलस्य निष्क्वाथस्तैलं मागधिका मधु ।
ससैन्धवः समधुकः सिद्धबस्तिरिति स्मृतः ॥७८॥
॥ सिद्धबस्तिः" ॥
(शार्ङ्गधर : उत्तरखण्ड : ६ : २२-३६)

*Siddha Basti*

The decoction of *pañcamūla, pippalī,* honey, *saindhava* and *yaṣṭimadhu* should be mixed together and used for enema. This is called *Siddha basti.*

'स्नेहं[४०] गुडो मांसरसः पयश्च
अम्लानि मूत्रं मधुसैन्धवम् च ।
ये तान्यनुक्तान्यपि दापयेत
निरूहे योगे मदनं फलं च ॥७९॥
लवणं कार्षिकं दद्यात्फलमेकं तु मादनम् ।
वाते गुडः सिता पित्ते कफे सिद्धार्थकादयः ॥८०॥

*Preparation of Recipes for Basti*

In the recipe for *basti* (enema), the physician should add *sneha* (oil, etc.), jaggery, meat soup, milk, juice of sour fruits, urine, honey and rock-salt. Other drugs, not mentioned in the recipe but required for the patient, can also be added to the recipe. The dose of rock-salt should be one *karṣa*. One fruit of *madana* may also be added to the recipe. For *vātika* diseases, jaggery; for *paittika* diseases, sugar; and for *kaphaja* diseases, mustard, etc., should be added to the recipes.

सैन्धवाक्षं समादाय शताह्वाक्षसमन्वितम् ।
गोमूत्रस्य पलान्यष्टौ अम्लीकायाः पलद्वयम् ॥८१॥
गुडस्य तु पले द्वे च सर्वमालोड्य यत्नतः ।
वस्त्रपूतं सुखोष्णं च बस्तिं दद्याद्विचक्षणः ॥८२॥
शूलविष्टम्भमानाहमूत्रकृच्छ्रं च दारुणम् ।
वृद्ध्युदावर्तगुल्मादीन्सद्यो हन्यान्निषेवितः ॥८३॥
॥ क्षारबस्तिः" ॥

***Kṣāra Basti (Alkali Enema)***

One *akṣa* of *saindhava*, one *akṣa* of *satāhvā*, eight *palas* of cow's urine, two *palas* of *amlikā* and two *palas* of jaggery should be mixed together and churned carefully. This should then be strained through a cloth, and while luke-warm, should be administered for enema by an expert physician. It instantaneously cures colic pain, constipation, flatulence, serious type of dysuria, hydrocele, *udāvarta* (upward movement of flatus in the abdomen), *gulma* (phantom tumour), etc.

स्नानमुष्णोदकैः कुर्याद्दिवास्वप्नमजीर्णता ।
वर्जयेदपरं सर्वमाचरेत्स्नेहबस्तिवत् ॥८४॥

***Regimens for Nirūha***

The patient, after *nirūha basti* should take bath in warm water, should avoid sleep during day time and indigestion. All other prohibitions prescribed for *anuvāsana basti* should also be followed.

इति श्रीमहाराजाधिराजश्रीटोडरमल्लविरचिते टोडरानन्दे
आयुर्वेदसौख्ये बस्तिविधिनिरूहणयुक्तरसबस्तिकथनं
नाम द्व्यशीतितमो हर्षः ॥

Thus, ends the 82nd chapter dealing with the process of administering *basti, nirūha* and *yuktarasa* types of enema in the *Āyurveda saukhya* of *Ṭodarānanda* composed by the great King Ṭodaramalla.

## NOTES AND REFERENCES

१. (क) This is the beginning of the eightly sixth chapter of *Āyurveda saukhya* in *Ṭoḍarānanda* and invocation reads as follows :

"ब्रजांगनाय हि विधाय लक्ष्यं प्राणप्रियं दूतमलिप्रकल्य ।
प्रेमान्तराः प्रोचुरथो सदुक्तैः कृपां सकृष्णः कुरुतान्नरेन्द्रे ।"

(ख) "ब्रजांगनाय ....... नरेन्द्रे" पाठोऽयं चतुर्थषष्ठपुस्तकयोः नोपलभ्यते ।

२. (क) .संज्ञिकः इति पंचमपुस्तके पाठः ।

(ख) .नामकः इति आकरे पाठः ।

३. (क) शोथ. इति षष्ठपुस्तके पाठः ।

(ख) शोक. इति आकरे पाठः ।

४. आतुराङ्गुष्ठमानेन इति पंचमपुस्तके पाठः ।

५. वंधये तत्र वर्त्यं इति षष्ठपुस्तके पाठः ।

६. मलः इति षष्ठपुस्तके पाठः ।

७. (क) 'दिवा ..... नुवासयेत्' पाठोऽयं षष्ठपुस्तके नोपलभ्यते ।

(ख) दिवसान्ते वसन्ते इति आकरे पाठः ।

८. 'रूक्षं. ...... .नुवासयेत्' पाठोऽयं पंचमपुस्तके अधिकमुपलभ्यते ।

९. भ्रमातिसार. इति चतुर्थपुस्तके पाठः ।

१०. पलाद्यर्द्धेन इति पंचमपुस्तके आकरे च पाठः ।

११. 'शताह्वा. ....... लाघवे' पाठोऽयं षष्ठपुस्तके नोपलभ्यते ।

१२. जात व लाय च इति पंचमपुस्तके पाठः ।

१३. वामपार्श्वे वा इति प्रथमपुस्तके पाठः ।

१४. (क) 'पीडयेद् ...... कारयेत्' पाठोऽयं प्रथमपुस्तके नोपलभ्यते ।

(ख) धारयेत् इति षष्ठपुस्तके पाठः ।

१५. वस्त्रे इति प्रथमपुस्तके पाठः ।

१६. प्राणे हितः स्नेहः उत्तानो इति चतुर्थषष्ठपुस्तकयोः पाठः ।

१७. (क) क्षिपेत तः इति पंचमपुस्तके पाठः ।

(ख) शुभः इति षष्ठपुस्तके पाठः ।

१८. जाने इति प्रथमपुस्तके पाठः ।

१९. शीघ्रं इति पंचमपुस्तके पाठः ।

२०. तथा शैथिल्यमाध्मानशूलं श्वासंश्च इति पंचमपुस्तके पाठः ।

२१. 'पक्वाशये ...... जायते' पाठोऽयं षष्ठपुस्तके नोपलभ्यते ।

२२. आनायते इति पंचमपुस्तके आकरे च पाठः ।

२३. द्राभ्यां इति पंचमपुस्तके पाठः ।

२४. परिहाराश्च कृत्स्नशी इति षष्ठपुस्तके पाठः ।

२५. कुडवस्द्वयं इति चतुर्थषष्ठपुस्तकयोः पाठः ।

२६. मूर्च्छातृषोदरानाह. इति चतुर्थषष्ठपुस्तकयोः पाठः ।

२७. (क) वृद्धचवृक्षुरमन्दाग्नि. इति प्रथमपुस्तके पाठः ।

(ख) वृत्यतिक्षधमन्दाग्नि. इति षष्ठपुस्तके पाठः ।

२८. .संयुतै इति चतुर्थषष्ठपुस्तकयोः पाठः ।

२९. 'यस्य ........ तमादिशेत्' पाठोऽयं चतुर्थषष्ठपुस्तकयोः नोपलभ्यते ।

३०. .विधितायुह्या इति षष्ठपुस्तके पाठः ।

३१. स्नेहः स एकः इति षष्ठपुस्तके पाठः ।

३२. 'पलशुक्तिकर्ष. ....... वैतरणा बस्तिः' पाठोऽयं प्रथमपंचमपुस्तकयोः नोपलभ्यते ।

३३. .बस्तिः इति पंचमपुस्तके पाठः ।

३४. .बस्तिः इति पंचमपुस्तके पाठः ।

३५. .बस्तिः इति पंचमपुस्तके पाठः ।

३६. .वस्तिः इति पंचमपुस्तके पाठः ।

३७. कफेन त्रिफलं क्षौद्रं इति षष्ठपुस्तके पाठः ।

३८. युक्तरथो इति पंचमपुस्तके पाठः ।

३९. युक्तरथबस्ति इति पंचमपुस्तके पाठः ।

४०. "स्नेहं ...... हन्यानिषेवितः ॥क्षारबस्तिः॥" पाठोऽयं प्रथमपंचमपुस्तकयोः नोपलभ्यते ।

# CHAPTER XV

## ॥ अथोत्तरबस्तिः[1] ॥

*(Urethral and Vaginal Douche)*

अतः परं प्रवक्ष्यामि बस्तिमुत्तरसंज्ञितम् ।
द्वादशाङ्गुलकृन्नेत्रं मध्ये च कृतकर्णिकाम् ।
मालतीपुष्पवृंताभं छिद्रं सर्षपनिर्गगम् ॥१॥

*Nozzle for Adult Males*

After the description of *anuvāsana* and *nirūha* types of enema, now *uttara basti* (urethral and vaginal douches) will be described. Its nozzle should be 12 *angulas* in length. In its centre, there should be a *karṇikā* (ring to facilitate tying). In shape, it should be like the stalk of the *mālatī*-flower and inside the nozzle there should be a hole enabling a mustard seed to pass through.

पंचविंशतिवर्षाणां मध्ये मात्रा द्विकार्षिकी ।
तदूर्ध्वं पलमात्रा च स्नेहस्योक्ता भिषक्वरैः ॥२॥

### *Dose of Oil for Adult Male*

The quantity of medicated oil, to be administered in *uttara basti,* should be two *karṣas* if the patient is below 25 years of age and if he is above this age, then the quantity of oil should be one *pala* according to expert physicians.

अथास्थापनशुद्धस्य तृप्तस्य स्नानभोजनैः ।
स्थितस्य जानुमात्रे च पीढे त्विष्यशलाकया ॥३॥
स्निग्धया मेढ्रमार्गं च ततो नेत्रं नियोजयेत् ।
शनैः शनैः घृताभ्यक्तं मेढ्ररन्ध्रेङ्गुलानि षट् ॥४॥
ततो[2] वा पीडयेद्बस्तिं शनैर्नेत्रं च निर्हरेत् ।
ततः प्रत्यागते स्नेहे स्नेहबस्तिक्रमो हितः ॥५॥

### *Method of Administration*

The patient, whose body has been cleansed by the administration of *nirūha basti* and who is satisfied with bath and meals, should be made to sit over a table (stool) which should be high up to the knee joint of the patient. Through a greased probe, the direction of the urethral passage should first of all be ascertained. Thereafter, the nozzle smeared with ghee, should be gradually inserted upto the length of six *aṅgulas* in the urethra. Then the enema (douche) sac should be gently pressed to enable the medicated oil enter into the bladder through the urethra. The nozzle should then be gently removed from the urethra. After the medicated oil comes out of the urethra, the patient should be provided with regimens like those prescribed for *anuvāsana basti.*

स्त्रीणां कनिष्ठिकामूलं नेत्रं कुर्याद्दशाङ्गुलम् ।
मुद्गः[3] प्रवेश्य[4] योग्यं च योन्यंतश्चतुरङ्गुलम् ॥६॥

### *Nozzle for Vaginal Douche*

The nozzle for vaginal douche should have the thickness of the little finger. It should be ten *aṅgulas* in length. The hole inside the nozzle should allow a seed of *mudga* to pass.

द्व्यङ्गुलं मूत्रमार्गे[1] च सूक्ष्मं नेत्रं नियोजयेत् ॥७॥

*Nozzle for Female Urethra*

The nozzle for *uttara basti* in the female urethra should be two *aṅgulas* in length and it should be very thin.

मूत्रकृच्छ्रविकारेषु बालानां त्वेकमंगुलम् ।
शनैर्निष्कंपमाधेयं सूक्ष्मं नेत्रं विचक्षणैः ॥८॥

*Nozzle for Infants*

For giving *uttara basti* to infants in the case of their dysuria, the length of the nozzle should be one *aṅgula* and it should be very thin. Such a nozzle should be inserted into the infant's urethra very slowly without any trembling of hands by an expert.

योनिमार्गेषु नारीणां स्नेहमात्रा द्विपालिकी ।
मूत्रमार्गे पलोन्मानां बालाणां च द्विकार्षिकी ॥९॥

*Dose of Oil for Females and Infants*

For vaginal douche, two *palas* of medicated oil should be used. For douching through the female urethra, the dose of the oil should be one *pala*, and for infants, the dose of oil should be two *karṣas*.

उत्तानायै स्त्रियै दद्यादूर्ध्वजानैर्विचक्षणैः[६] ।
अप्रत्यगाकृति[७] भिषक् बस्तिरुत्तरसंज्ञितः ॥१०॥
'भूयो[८] बस्तिं विदध्यात्र संयुक्तैः शोधनैर्गणैः ।
फलवर्तिं विदध्याद्वा योनिमार्गे दृढां भिषक् ॥११॥
सूत्रैर्विनिर्मितां स्निग्धां शोधनद्रव्यसंयुताम्' ।
दह्यमाने तथा बस्तौ दद्याद्बस्ति विशारदः ।
क्षीरवृक्षकषायेण पयसा शीतलेन च ॥१२॥

*Method of Administering Vaginal Douche*

The lady should be made to lie on her back and keep her knee joints folded and raised. Then the vaginal douche should be administered. If the oil given through the douche does not come out, then another *uttara basti* containing drugs belonging to *Śodhana gaṇa* should be administered. Alternatively, a hard *phala varti* (suppository) should be tied through a thread, made oily and inserted into the vaginal tract, [keeping the other end of the thread outside]. This suppository should be made of drugs belonging to *Śodhana* group. If there is burning sensation in the vaginal canal, then *uttara basti* with the decoction of *kṣīrī vṛkṣas* and cold milk should be administered.

बस्तिं शुक्ररुजः[९] पुंसां स्त्रीणामार्त्तवजां रुजः ।
हन्यादुत्तरबस्तिस्तु[१०] नोचिता मेहिनां क्वचित्" ॥१३॥

(शार्ङ्गधर : उत्तरखण्ड : ७ : १-१४)

### Effects of Uttara Basti

*Uttara basti* (vaginal and urethral douches) cures seminal diseases in males and menstrual disorders (including those of ova) in females. It should not be administered to a patient suffering from *meha* (obstinate urinary disorders including diabetes).

"सम्यक्दत्तस्य लिंगाणां व्यापदक्रम एव च ।
बस्तेरुत्तरसंज्ञस्य समानं स्नेहबस्तिना ॥१४॥

Signs of appropriate administration, likely complications and their management in respect of both *anuvāsana basti* and *uttara basti* are similar.

घृताभ्यक्ते[११] गुदे क्षेप्या श्लक्ष्णा स्वांगुष्ठसन्निभा[१२]।
मलप्रवर्त्तिनी ह्येषा फलवर्त्तिश्च सा[१३] स्मृता ॥१५॥
॥ इति फलवर्त्तिः" ॥

(शार्ङ्गधर : उत्तरखण्ड : ७ : १७-१८)

### Suppository

A thick pill of the size and shape of the thumb of the patient which is smeared with ghee and made hard as well as smooth (*ślakṣṇā*) is called *Phala vartti*. When inserted into the anus, it causes evacuation of stool.

इति श्रीमहाराजाधिराजश्रीटोडरमल्लविरचिते टोडरानन्दे आयुर्वेदसौख्ये निदानरोगपरीक्षाचिकित्सा[४]कथनं नाम त्र्यशीतितमो हर्षः ॥

'रामजी'[१५]

॥ श्री रामचन्द्राय नमः' ॥

Thus, ends the 83rd Chapter dealing with the diagnosis of diseases, method of examination of patients and treatment of diseases in the *Āyurveda saukhya* of *Ṭoḍarānanda* composed by the great King Ṭoḍaramalla.

[This colophon is for the entire section of the work dealing with the diagnosis and treatment of diseases of all types and not for this chapter alone.]

## NOTES AND REFERENCES

१. (क) This is the beginning of the eighty seventh chapter of *Āyurveda saukhya* in *Ṭoḍarānanda* and invocation reads as follows :

"यमुद्भवो वोधयदुत्थितानां गोबिन्दविश्लेषकृषीतांगम् ।
गोपांगनानां हृदि वर्त्तमानं प्रवर्त्ततां श्री नृपटोडरस्य" ॥

(ख) "यमुद्भवो ....... नृपटोडरस्य" पाठोऽयं षष्ठपुस्तके नोपलभ्यते ।

२. ततोऽवपीडयेद्वस्तिं इति आकरे पाठः ।

३. (क) मुहुः इति प्रथमपुस्तके पाठः ।

(ख) मुद्गप्रवेशं इति आकरे पाठः ।

४. प्रवेशं इति चतुर्थषष्ठपुस्तकयोः पाठः ।

५. मार्गेण सूक्ष्मनेत्रं प्रयोजयेत् इति षष्ठपुस्तके पाठः ।

६. .जान्वै विचक्षणः इति आकरे पाठः ।

७. (क) अप्रत्यागच्छति भिषग्बस्तावुत्तरसंज्ञिते इति आकरे पाठः ।

(ख) अपत्यगागवति भिषक् व शोधनद्रव्यसंयुतां इति षष्ठपुस्तके पाठः ।

८. 'भूयो ....... .संयुताम्' पाठोऽयं षष्ठपुस्तके नोपलभ्यते ।

९. शुक्ररजपुंसो इति षष्ठपुस्तके पाठः ।

१०. .स्तनो. इति षष्ठपुस्तके पाठः ।

११. घृतत्यक्ते इति षष्ठपुस्तके पाठः ।

१२. .लक्षणस्वां. इति षष्ठपुस्तके पाठः ।

१३. प्रशस्यते इति चतुर्थषष्ठपुस्तकयोः पाठः ।

१४. The colophon appears to be misleading.

१५. 'रामजी ........ नमः' पाठोऽयं चतुर्थपुस्तके अधिकमुपलभ्यते ।

# CHAPTER XVI

## ।। अथ शोणितस्रावविधिः ।।

## *(Blood-Letting Therapy)*

"शोणितं स्रावयेज्जन्तोरामयं प्रसमीक्ष्य च ।
प्रस्थं प्रस्थार्द्धकं वापि प्रस्थार्द्धार्द्धमथापि वा ।।१ ।।

### *Quantity of Blood to be Removed*

Depending upon the nature of the disease, one, half or quarter *prastha* of blood should be removed from the body of the patient.

"शरत्काले स्वभावेन कुर्याद्रिक्तस्रुतिं नरः ।
त्वग्दोषग्रन्थिशोथाद्याः न स्यूः रक्तस्रुतेर्यतः"[२] ।।२ ।।

(योगरत्नाकर : पृष्ठ १८०)

### *Suitable Season*

As a preventive measure, blood-letting therapy should be administered to a healthy (normal) person during the autumn season. Blood-letting therapy prevents the occurrence of skin diseases, *granthi* (enlarged glands) oedema, etc.

मधुरं वर्णतो रक्तमशीतोष्णं तथा गुरुः ।
शोणितं स्निग्धं विस्रं स्याद्विदाहश्चास्य पित्तवत् ॥३॥

*Characteristics of Normal Blood*

Blood, normally has the following characteristic features :

(1) It is sweet in taste and red in colour;
(2) it is neither hot nor cold;
(3) it is heavy and unctuous;
(4) in smell, it is *visra* (like the smell of meat); and
(5) its *vidāha* (metabolic transformation) takes place like that of *pitta*.

विस्रता द्रवता रागश्चलनं विलयं[३] तथा ।
भूम्यादिपंचभूतानामेते रक्तगुणस्मृताः ॥४॥

*Properties of Five Mahābhūtas*

Presence of five *mahābhūtas* (basic elements) is indicated by the following attributes of the blood :

| | *Mahābhūtas* | *Attributes of blood* |
|---|---|---|
| 1. | *Pṛthvī* | *visratā* (fleshy smell) |
| 2. | *Ap* | *dravatā* (liquidity) |
| 3. | *Tejas* | *rāga* (red colour) |
| 4. | *Vāyu* | *calana* (mobility) |
| 5. | *Ākāśa* | *vilaya* (nature of getting mixed up with others quickly). |

रक्ते दुष्टे वेदना स्यात्पाको दाहश्च जायते ।
[४]रक्तमण्डलताकण्डूशोथस्यात्पिडिकोद्भवः ॥५॥

*Signs of Blood-Vitiation*

If the blood is vitiated, then the patient suffers from pain, suppuration, burning sensation, red patches over the skin, itching oedema and pimples.

वृद्धे रक्ताङ्गनेत्रत्वं शिराणां पूर्णता तथा ।
गात्राणां गौरवं निद्रा मदो दाहश्च जायते[१] ॥६॥

### *Signs of Increased Quantity of Blood*

If the quantity of blood is increased (aggravated), then patient suffers from redness of the body and eyes, fullness of veins, heaviness of the body, excessive sleep, *mada* (intoxication) and burning sensation.

क्षीणेऽम्लमधुराकांक्षा मूर्च्छा च त्वचि रूक्षता ।
शैथिल्यं च शिराणां च वातादुन्मार्गगामिता ॥७॥

### *Signs of Decreased Quantity of Blood*

Diminution of the quantity of blood produces the following signs and symptoms :

(1) The patient desires to take more of sour and sweet things;
(2) fainting, dryness of the skin and slothness (looseness) of the vessels; and
(3) because of aggravated *vāyu* associated in this condition, blood moves upwards (*unmārga gāmitā*).

अरुणं फेनिलं रूक्षं परुषं तनु शीघ्रगम् ।
अस्कन्धसुचिनिस्तोदि[५,६] रक्तं स्याद्वातदूषितम् ॥८॥

### *Vitiation of Blood by Vāyu*

If blood is vitiated by *vāyu*, then it becomes reddish in colour, frothy, ununctuous, rough to touch, thin and quick in mobility. It does not get coagulated and the patient feels pain as if pricked by needles.

पित्तेन पीतं हरितं नीलं श्यावं च विस्रकम् ।
अस्कन्द्युष्णं मक्षिकाणां पिपीलि(का)नामनिष्टकम् ॥९॥

### *Vitiation of Blood by Pitta*

If blood is vitiated by *pitta*, then it becomes yellow, green, blue or brownish black in colour. It bleeds profusely and does not get coagulated. It becomes hot to touch and it is not liked by flies and ants.

शीतलं बहलं स्निग्धं गैरिकादकसन्निभम् ।
मांसपेशीप्रभं स्कंदी मन्दगं कफदूषितम् ॥१०॥

*Vitiation of Blood by Kapha*

If the blood is vitiated by *kapha*, then it is cold to touch, thick and unctuous. In colour, it looks like the solution of *gairika* (red ochre) or muscle tissue. It gets coagulated quickly and it moves very slowly.

'द्विदोषदुष्टं" संसृष्टं त्रिदुष्टं पूतिगन्धकम्' ।
सर्वलक्षणसंयुक्तं काञ्जिकाभं च जायते ॥११॥

*Vitiation by Two or Three Doṣas*

If the blood is vitiated by two of the aggravated *doṣas*, then signs of both these *doṣas* will appear in the blood. If it is vitiated by all the three *doṣas* together, then it gives out putrid odour and produces signs of all the three *doṣas*. In addition, it appears like *kāñji* (a preparation of sour drink).

विषदुष्टं भवेत्श्यावं नासिकोन्मार्गगं तथा ।
विस्रं काञ्जिकसंकाशं सर्वकुष्ठकरं तथा ॥१२॥

*Vitiation of Blood by Poisons*

If blood is vitiated by poisons, then it becomes brownish black in colour; bleeding takes place through nostrils; it bears fleshy smell; it looks like *kāñji* (a preparation of sour drink) and causes all types of *kuṣṭha* (obstinate skin diseases including leprosy).

इन्द्रगोपप्रभं ज्ञेयं प्रकृतिस्थमसंहतम् ॥१३॥

*Characteristics of Normal Blood*

The colour of natural or normal blood is like that of *indragopa* (the insect cochineal) and it is not of high density.

शोथे दाहेऽंगपाके च रक्तवर्णेऽसृजः स्रुतौ ।
"वातरक्ते तथा कुष्ठे सपीडे दुर्जयेऽनिले ॥१४॥
पाणिरोगे श्लीपदे च विषदुष्टे च शोणिते ।
ग्रन्थ्यर्बुदापचीक्षुद्ररोगरक्ताधिमन्थिषु ॥१५॥

विदारीस्तनरोगेषु गात्राणां सादगौरवे ।
रक्ताभिष्यन्दि तन्द्रायां पूतिघ्राणास्यदेहके ॥१६॥
यकृत्प्लीहविसर्पेषु विद्रधौ पिडिकोद्गमे ।
कर्णौष्ठघ्राणवक्त्राणां पाके दाहे शिरो रुजि ।
उपदंशे रक्तपित्ते रक्तस्रावः प्रशस्यते" ॥१७॥

(योगरत्नाकर : पृष्ठ १८0)

### *Patients Suitable for Blood-Letting Therapy*

Blood-letting therapy is useful for patients suffering from oedema, burning sensation, suppuration of limbs, red colouration of the skin, bleeding from different parts of the body, *vāta rakta* (gout), *kuṣṭha* (obstinate skin diseases including leprosy), *piḍaka* (pimples), serious type of aggravated *vāyu*, diseases of hands, elephantiasis, poisoning of blood, *granthi* (lymphadenitis), *arbuda* (tumours), *apacī* (tubercular lymphadenitis), *kṣudra roga* (minor disease), *raktādhimantha* (*raktaja* type of glaucoma), *vidārikā* (a popular growth in the axillae and groins), breast-diseases, prostration and heaviness of the body, conjunctivitis caused by the vitiation of blood, drowsiness, putrid smell coming out of nose, mouth and body, diseases of liver and spleen, erysipelas, abscess, pimples, suppuration of ears, lips, nose and mouth, burning sensation, headache, *upadaṃśa* (syphilis) and *raktapitta* (a disease charaterised by bleeding from different parts of the body).

एषु रोगेषु शृंगैर्वा जलौकालाबुकैरपि ।
अथवापि शिरामोक्षैः कुर्याद्रक्तस्रुतिं नरः ॥१८॥

### *Modes of Administering Blood-Letting Therapy*

In the above mentioned diseases, blood-letting therapy should be administered by the application of *śṛṅga* (horn), *jalaukā* (leeches) or *alābu* (gourd-fruit) or by venesection.

न कुर्वीत शिरामोक्षं कृशस्यातिव्यवायिनः ।
क्लीबस्य भीरोर्गर्भिण्याः सूतिकापाण्डुरोगिणाम् ॥१९॥

पंचकर्मविशुद्धस्य पीतस्नेहस्य चार्शसाम् ।
सर्वाङ्गशोथयुक्तानामुदरिश्वासकासिनाम् ॥२०॥
छर्द्यतीसारयुष्टानामतिस्विन्नतनोरपि ।
ऊनषोडशवर्षस्य गतसप्ततिकस्य च ।
आघातस्रुतरक्तस्य शिरामोक्षो न शस्यते ॥२१॥

*Contra-Indications of Blood-letting Therapy*

The following types of patients are not suitable for blood-letting therapy :

(1) Persons who are emaciated and who indulge in excess of sex;
(2) persons suffering from impotency and those who are scared of such therapies;
(3) pregnant women and ladies after delivery;
(4) those suffering from *pāṇḍu* (anemia);
(5) those whose bodies are cleansed by the administration of *pañca karma* therapies and those who have taken oleation therapy;
(6) those suffering from piles, general anasarca, *udara* (obstinate abdominal diseases including ascites), asthma, cough, vomiting and diarrhoea;
(7) those who have received fomentation therapy in excess;
(8) persons below the age of 16 and above the age of 70; and
(9) those who have bleeding because of injury.

एषां चात्ययिके रोगे जलौकाभिस्तु निर्हरेत् ।
तथापि विषयुष्टानां शिरामोक्षोऽपि शस्यते ॥२२॥

In the case of emergency, patients of the above categories can be given blood-letting therapy by the application of leeches. In the case of afflictions by poisons, even the above mentioned categories of patients can be given blood-letting therapy by venesection.

गोशृंगेन जलौकाभिरलाबूभिरपि त्रिधा ।
वातपित्तकफैर्दुष्टं शोणितं स्रावयेद्बुधः ॥२३॥

द्विदोषाभ्यां तु संदुष्टं त्रिदोषैरपि दूषितम् ।
शोणितं स्रावयेद् युक्त्या शिरामोक्षैः पदैस्तथा ॥२४॥

*Different Modes of Blood-letting*

Blood-letting therapy should be administered with the help of cow's horn, leeches and *alābu* (gourd) to correct the vitiation of blood by *vāyu*, *pitta* and *kapha* respectively. If the blood is vitiated by two *doṣas* or three *doṣas* together, then blood-letting therapy should be performed by either venesection or by *[kāka]pada* (scratching).

गृह्णाति शोणितं शृङ्गं दशाङ्गुलमितं बलात् ।
जलौकाहस्तमात्रं तु तुम्बं[१०] च द्वादशाङ्गुलम् ।
पदमंगुलमात्रस्य शिरा सर्वाङ्गशोधिनी ॥२५॥

*Area of Effect*

With the help of horn, one can take out vitiated blood from an area of ten *aṅgulas*; with leeches, from the area of one *hasta*; by *tumbī* (*alābu* or gourd), from twelve *aṅgulas*; by *kākapada* (scratching), from an area of only one *aṅgula* and by venesection, one can take out vitiated blood from all over the body.

शीते निरन्ने मूर्च्छार्तिनिद्राभीतिमदश्रमैः[११] ।
युतानां न स्रवेद्रक्तं तथा विण्मूत्रसंगिनाम् ॥२६॥

*Factors Prohibiting Bleeding*

By the administration of blood-letting therapy, bleeding does not take place because of the following factors :

(1) In winter when it is cold;
(2) if the patient is on fast;
(3) if the patient is suffering from fainting or is excessively sleepy or if he is scared;
(4) if he is suffering from intoxication or is fatigued; and
(5) if there is obstruction to the passage of stool and urine

अप्रवर्त्तिनि[१२] रक्ते च कुष्ठत्रिकटुसैन्धवैः ।
मर्दयेद् व्रणवक्त्रं च तेन सम्यक् प्रवर्त्तते ॥२७॥

तस्मान्न शीते नात्युष्णे न स्विन्ने नातितापिते ।
पीत्वा यवागूं तृप्तस्य स्रावयेत्शोणितं बुधैः ॥२८॥

*Measures to Induce Bleeding*

If by the administration of blood-letting therapy, bleeding does not take place, then the mouth (opening) of the cut surface should be rubbed with the powders of *kuṣṭha, śuṇṭhī, pippalī, marica* and *saindhava.* This facilitates proper bleeding.

Therefore, blood-letting therapy should not be administered when it is very cold or very hot, when the patient is perspiring and when the patient is excessively exposed to the heat of fire or sun. He should be made to take *yavāgū* (gruel) in sufficient quantity till he feels satisfied and only after that blood-letting therapy should be administered.

अतिस्विन्नस्योष्णकाले तथैवातिशिराव्यधात् ।
अतिप्रवर्त्तते रक्तं तत्र कुर्यात्प्रतिक्रियाम् ॥२९॥

*Causes of Excessive Bleeding*

If the patient is having excessive perspiration, if the season is hot and if the vein is cut in excess, then there will be profuse bleeding and it should be corrected.

अतिप्रवृत्ते रक्ते च लोध्रसर्ज्जरसाञ्जनैः ।
यवगोधूमचूर्णैर्वा धवधन्वनगैरिकैः ॥३०॥
सर्पनिर्म्मोकचूर्णैर्वा भस्मना क्षौमवस्त्रयोः ।
मुखं व्रणस्य बध्वा च शीतैश्चोपचरेद् व्रणम् ॥३१॥
विध्येदूर्ध्वं शिरां तां वा दहेत् क्षारेण वाग्निना ।
व्रणं कषायः[१३] संधत्ते रक्तं स्कन्दयते[१४] हिमम् ।
व्रणास्यं पाचयेत् क्षारैदहैः संकोचयेत् शिराम् ॥३२॥

*Measures to Check Excessive Bleeding*

If there is excessive bleeding while administering blood-letting therapy, then following measures should be adopted :

(1) The powders of *lodhra, sarjarasa* and *añjana* or the powder of *yava* and *godhūma* or the powders of *dhava, dhanvana* and *gairika* or the powder of the slough of the snake or the ash of burnt silken cloth should be used for packing the mouth (opening) of the cut surface and tied with the help of a bandage;

(2) the patient should be given cooling therapies and cooling drugs should be applied over the cut surface;

(3) the vein should be incised again at a higher level;

(4) the opening (cut surface) of the vein should be cauterised with alkalies or fire (red hot iron rod).

Application of cool and astringent decoction on the cut surface obstructs bleeding and causes coagulation of the blood. By the application of alkalies, the cut surface of the vein gets inflammed and cauterisation with the help of a red hot iron rod causes contraction of the vascular wall which leads to stoppage of bleeding.

स यथाह

वामाण्डशोथे दक्षस्य करस्यांगुष्ठमूलजाम् ।
दहेच्छिरां व्यत्यये च वामाङ्गुष्ठशिरां दहेत् ।
शिरादाहप्रभावेन मुष्कशोथः प्रणश्यति ॥३३॥

### *Selection of Sites for Cauterisation Therapy*

If there is swelling in the left testicle, then cauterisation should be performed on the vein over the right thumb of the patient. Conversely, if there is swelling in the right testicle, then the vein over the left thumb should be cauterised. Because of the cauterisation of these vessels testicular swelling gets cured.

विषूच्यां पार्ष्णिदाहेन जायतेग्नेः प्रदीपनः ।
संकुचंति यतस्तेन रसश्लेष्मवहा शिराः ॥३४॥

In choleric diarrhoea, cauterisation should be performed over the calcaneum region (*pārṣṇi*). It stimulates the power of digestion because the channels carrying *rasa* (chyle) and *kapha* get contracted as a result of this cauterisation.

यदा वृद्धिः यकृत्प्लीह्नोः शिशोः संजायतेसृजः ।
तदा तत्स्थानदाहेन संकुचंत्यसृजः शिराः ॥३५॥

When the child suffers from enlarged liver and spleen because of the accumulation of excess of blood in these organs, then cauterisation should be performed on the skin over these viscera. It causes contraction of vessels supplying blood to these organs and cures the patient.

रक्तदुष्ट्यवशिष्टेऽपि व्याधिर्नैव प्रकुप्यति ।
अतः[१५] स्थैर्यं[१६] सावशेषं रक्तं नातिक्रमो हितः ॥३६॥

*Limit of Blood-Letting Therapy*

Even if after the blood-letting therapy some residual vitiated blood remains in the body, it does not aggravate the disease. Therefore, this residual blood (vitiated) should be allowed to remain in the body and it is useful if the physician does not exceed the limit.

आंध्यमाक्षेपकं तृष्णां तिमिरं शिरसो रुजाम् ।
पक्षाघातं श्वासकासौ हिक्कां दाहं च पाण्डुताम् ।
कुरुतेऽतिस्रुते[१७] रक्तं मरणं वा करोति च ॥३७॥

*Signs of Excessive Bleeding*

If excess of blood is taken out by the blood-letting therapy, then the patient suffers from blindness, *ākṣepaka* (convulsions), thirst, *timira* (appearance of blackness in front of the eyes), headache, paralysis, asthma, cough, hiccup, burning sensation and anemia. Such excessive bleeding may even cause death of the patient.

देहस्योत्पत्तिरसृजाद् देहस्तेनैव धार्यते ।
विना तेन व्रजेज्जीवो रक्षेद्रक्तमतो बुधः ॥३८॥

*Need for Protecting Blood*

The body of living being is created and sustained by blood, and without blood, the living being succumbs to death. Therefore, a wise person should always protect blood and prevent excessive bleeding.

शीतोपचारैः कुपिते स्रुतरक्तस्य मारुते ।
कोष्णेन सर्पिषा शोथं सव्यथं परिषेचयेत् ॥३९॥

*After Care*

After blood is taken out by blood-letting therapy, the patient is given cooling regimens. This may cause aggravation of *vāyu*. In such an event, the swelling and pain in the site of venesection should be treated by the sprinkling of luke warm ghee over the affected part.

क्षीणस्यैनं शशोरभ्रहरिणछागमांसजाः ।
रसः समुचितः पाने क्षीरं वा षष्टिका हिताः ॥४०॥

If the patient becomes emaciated after the blood-letting therapy, he should be given the soup of the meat of rabbit, sheep, deer or goat in appropriate quantity. Such a patient should also be given milk along with *ṣaṣṭika* type of rice in his meals.

पीडाशान्तिर्लघुत्वं च व्याधेरुद्रेकसंक्षयः[१८] ।
शोथहानिः[१९] भवेच्चिह्नं सम्यग्विस्राविते‍ऽसृजि ॥४१॥

*Signs of Appropriate Blood-Letting*

If blood-letting therapy is administered appropriately, then the patient gets relief from pain, feels lightness in his body, alleviation of acuteness of the manifested disease and diminution of oedema.

व्यायाममैथुनं क्रोधशीतस्नानप्रवातकान् ।
एकाशनं दिवानिद्रां क्षाराम्लकटुभोजनम् ।
शोकं वादमजीर्णं च त्यजेदाबलदर्शनात्' ॥४२॥

(शार्ङ्गधर : उत्तरखण्ड : १-४५)

*Prohibitions*

After the administration of blood-letting therapy, the patient should avoid physical exercise, sexual intercourse, anger, cold bath, exposure to strong wind, taking food only once per day, sleep during the day time, intake of alkaline, sour and pungent food, grief, attending debates and indigestion (intake of heavy food) till he regains his normal strength.

अथ रक्तावसेचनार्थं जलौकसां परीक्षा लिख्यते ॥४३॥

*Application of Leeches for Blood-Letting*

Now, application of leeches for the blood-letting therapy will be described.

"ता द्वादशस्तासां, सविषाः षट्, तावंत्येव निर्विषाः ॥४४॥

*Variety of Leeches*

Leeches are of twelve varieties; six of them are poisonous and the remaining varieties are nonpoisonous.

तत्र सविषाः - कृष्णा कर्बुरा अलगर्दा ।
इन्द्रयुधा सामुद्रिका गोचन्दना चेति ॥४५॥

*Poisonous Leeches*

Six varieties of poisonous leeches are called *Kṛṣṇā, Karburā, Alagardā, Indrayudhā, Sāmudrikā* and *Gocandanā.*

तासु अञ्जनचूर्णवर्णाः पृथुशिराः कृष्णाः, वर्मिमत्स्यायता च्छिन्नोन्नतकुक्षिः कर्ब्बुराः, रोमशाः महापार्श्वाः कृष्णमुख्यालगर्दाः, इन्द्रयुधावदूर्ध्वराजिभिश्चित्रिताः इन्द्रयुधाः, ईषदसितपीतिकाः विचित्रपुष्पाकृतिचित्राः सामुद्रिकाः, गोवृषणवदधोभागे द्विधाभूताकृतिरणुमुखी गोचन्दना चेति ॥४६॥

*Characteristic Features of Poisonous Leeches*

Poisonous varieties of leeches have the following characteristic features :

(1) *Kṛṣṇā* : This type of leech is black in colour like the collyrium powder and it has prominent veins in the body.
(2) *Karbburā* : This type of leech is flat in shape like a fish called *varmi*; its belly is scratched and elevated.
(3) *Alagardā* : This type of leech is hairy with expanded sides and its mouth is black in colour.
(4) *Indrāyudhā* : This type of leech is like rainbow in colour and spotted with patches at its back.
(5) *Sāmudrikā* : This type of leech is slightly black and yellow in colour and spotted with variegated colours like a flower.
(6) *Gocandanā* : This type of leech has a belly which is divided into two segments like the scrotum of a bull and it has a thin mouth.

ताभिर्दष्टे पुरुषे दंशे श्वयथुरतिमात्रं कण्डूर्मूर्च्छा ज्वरो
दाहश्छर्दिर्मदः सदनमिति लिङ्गानि भवन्ति ॥४७॥
तत्र महागदः पानालेपननस्यकर्मादिषूपयोज्यः[२०] ॥४८॥
इन्द्रायुधादष्टमसाध्यम् ॥४९॥
इत्येता सविषाः सचिकित्सिता व्याख्याताः ॥५०॥

(सुश्रुत : सूत्रस्थान : १३ : १०-११)

तद्दुष्टलिङ्गं तु असाध्यसर्पदष्टविषवेगविज्ञाने च द्रष्टव्यम् ॥५१॥

### Signs and Management of Poisonous Leech Bite

If a person is afflicted with the bite by poisonous leeches, then he suffers from oedema and excessive itching at the site of bite, fainting, fever, burning sensation, vomiting, intoxication and prostration.

For such patients, the recipe called *Mahāgada* should be used for internal intake, external application, inhalation therapy, etc. If, however, he is bitten by *Indrāyudha* type of leech, then he is incurable.

Thus, the characteristic features of poisonous leeches and the treatment of ailments caused by their bite are explained.

For further details about the signs and symptoms caused by the bite of poisonous leeches, one should refer to the section dealing with the incurable types of snake bites.

'अथ[21] निर्विषा :

कपिला, पिङ्गला, शङ्कुमुखी, मूषिका, पुण्डरीकमुखी, सावरिका चेति ॥५२॥

*Nonpoisonous Leeches*

Six varieties of nonpoisonous leeches are (1) *Kapilā*, (2) *Piṅgalā*, (3) *Śaṅkumukhī*, (4) *Mūṣikā*, (5) *Puṇḍarīkamukhī* and (6) *Sāvarikā*.

तत्र मनःशिलारञ्जिताभ्यामिव पार्श्वाभ्यां पृष्ठे स्निग्धा मुद्गवर्णा कपिला; किंचिद्रक्ता वृत्तकाया पिङ्गाऽऽशुगा च पिङ्गला; यकृद्वर्णा शीघ्रपायिनी दीर्घतीक्ष्णमुखी शङ्कुमुखी; मूषिकाकृतिवर्णानिष्टगन्धि च मूषिका; मुद्गवर्णा पुण्डरीकतुल्यवक्त्रा पुण्डरीकमुखी; स्निग्धा पद्मपत्रवर्णाऽष्टादशाङ्गुलप्रमाणा सावरिका, सा च पश्वर्थे; इत्येताः अविषा व्याख्याताः ॥५३॥

*Characteristic Features of Nonpoisonous Leeches*

Nonpoisonous varieties of leeches have the following characteristic features :

(1) *Kapilā* : Its sides are red in colour as if smeared with *manaḥśilā*. Its back is smooth having the colour of that of *mudga*.

(2) *Piṅgalā* : It is reddish in colour and round in shape. It is pink and exceedingly mobile.

(3) *Śaṅkumukhī* : It is like liver in colour. It sucks blood very fast. Its mouth is long and pointed.

(4) *Mūṣikā* : In shape and colour, it is like a mouse. It produces foul smell.

(5) *Puṇḍarīkamukhī* : In colour, it is like *mudga* and its mouth is like a lotus flower.

(6) *Sāvarikā* : It is unctuous and in colour, it is like a lotus leaf. It is ten *aṅgulas* in length. It is generally used for blood-letting therapy of animals.

Thus, the nonpoisonous varieties of leeches are described.

तासां यवनपाण्ड्यसह्यपौतनादीनि क्षेत्राणि; तेषु महाशरीरा बलवत्यः शीघ्रपायिन्यो महाशनाः निर्विषाश्च विशेषेण भवन्ति ॥५४॥

### *Habitat of Nonpoisonous Leeches*

Normally, these nonpoisonous varieties of leeches are available in the regions of *Yavana* (Turkey), *Pāṇḍya* (a region in South India), *Sahya* (the mountainous region located south of the river Narmadā) and *Pautana* (region around Mathurā). The leeches available in these regions are of stout physique and strong. They suck very quickly large quantity of blood and these are exceedingly nonpoisonous.

तत्र, सविषमत्स्यकीटदर्दुरमूत्रपुरीषकोथजाताः कलुषेऽम्भस्सु च सविषाः; पद्मोत्पलनलिनकुमुदसौगन्धिककुवलयपुण्डरीकशैवल-कोथजाता विमलेष्वम्भसु च निर्विषाः ॥५५॥

भवति चात्र

क्षेत्रेषु विचरन्त्येताः सलिलाढ्यसुगन्धिषु ।
न च संकीर्णचारिण्यो न च पङ्केशयाः सुखाः ॥५६॥

### *Effect of Habitat on Nature of Leeches*

Leeches living in polluted water and in the surrounding of poisonous fish, insects, frogs and mud containing urine and stool are poisonous. Those living in clean water and in the surrounding of *padma, utpala, nalina, kumuda, saugandhika, kuvalaya, pauṇḍarīka* and mud containing *śaivāla* are nonpoisonous.

Thus it is said : Those leeches who move in plenty of aromatic water, who do not live in polluted water and who do not sleep in mud are useful for application in the blood-letting therapy.

तासां ग्रहणमार्द्रचर्मणा, अन्यैर्वा प्रयोगैर्गृह्णीयात् । अथैनां नवे महति घटे सरस्तडागोदकपङ्कमावाप्य निदध्यात्; भक्ष्यार्थे चासामुपहरेच्छैवलं वल्लूरमोदकांश्च कन्दांश्चूर्णीकृत्य; शय्यार्थं तृणमौदकानि च पत्राणि; त्र्यहात्र्यहाच्चाभ्योऽन्यज्जलं भक्ष्यं च दद्यात्; सप्तरात्रात् सप्तरात्राच्च घटमन्यं संक्रामयेत् ॥५७॥

### *Collection and Storage of Leeches*

These nonpoisonous leeches should be collected through a wet leather or by such other means. These are to be kept in a new earthen jar containing water and mud collected from a lake or pond. For their food moss, powder of dry-meat and powder of roots of aquatic plants should be kept in the jar. Grass and leaves of aquatic plants should be kept in the jar to facilitate their sleeping over them. Every third day, the water and food ingredients should be changed and fresh water and food ingredients should be given kept in the jar. Every seventh day, fresh jar should be used in the place of the old one.

भवति चात्र

स्थूलमध्याः परिक्लिष्टा पृथ्व्यो मन्दविचेष्टिताः ।
अग्राहिण्योऽल्पपायिन्यः सविषाश्च न पूजिताः ॥५८॥

***Unsuitable Leeches***

Thus it is said : Leeches having a bulky middle part of the bod' fatigued ones, those who have grown fatty, those having sluggishness i movement, those who do not suck blood or suck blood only in sma quantity and the poisonous ones are not suitable for application in bloo letting therapy.

'अथ जलौकोवसेकसाध्यव्याधितमुपवेश्य संवेश्य वा, विरूक्ष्य चास्य तमवकाशं मृद्गोमयचूर्णैर्यद्यरुजः स्यात् । गृहीताश्च[२] ताः सर्षपरजनीकल्कोदकप्रदिग्धगात्राः सलिलसरकमध्ये मुहूर्तं स्थिता विगतक्लमा ज्ञात्वा ताभी रोगं ग्राहयेत् । श्लक्ष्णशुक्लार्द्रपिचुप्लोतावच्छन्नां कृत्वा मुखमपावृणुयात्; अगृह्णन्त्यै क्षीरशोणितबिन्दुं दद्यात्, शस्त्रपदानि वा कुर्वीत; यद्येवमपि न गृह्णीयात्तदाऽन्यां ग्राहयेत् ॥५९॥

***Method of Leech Application***

The patient suffering from the disease which is curable by leecl application type of blood-letting therapy, should be made to sit or lie down. The skin of the area from where blood is to be taken out should be made rough by rubbing with the powder of earth or cow-dung cake if that is not painful. [If there is pain, then the area should be just cleaned by a cotton swab gently.) The leech should then be caught [through forceps or any other suitable implement] and smeared with the paste of mustard and turmeric mixed with water. Then it should be kept inside a vessel containing water for some time till it becomes free from fatigue [becomes active]. Then this leech should be applied over the selected part of the skin and when it starts sucking, its mouth should be covered with a smooth, white and wet swab of cotton or cloth. If it does not suck blood, then in that part of the skin, a drop of milk or blood should be dropped or it should be slightly scratched. If inspite of these measures, the leech does not suck blood, then another leech should be used for this purpose.

यदा च निविशतेऽश्वसुखदाननं कृत्वोन्नम्य च स्कन्धं तदा जानीयाद्गृह्णातीति; गृह्णन्तीं चार्द्रवस्त्रावच्छन्नां धारयेत्[२३] ॥६०॥

When the leech lies over the skin with its mouth protruded like the hoof of a horse and its neck is swollen, then it should be determined that the leech has started sucking blood. This sucking leech should then be covered with a wet cloth.

दंशे तोदकण्डूप्रादुर्भावैर्जानीयाच्छुद्धमियमादत्त इति; शुद्धमाददानामपनयेत्; अथ शोणितगन्धेन न मुञ्चेन्मुखमस्याः सैन्धवचूर्णेनावकिरेत् ॥६१॥

While the leech is sucking blood, if the patient gets pain and itching sensation, then it should be determined that it is sucking pure blood, and at that time, the leech should be removed from the skin. If because of the attracting smell of the blood, the leech does not leave the skin then *saindhava* powder should be sprinkled over it.

'अथ[२४] पतितां तण्डुलकण्डनप्रदिग्धगात्रीं तैललवणाभ्यक्तमुखीं वामहस्ताङ्गुष्ठाङ्गुलीभ्यां गृहीतपुच्छां दक्षिणहस्ताङ्गुष्ठाङ्गुलीभ्यां शनैः शनैरनुलोममनुमार्जयेदामुखात्, वामयेत् तावद्यावत् सम्यग्वान्तलिङ्गनीति । सम्यग्वान्ता सलिलसरके न्यस्ता भोक्तुकामा सती चरेत् । या सीदती न चेष्टते सा दुर्वान्ता,

तां पुनः सम्यग्वामयेत् । दुर्वान्ताया व्याधिरसाध्य इन्द्रमदो नाम भवति । अथ सुवान्तां पूर्ववत् सन्निदध्यात् ॥६२॥

When the leech falls down from the place of bite, its body should be smeared with the coarse powder of rice and its mouth should be smeared with salt and oil. It should be caught at its tail with the left hand and with the fingers of the right hand, it should be gradually squeezed with pressure downwards towards the mouth. Thus, the leech will vomit out the blood. The squeezing should be continued till signs and symptoms of proper emesis appear in the leech. After proper emesis, the leech should be kept in a vessel containing water and it will start moving inside water in search of food. If it lies lazy and does not move, then it has not vomited out the polluted blood properly. It should then be squeezed again for emesis. If proper vomiting has not taken place, then the leech suffers from a disease called *indramada*. After proper vomiting, the leech should be kept in the jar as before.

शोणितस्य योगायोगानवेक्ष्य शतधौतघृताभ्यङ्गः, तत्पिचुधारणं वा; जलौकोव्रणान् मधुनाऽवघट्टयेत्, शीताभिरद्भिः परिषेचयेद्बध्नीत वा, कषायमधुरस्निग्धशीतैश्च प्रदेहैः प्रदिह्यादिति ॥६३॥

*After Care*

After the blood-letting has taken place, the physician should ascertain if it has been done properly or improperly. If it is properly done, then the skin surface should be smeared with *Śatadhauta ghṛta* or it should be covered with a cotton swab smeared with this medicated ghee. If less of blood is sucked by the leech, then the site of bite in the skin should be rubbed with honey. If excess of blood is sucked by the leech, then the area should be sprinkled with cold water or tied with a bandage, and over the skin, paste of astringent, sweet, unctuous and cooling drugs should be applied.

भवति चात्र

"क्षेत्राणि ग्रहणं जातीः पोषणं सावचारणम् ।
जलौकसां च यो वेत्ति तत्साध्यान् स जयेद्गदान्" ॥६४॥

(सुश्रुत : सूत्रस्थान : १३ : १४-२४)

***Expertise of Physician***

A physician, who is well versed with the habitat, method of collection, different types, nourishment and method of application of leeches, becomes capable of curing diseases amenable to the therapy of leech application.

इति श्रीमहाराजाधिराजश्रीटोडरमल्लविरचिते टोडरानन्दे आयुर्वेदसौख्ये शोणितस्रावविधिकथनं[१५] नामैकाशीतितमो हर्षः ॥

Thus, ends the 81st chapter describing the method of administering blood-letting therapy in *Āyurveda saukhya* of *Ṭoḍarānanda* composed by the great King Ṭoḍaramalla.

## NOTES AND REFERENCES

१. (क) This is the beginning of the eighty chapter of *Āyurveda saukhya* in *Ṭoḍarānanda* and invocation reads as follows :
"य उद्धवेनात्महितेन पित्तोर्मित्रेण तापं विजहौ मुरारी ।
स्वकीयविश्लेषनवंधुनोतु तापत्रयं टोडरमल्लभूपे" ॥

(ख) 'य ...... भूपे' पाठोऽयं चतुर्थषष्ठपुस्तकयोः नोपलभ्यते ।

२. रक्तसृजो यतः इति आकरे पाठः ।

३. (क) विलम्बं गतिः इति चतुर्थपुस्तके पाठः ।

(ख) स्वलंगति इति षष्ठपुस्तके पाठः ।

(ग) विलयस्तथा इति आकरे पाठः ।

४. 'रक्तमण्डलता ....... जायते' पाठोऽयं पंचमपुस्तके अधिकमुपलभ्यते ।

५. अस्कन्दिसुचि इति पंचमपुस्तके आकरे च पाठः ।

६. विस्राविं इति आदर्शपुस्तकेषु पाठः ।

७. 'द्विदोषदुष्टं ...... पूतिगन्धकम्' पाठोऽयं चतुर्थपुस्तके नोपलभ्यते ।

८. .युक्तानांमति. इति चतुर्थषष्ठपुस्तकयोः पाठः ।

९. विषयुक्तानां इति पचमपुस्तके पाठः ।

१०. तुम्बि इति षष्ठपुस्तके पाठः ।

११. .मदभ्रमे इति षष्ठपुस्तके पाठः ।

१२. अप्रवर्तितरक्ते इति आकरे पाठः ।

१३. कषायं इति षष्ठपुस्तके पाठः ।

१४. स्कन्धयते इति षष्ठपुस्तके पाठः ।

१५. अन्तं स्थेयं इति प्रथमपुस्तके पाठः ।

१६. स्राव्यं इति आकरे पाठः ।

१७. कुरुतेऽतिस्रुतं इति प्रथमपुस्तके आकरे च पाठः ।

१८. रुद्वेगसंक्षये इति षष्ठपुस्तके पाठः ।

१९. (क) मनः स्थं भवेच्चिह्नं इति पंचमपुस्तके पाठः ।
(ख) मनः स्वास्थ्यं इति आकरे पाठः ।

२०. पानालेपनभ्यकरणादिषूपयोज्यः इति प्रथमपुस्तके पाठः ।

२१. 'अथ ..... संक्रामयेत्' पाठोऽयं पंचमपुस्तके नोपलभ्यते ।

२२. 'अथ जलौकसौ मुद्गकल्कसंयुतेन बहिः प्रक्षाल्यातः' पाठोऽयं प्रथमपुस्तके अधिकमुपलभ्यते ।

२३. कृत्वा धारयेत् इति आकरे पाठः ।

२४. 'अथ ....... सन्निदध्यात्' पाठोऽयं प्रथमपंचमपुस्तकयोः नोपलभ्यते ।

२५. शोणितस्रावविधिनामैकाशीतितमो हर्षः इति चतुर्थपुस्तके पाठः ।

# INDEX I
## (Authors and Books Quoted)

# INDEX II
## (Names of Recipes Described in the Book)

# INDEX III
## (Names of Drugs, etc. Used in the Book)

# INDEX IV
## (Glossary of Technical Terms)

*Abhicāra*, 4, 56
Infliction of spells.

*Abhiṣyandī*, 258, 265, 280
Food which obstructs the channels of circulation.

*Abhyaṅga*, 26, 28, 157
Massage.

*Acaraṇā* [*yoni*], 24
N. of a disease of female genital tract, in which woman gets orgasm before the man during sexual intercourse.

*Accha sneha*, 252
Pure fat not mixed with any drug.

*Āḍhaka(s)*, 16, 59, 2[illegible]
Unit of measurement. Four *prasthas* make one *āḍhaka* which is equivalent to 3. 072 kg. or ltr.

*Adhijihvā*, 297
Enlarged adenoid glands.

*Āgantavaḥ*, 185
Extraneous factors.

*Āgantuja*, 185
Caused by the extraneous factors.

*Āgneya*, 120
South-east direction.

*Agni*, 202
Power of digestion and metabolism.

*Ahiṇḍikā*, 92
Marasmus, also called *bāla śoṣa*.

*Ahipūtanā*, 86
N. of a children's disease. Ref. Glossary in p. 559 of diagnosis and Treatment of Diseases, Part-7.

*Ahṛdya*, 216
Which is not congenial for the heart or the mind.

*Aiśānya*, 119
North-eastern direction.

*Ajagāallikā*, 86
N. of a *kṣudra roga* (minor-disease). Ref. Glossary in p. 559 of Diagnosis and Treatment of Diseases, Part-7.

*Ākāśa* [*mahābhūta*], 349
Ether; One of the five basic elements (*pañca mahābhūtas*). Ref. Glossary in page 610 (*mahābhūta*) of Basic Principles of Ayurveda.

*Akṣa*, 6, 204, 231. 252, 336, 339
Unit of weight, approx. 12 Gm. This term is used as syn. of *bibhītaka* (*Terminalia belerica* Roxb.). Weight of the fruit of this plant is also implied by this term.

*Ākṣepaka*, 357
Convulsion.

*Alagarda*, 359, 360
A variety of poisonous leeches.

*Āma*, 66
Immature stage when there is beginning of the swelling, 305
Product of improper digestion and metabolism. Ref. Glossary in page 587 of Basic Principles of Ayurveda.

*Āmavāta*, 55, 334
Rheumatism.

*Amla pitta*, 59, 207, 227
Hyper-acidity.

*Ānāha*, 51
Abdominal distension.

*Aṇḍinī* [*yoni*], 24, 25
N. of a disease of female genital tract in which a resultant change apears in a young woman after

sexual intercourse with a person having robust body.

*Anāmaka*, 93, 94
Anal ulcer.

*Andha pūtanā*, 89
Seizure by an evil spirit called Andha pūtanā.

*Aṅgas*, 185
Limbs.

*Aṅgulas*, 155, 269, 284, 322, 323, 343, 354, 361
Finger-breadth or unit of measurement equivalent to ½" approx. Ref. Glossary in p. 587 of Diagnosos and Treatment of Diseases in Ayurveda, Part-I.

*Añjana*, 156, 157, 174
Collyrium.

*Anna*, 185
Food ingredients.

*Annāda*, 82
A stage of a child when he or she depends upon cereals for nourishment.

*Annamada*, 145
Feeling of intoxication after the intake of food.

*Anulepana*, 173, 179
Pastes of aromatic items or drugs used for external application.

*Anupāna*, 252
Post-prandial drink.

*Anuvāsana*, 280, 320, 321, 323, 325, 326, 329, 332, 342

*Anuvāsana basti*, 320, 321, 323-325, 327-329, 331, 333, 339, 342, 345
A type of medicated enema prepared with oil, etc. Ref. Glossary in p. 591 of Basic Principles of Ayurveda.

*Ap*, 349
Water; one of the five basic elements (*pañca mahābhūta*) composing universe. Ref. *Mahābhūta* in Glossary in p. 610 of Basic Principles of Ayurveda.

*Apacī*, 352
Tubercular lymphadenitis.

*Apatantraka*, 271
Convulsion.

*Āranāla*, 55
A type of sour-vinegar.

*Arbuda*, 352
Tumour.

*Arddhāvabhedaka*, 273, 274
Hemicrania.

*Arśas*, 311
Polyp or piles.

*Asṛgdara*, 2
Menorrhagia.

*Āsthāpana*, 330
Syn. of *nirūha basti* (one of the two types of medicated enema). Ref. Glossary in p. 593 of Basic Principles of Ayurveda.

*Atharvāṇas*, 185
Followers of the *Atharva-veda*.

*Aticaraṇā [yoni]*, 24
N. of a disease of female genital tract in which woman gets orgasm after repeated sexual intercourse.

*Atyānandā [yoni]*, 23
A disease of female genital tract in which woman does not draw satisfaction even after sexual intercourse.

*Avabāhuka*, 275
Pain in the root of arm.

*Avapīḍa*, 269, 270

*Avapīḍa nasya*, 269, 270
A type of inhalation therapy in which medicine is administered through pressure.

*Bāhya*, 66
External.

*Bāhya vidradhi*, 66
External abscesses or swollen growths.

*Bāla*, 82
Infancy.

*Bāla graha(s)*, 286
Seizure of a child by evil spirits.

*Bāla śoṣa*, 92
Marasmus.

*Bali*, 114-126, 173, 239
Sacred sacrifice or sacrificial food.

*Bharaṇī*, 141
N. of a constellation.
*Basti*, 26, 320, 321, 324, 326, 329, 334, 336-338
Enema can.
Medicated enema therapy, 322
Urinary bladder, 322
*Bhasma*, 92
Calcined powder of metals, minerals, etc. Ref. Glossary in p. 597 of Basic Principles of Ayurveda.
*Bhogi*, 140, 141
A type of snake having hood.
*Bhramara*, 202
Black-bee.
*Bhṛṅgarāja* 174
N. of a bird.
*Bīja*, 22
Sperm and ovum (lit. seed).
*Bījaka*, 36
An abnormal foetal presentation in the genital tract.
*Bījas*, 163
Seed-letters.
*Bindu*, 275
Drop.
*Brāhmaṇas*, 116-126
One of the upper cast of the Hindus.
*Bṛṃhaṇa*, 267, 335
Therapy which produces nourishing effect.
*Bṛṃhaṇa nasya*, 272, 273
Inhalation therapy which produces nourishing effect.
*Bṛṃhaṇa*, 281, 284
*Bṛṃhaṇa dhūma*, 281
A type of smoking therapy which produces nourishing effect.
*Cakora*, 174
N. of a bird; known as Greek partridge.
*Cālana*, 349
Mobility.
*Chatra*, 235
Parasol-shaped hive.
*Cyavana mantra*, 45
A sacred incantation which is recited for the consecration of the water. This water is given to the enceinte for drinking which helps in easy delivery.
*Dāha*, 112, 165
Cauterisation.
*Dantakāṣṭha*, 175, 178
Twig used for brushing teeth.
*Darvīkara*, 141
A type of snake having hood.
*Devas*, 210
Demons.
*Dhāroṣṇa*, 219
Freshly collected warm milk.
*Dhātrī*, 69
Wet-nurse.
*Dhātus*, 112, 151
Tissue elements.
*Dhātu*, 153
Minerals.
*Dhātuviṣa*, 153
Poisonous minerals.
*Dhvajabhaṅga*, 217
Non-erection of penis.
*Dīpataila*, 167
Oil collected from a burning lamp. It is also a name of a recipe.
*Doṣas*, 9, 25, 56, 57, 61, 65, 69-71, 85, 112, 140, 147, 151, 185, 225, 251, 254, 263,, 266, 268-273, 281, 286-289, 295, 298, 309, 330, 333-335, 337, 351, 354
Factors responsible for the regulation of all the functions of the body. These are three in number, namely, *vāyu*, *pitta* and *kapha*. Ref. Glossary in p. 601 of Basic Prinsciples of Ayurveda.
*Soṣahara*, 334
Elimination of *doṣas*.
*Dravatā*, 349
Liquidity.
*Droṇa*, 75, 231
Unit of weight. Approx. 12.288 kg./ltrs.

*Pīḍakā*, 352
Pimples.

*Pilipicchikā*, 125
N. of an evil goddess.

*Piṅgalā*, 361
N. of a variety of non-poisonous leeches.

*Piśācas*, 111, 286
N. of an evil spirit, specially a class of demons fond of flesh.

*Pitṛpakṣa*, 141
Fortnight when oblations are offered to manes.

*Pitta*, 10, 11, 23, 25, 26, 54, 56, 59, 61, 67, 70, 71, 83, 103, 140, 141, 144, 162, 209, 229, 251, 262, 265, 267, 273, 274, 287, 289, 297, 300, 303, 305, 307, 309, 333, 349, 350. 354
One of the three *doṣas* – the others being *vāyu* and *kapha*. For details, Ref. Glossary in p. 616 of Basic Principles of Ayurveda, 312, 332
Bile.

*Pittaja*, 65
Diseases caused by aggravated *pitta*.

*Pittagata* poison, 162
Affliction of *pitta* by the poison.

*Pittala*, 28
Diseases caused by the aggravation of *pitta doṣa*.

*Pittalā* [*yoni*], 23
N. of a disease of female genital tract in which patient suffer from excessive burning sensation and suppuration in the genital tract associated with high fever.

*Pitta-rogas*, 59
Diseases caused by aggravated *pitta*.

*Pothakī*, 83, 109
N. of an eye-disease characterised by the appearance of hard papules of the size of mustard seed inside the eyelids.

*Pradara* [*kaphaja* type of], 6
Menorrhagia or foul smelling discharge from the female genital tract caused by the vitiation of *kapha*.

*Pradhamana*, 269, 270

*Pradhama nasya*, 269, 270
A type of inhalation therapy in which medicine is administered by blowing powdered drug into the nostrils.

*Prahara*, 238
Unit of measurement of time; equivalent to three hours.

*Pralepa*, 26
External application of drugs in the form of paste.

*Prameha*, 16, 59, 141, 225, 282, 307, 331
Obstinate urinary disorders including diabetes.

*Praṇava oṃ*, 163
Ref. Glossary in p. 614 of Basic Principles of Ayurveda.

*Prasannā*, 27
A type of wine.

*Prasraṃsinī* [*yoni*], 23
N. of a disease of female genital tract associated with excruciating pain during menstruation and delivery.

*Prasṛt(i)*, 206, 209, 210, 336, 337
Unit of measurement; Approx. 96 Gms./ml.

*Prastha*, 9, 11, 15, 16, 55, 59, 74, 78, 110, 222, 224, 231, 233, 299, 300, 330, 348
Unit of measurement ; Approx. 768 Gms./ml.

*Pratikhura*, 36
An abnormal foetal presentation in genital tract. In this stage, foetus obstructs the cervical opening of the uterus with its limbs projecting out through the vaginal canal like the hoof of horse.

*Pratimarśa*, 272, 275, 276

*Pratimarśa nasya*, 272, 275, 276
A type of inhalation therapy.

*Pratisāraṇa*, 290, 291
Rubbing of drugs.

*Pratiśyāya*, 267
Coryza.

*Pravāhikā*, 305

the body.

*Recana [nasya]*, 266, 268, 169, 273, 286
Inhalation therapy which causes elimination of *doṣas* from the head.

*Revatī [graha]*, 88
N. of an evil spirit.

*Ropaṇa [gaṇḍūṣa]*, 287
A variety of *gaṇḍuṣa* (rinsing the mouth with mouthful of decoction) which helps in healing ulcers.

*Rūkṣa*, 256
Ununctuous.

*Rūkṣaṇa*, 257
Drying therapy.

*Sahya*, 362
The mountanous region located in the south of the river Narmadā.

*Śakuni*, 88
N. of an evil spirit.

*Śakuni graha*, 88
Afflictions by an evil spirit called Śakuni.

*Śamana*, 335
Alleviation therapy.

*Śamana [dhūma]*, 281, 284, 285
A type of smoking therapy which causes alleviation of *doṣas*.

*Śamana [gaṇḍūṣa]*, 286, 287
A variety of *gaṇḍūṣa* (rinsing of mouth with mouthful of decoction) which helps in alleviating *doṣas*.

*Saṃśamana*, 254, 334
Alleviation of aggravated *doṣas*.

*Saṃśśodhana*, 254, 295
Elimination or purification.

*Saṃodhana [gaṇḍūṣa]*, 287
A variety of *gaṇḍūṣa* which helps in alleviating *doṣas*.

*Sāmudrikā*, 359, 360
A variety of poisonous leeches.

*Śaṇa(s)*, 72, 233, 269, 272
Unit of weight; approx. 3 Gm./ml.

*Śaṇḍī [yoni]*, 24, 25
N. of a disease of female genital tract in which woman does not get menstruation, whose breasts are not developed and whose genital tract remains rough during sexual intercourse.

*Saṅgrahaṇī*, 59
Sprue syndrome.

*Saṅkaras*, 185
Mixed breed offsprings.

*Śaṅkha*, 127
Conch-shell.

*Saṅkīlaka*, 36
An abnormal presentation of the foetus in the genital tract. In this condition, the cervical opening of the uterus gets obstructed by the back, hands, legs and head like a peg.

*Śaṇmukhī*, 361
A variety of non-poisonous leeches.

*Sannipāta*, 61, 270
Simultaneous vitiation of all the three *doṣas*.

*Sānnipātika*, 2, 3, 7, 25, 26, 66
Diseases caused by the simultaneous vitiation of all the three *doṣas*.

*Sānnipātika asṛgdara*, 3
Menorrhagia caused by the simultaneous vitiation of all the three *doṣas*.

*Sānnipātika yonikanda*, 26
Prolapse of female genital tract caused by the simultaneous vitiation of all the three *doṣas*.

*Sānnipātika yoniroga*, 25
Diseases of female genital tract caused by the simultaneous vitiation of all the three *doṣas*.

*Sāra*, 138, 153
Heart wood.

*Śaṣkulikās*, 121
A type of food preparation.

*Sātmya*, 254
Assimilation of any therapy or food ingredient into the body. Therefore, it does not work as a therapy.

*Sauvīra(ka)*, 67, 246

A type of vinegar.

*Sāvarikā*, 361
A variety of non-poisonous leeches.

*Savraṇa śukla*, 207
Corneal ulcer.

*Śayyā*, 179
Bed.

*Seka*, 28
Sprinkling of drugs over the body.

*Śikhodgama*, 83
Apearance of crest or comb.

*Śirāmarma*, 141
Vital spot in the body having the predominance of vessels.

*Śirastrāṇa*, 181
Umbrella.

*Śirobhyaṅga*, 180
Oil used for the massage of head.

*Sīt*, 168
Cooing sound.

*Śīta pūtanā*, 89
Seizure by an evil spirit called Śīta Pūtanā.

*Skanda*, 87
N. of an evil spirit.

*Skanda graha*, 87
Affliction by an evil spirit called Skanda.

*Skandāpasmāra*, 87
Epileptic fits caused by the affliction by an evil spirit called Skanda.

*Ślakṣṇā*, 345
Smooth.

*Śleṣmalā [yoni]*, 24
N. of a female disease in which woman's genital tract is slimy, itchy and excessively cold.

*Snaihika [gaṇḍūṣa]*, 286, 287
A type of *gaṇḍūṣa* (rinsing the mouth with mouthful decoction) which produces oleating effect.

*Snaihika nasya*, 270
A type of inhalation therapy which produces oleating effect.

*Snāna*, 180
Bath-water.

*Sneha*, 251
Oleation therapy, 6, 258, 324, 333, 338
Fat which includes ghee, oil, *vasā* (muscle fat) and bone-marrow.

*Snehana [dhūma]*, 281, 285
Smoking therapy which produces oleation. It is syn. of *bṛṃhaṇa dhūma* (nourishing smoking therapy).

*Snehana [nasya]*, 266, 272, 273, 275, 276
Inhalation therapy which produces oleating effect.

*Śodhana*, 281
Cleansing therapy. This is a syn. of *recana dhūma* (smoking therapy which causes elimination of *doṣas* from the body).

*Śodhana [gaṇḍūṣa]*,
A type of *gaṇḍūṣa* (gargling) which eliminates *doṣas* from the body.

*Soma*, 5
N. of a disease; Polyuria.

*Somaroga*, 3-5, 12, 13, 59
Polyuria.

*Śrāvaṇa*, 72
N. of a month according to Hindu calender. According to English calender, this is a period about 15 July to 15 August.

*Śṛṅga*, 352
Horn.

*Śṛṅgāṭaka*, 278
Upper part of the nasal passage.

*Śrutidhara*, 78
One who can retain in memory whatever he hears.

*Stanakīla*, 56
Polyp-like growth in the breast.

*Stanya*, 70
Breast-milk.

*Sthagikā*, 151
A type of bee.

*Sthalī*, 188
Open space of sitting together.

*Sthāpana*, 330
A therapy which helps in maintaining the homeostasis of

*doṣas* and *dhātus* (tissue elements)

*Sthāvara*, 163
Inanimate objects.

*Sthāvara viṣa*, 136, 137, 152, 153
Posion derived from inanimate objects.

*Sūcīmuk[illegible]*, 25
The woman whose vaginal tract is very narrow.

*Sugrīva mantra*, 127
A sacred incantation. Recitation of this incantation alleviates the effects of evil spirits.

*Śukanikā*, 120
N. of an evil goddess.

*Śukti*, 278
Snail, 334
Unit of weight and measurement; Approx. 24 Gm./ml.

*Sunandā*, 116
N. of an evil goddess.

*Śūnyatā mantra*, 155
A sacred incantation, recitation of which makes a person free from poison.

*Sūryāvartta*, 273, 274
Headache which increases in accordance with the movement of sun in the sky.

*Śuṣka Revatī*, 121
N. of an evil goddess.

*Sūtikā*, 51, 52
Puerperal, 123
N. of an evil goddess.

*Svara*, 202
Voice.

*Svara kṣaya*, 59
Diminution of voice.

*Svastika(s)*, 116-118, 120, 121
A type of *yantra*.

*Takṣaka*, 154, 161
A type of celestial snake.

*Tālu*, 93, 99
Anterior fontanel.

*Tālu kaṇṭaka*, 85
A children's disease occurs in the palatal muscles of the child and caused by the aggravation of *kapha*.

*Tālu pāta*, 85, 104
A children's disease in which the palate of the child hangs down.

*Tamaka*, 107
A type of asthma.

*Ṭaṅka*, 257
Unit of weight, approx.

*Tantra*, 45
Powerful spell.

*Tanutra*, 179
Mystic amulet or protecting jacket.

*Tāpa*, 262
Heat of fire.

*Tarkū*, 90
Spinning spindle.

*Tarpaṇa*, 282
Nourishing therapy.

*Tejas*, 349
Fire. One of the five basic elements (*pañca mahābhūtas*) composing universe. Ref. Glossary in p. 610 (*mahābhūta*) of Basic Principles of Ayurveda.

*Tīkṣṇa*, 34, 328
Drug or therapy having sharp attribute, 268, 269
Pungent or sharp effect, 281, 284
Sharp. Syn. of *recana dhūma* (smoking theraphy which causes elimination of *doṣas* from the body).

*Timira*, 207
Cataract, 357
Appearance of blackness of front in the eyes.

*Tīrtha*, 188
Steps leading to a water reservoir.

*Tridoṣa*, 56
Collective name for three *doṣas* namely *vāyu, pitta* and *kapha*.

*Tulā*, 59
Unit of weight; aprox. 4.800 kg./ltr

*Tak-sāra-niryāsa viṣa*, 153
Plants whose bark, heart-wood and resins are poisonous.

*Uccitiṅga*, 149

Disease of female genital tract caused by the aggravation of *vāyu*.

*Vāyavya*, 124
North-west direction.

*Vāyu*, 2, 3, 10, 15, 22, 25, 26, 35, 36, 50, 51, 52, 54, 56, 59, 61, 70, 73, 75, 85, 97, 104, 140, 144, 163, 209, 252, 261, 262, 267, 273, 274, 280, 283, 287, 300, 302, 307, 309, 311, 321, 333, 350, 352, 354, 358
One of the three *doṣas*; other two being *pitta* and *kapha*. Ref. *vāta* in p. 625 of Glossary of Basic Principles of Ayurveda.

*Vāyu*, 312
Flatus.

*Vāyu* [*mahābhūta*], 349
One of the five basic element (*pañca mahābhūtas*) composing universe. Ref. *mahābhūta* in p. 610 of Glossary in Basic Principles of Ayurveda.

*Vāyugata* poison, 163
*Vāyu* afflicted by poison.

*Vāyu-kapha*, 70
Simultaneous vitiation of *vāyu* and *kapha*.

*Vāyu-pitta*, 70
Simultaneous vitiation of *vāyu* and *pitta*.

*Vedic mantras*, 185
Sacred incantations found in vedas.

*Veṇi*, 155
Breads of the hair.

*Vidagdha*, 66
A stage of disease when there is inflammation but no suppuration.

*Vidāha*, 349
Metabolic transformation.

*Vidārikā*, 296
A type of diabetic carbuncle, 352
A popular growth in the axillae and groins.

*Vidradhi(s)*, 66
Abscesses.

*Vilaya*, 349
Nature of getting mixed up with others quickly.

*Viplutā* [*yoni*], 22
Disease of female genital tract characterised by constant pain i the pelvic regoin.

*Virecaka nasya*, 269, 270
See *recana nasya*.

*Viruddhāśana*, 168
Intake of mutually contradictory food.

*Viṣa kanyā*, 169
A beautiful young girl whose body poisoned by gradual administration of small doses o poisons.

*Viṣama jvara*, 311, 331
Irregular fever.

*Visarpa*, 85
Erysipelas; N. of a skin disease in which skin becomes red like th colour of lotus; also called *mahāpadma*.

*Viṣkira*, 314, 315
Gallinacious birds.

*Visphoṭa*, 93
Pustular eruptions.

*Visra(tā)*, 349
Fleshy smell.

*Vivṛtā [yoni]*, 25
A female disease in which vagina tract of the woman is very wid

*Vraṇa basti*, 323
Douche for cleansing ulcers.

*Vraṇa dhūpana*, 281, 285
A type of smoking therapy administered for the fumigati of ulcers.

*Vraṇa nāḍī*, 284
See *vraṇa dhūpana*.

*Vṛṣya*, 230
Aphrodisiac.

*Vyaṅga*, 209, 243
Black pigmented patches in the face.

*Yakṣas*, 111
A class of demons.

*Yantra*, 45, 116-118, 120, 121, 237
Talishman used as amulet.

*Yāpya*, 146

Palliable disease, suppressible but not curable.

*Yava*, 269
One of the synonyms of barley; also used as the unit of weight equivalent to a grain of barley; approx.

*Yavāgū*, 255, 355
Thin gruel.

*Yavana* region, 362
Turkey.

*Yogavāhī*, 227
A drug or thing which enhances the effects of other added medicines.

*Yoni*, 15
Female genital tract including uterus.

*Yonikanda*, 25, 26
Prolapse of uterus. Some physicians interprete this term as a vaginal tumour or polyp.

*Yoniroga*, 22, 23, 25, 26, 28, 29, 61
Diseases of female genital tract.

*Yonivyāpat*, 26
Diseases of female genital tract.